Assessment and Remediation of Articulatory and Phonological Disorders

Parley W. Newman
Brigham Young University

Nancy A. Creaghead
University of Cincinnati

Wayne Secord
University of Cincinnati

Charles E. Merrill Publishing Company
A Bell & Howell Company
Columbus   Toronto   London   Sydney

Published by
Charles E. Merrill Publishing Company
A Bell & Howell Company
Columbus, Ohio 43216

This book was set in Baskerville
Production Coordinator: Linda Hillis Bayma
Cover Design: Cathy Watterson
Cover photo by Vivienne della Grotta

Library of Congress Catalog Card Number: 84-62599
International Standard Book Number: 0-675-20330-9

Printed in the United States of America

1 2 3 4 5 6 7 8 9—89 88 87 86 85

To
E. LeRoi Jones
R. Vernon Stroud
Doris Sarver White

Contents

PART III
SPECIFIC ARTICULATION TREATMENT PROGRAMS

14 A Distinctive-Feature Approach to
Articulation Therapy   383

Stephen E. Blache

Preface

This text was constructed with three major goals in mind. The first was to cover in a comprehensive way the work of the last 40 years in the service of people who find intelligible speech beyond their ability to master. This book explains traditional views toward articulation disorders and their treatment, behavioral management approaches with their greater efficiency, and, finally, current thinking and methods derived from the contributions of modern linguistics.

The second major goal was to provide a text that would emphasize treatment. Of the book's 14 chapters, 9 are fully developed discussions of remedial procedures by authors who in many cases actually developed them, or who are recognized experts in the method described. This work is thus a rich source on therapy. To our knowledge, no other text explicates fully between two covers the major current approaches for remediating disorders of articulation and phonology.

Finally, the editors hoped to collect in one volume the contributions of a number of authors who have achieved national recognition for their original works. The contributors to this volume have provided extensive service to the communicatively impaired.

The text also supplies foundation material for the presentations on treatment. The first of the book's three major sections provides the bases for understanding normal articulation and phonology. Chapter 1, an opening rationale with emphasis on communication, serves as a point of departure for subsequent chapters. In chapter 2, Nancy Creaghead and Parley Newman discuss phonetics and phonology. Chapter 3 by Creaghead reviews development of phonology in children. Chapter 4, also by Creaghead and Newman, treats assessment of articulatory and phonologic disorders.

The second major part of the book presents an overview of remediation methods. These are introduced in chapter 5 by Wayne Secord, who discusses traditional articulation therapy methods. Dr. Secord is a creative and productive worker in the fields of assessment and remediation.

In chapter 6, Donald E. Mowrer explains how a clinician can apply the power and efficiency of behavioral methods to the remediation of disorders of articulation and also how the clinician can write programs that paraprofessionals can follow. Dr. Mowrer has achieved national recognition for his many publications and other contributions to the amelioration of speech disorders through the application of behavioral management techniques.

In chapter 7, Nancy Creaghead provides an up-to-date explanation of linguistic approaches to articulation therapy and phonological disorders. Dr. Creaghead's ambitious work is in the mainstream of modern linguistic thought concerning the understanding and remediation of articulation and phonological disorders.

Chapter 8 by Gordon M. Low, Mildred T. Ravsten, and Parley W. Newman extends our perceptions of remediating articulation and phonology through the communicative power of peer interaction. This viewpoint takes into account current pragmatic approaches to understanding and remediating disorders of language. For a quarter of a century, Dr. Low has had the vision of communication as the overarching rubric embracing disorders of speech, language, hearing, reading, and learning and has applied this vision to the treatment of disorders of communication. Professor Ravsten, a former student of Dr. Low, has been importantly involved in the clinical application of this innovative approach.

In chapter 9, Harris Winitz provides an insightful and thought-provoking refocusing on the auditory channel in treating articulatory disorders. Dr. Winitz is a distinguished scholar who has earned the respect of members of the profession and leaders of the field, who see him as one of its truly significant contributors.

Considerations for organic disorders are explained in chapter 10 by Dorothy H. Air and Ann S. Wood. The special assessment and remediation procedures required for individuals with motor speech disorders and cleft palate are discussed by two authors who have served these clients in hospital and private-practice settings and are respected as experts by the members of their professional community.

Chapter 11 by Doris P. Bradley explains how traditional articulation treatment procedures can be applied systematically to correct multiple phoneme deficiencies simultaneously and efficiently. Dr. Bradley is well known for her many contributions to the welfare of the communicatively handicapped, not the least of which is her development of the multiphonemic approach.

In chapter 12, Alan J. Weston and John V. Irwin describe and update their paired-stimuli technique and provide an extensive data base that demostrates its effectiveness. An attractive feature of their approach is that aides and paraprofessionals can apply it, thus expediting the work of the clinician. Dr. Weston, an active member of the profession, was formerly a student of Dr. Irwin. Dr. Irwin is one of the great statesmen of the field. His long career is characterized by penetrating scholarship and high productivity in research and publication.

The method of meaningful minimal contrasts, created by Reuben Cooper and discussed in chapter 13, represents a bridge from traditional remedial techniques to the methods of contrasts emphasized in modern phonological literature. In this approach, the function of the phoneme in contrasting meaning is recognized as central to the process of human communication. Professor Emeritus Cooper is credited with a signal achievement in developing from that insight the application of meaningful minimal contrastive therapy.

A current application of distinctive-feature theory to the correction of articulation disorders is presented in chapter 14 by Stephen E. Blache. Dr. Blache has distinguished himself in the current professional literature by his innovative work in analyzing distinctive features and developing methods to teach them.

The authors of the various chapters of this book, then, are the creators of the procedures presented and are therefore authoritative on their topics. The procedures described represent major contemporary methods in dealing with the communication disorders of articulation and phonology. They also provide insights into the shape of the future in this field.

My coeditors and I take pride in bringing together the substantive works of creative scholars and clinicians in the field of speech-language pathology. We believe that what these writers have produced is not just another text on disorders of articulation and phonology, but a significant work that combines current impact with lasting value.

Parley W. Newman

Acknowledgments

It is obvious that a project such as this cannot be accomplished without the cooperation and help of many people. The following individuals have given us special help and support.

First, we want to thank our 11 contributors for their fine chapters and for their cooperation in getting them in their final and polished form.

There are a number of people from Charles E. Merrill who have provided special support for us. We appreciate the confidence placed in us by Marianne Taflinger who originally brought us under contract for this book. We especially thank Vicki Knight, our administrative editor, for her insistence on high quality and readability for the entire text and for her patience with us. She secured for us valuable help from our reviewers Gordon Blood, Richard Schwartz, Paul R. Hoffman, Marcia McMillan, Rebecca Leonard, Mary Louise Edwards, and Mary Elbert, who provided thorough and in-depth reviews which gave us excellent direction for our revisions. In addition, we have received valuable help from members of the editorial staff, including our copy editor, Anne Kantor, and our production coordinator, Linda Bayma.

We also thank Frances Margolin and Faughn Ashworth for their time and editorial assistance.

And finally, we all thank each other for time spent, support given, and an overall cooperative attitude which made difficult things easier.

1 Introduction

Speech is a creative communicative act. Through speech it is possible to convey an endless set of thoughts and ideas. Although speech is the most frequently used and most efficient manifestation of our communication system, it is estimated that approximately 10% of the population has some type of communication deficit involving speech, language, and/or hearing. It is further estimated that nearly 75% of these problems are articulatory disorders (Perkins, 1977). Given the prevalence of such problems, students and clinicians should be well prepared to provide effective assessment and remediation.

This is a book for that purpose, intended for both students in training in speech-language pathology and practicing clinicians. It is concerned with the nature and treatment of individuals who have articulation disorders, with a focus on treatment. While a number of approaches and methods have been commonly used in the treatment of articulation disorders, recent advances in the profession have changed our perceptions about articulation problems and

Parley W. Newman, Ph.D., is program chairman in the Area of Communicative Sciences and Disorders at Brigham Young University, Provo, Utah. **Gordon M. Low**, Ph.D., is a professor emeritus of communication disorders in the Department of Educational Psychology at Brigham Young University, Provo, Utah. **Nancy A. Creaghead**, Ph.D., is an associate professor of communication disorders at the University of Cincinnati. **Wayne A. Secord**, Ph.D., is an assistant professor of communication disorders at the University of Cincinnati.

have also helped to reshape our thinking about therapy. This is especially true for individuals who have severe articulation disorders.

The following story about a child named Sean provides background for discussion of changes in approach that have occurred in recent years. Sean was the first client of one of the authors of this text. The story of his treatment is a good example of a clinical approach used 15 years ago.

About 15 years ago, I was working as a speech-language pathologist (actually, they called me a speech therapist then) at Indian Springs Elementary School in Columbus, Ohio. It was my first real professional employment. In fact, I was only 2 months out of Ohio State University. I was green, a little scared, but honestly excited about doing something for which I had trained for so long. I was even going to be paid.

It was only my third or fourth day on the job. I was screening the kindergarten class for potential speech problems when I met 5-year-old Sean. Sometimes a decision whether to pass or fail a child in screening is a close call. Unfortunately, that was not the case with Sean. I couldn't understand anything he said, nor could his teacher or any of his classmates.

I had learned in my training how important it was to conduct a thorough diagnostic work-up, and so I did just that. I gathered a complete case history, including interviews with Sean's parents and his teacher. I even talked to the teacher of his sixth-grade brother to see if she could offer any insights. I could find nothing remarkable socially, educationally, medically, or even developmentally, except that Sean did not really begin talking until about age 2½.

I then gave Sean an audiometric screening and administered several formal and informal assessments, including the Templin-Darley Tests of Articulation, Peabody Picture Vocabulary Test, Preschool Language Scale, Utah Test of Language Development, Templin Picture Sound Discrimination Test, and Boston University Speech Sound Discrimination Test. I even remember conducting a more in-depth than usual oral examination thinking there might be some organic involvement, but I found none.

I considered the possibility of a language disorder. However, Sean's receptive language was well within the norms for his age, and although his many articulation errors made evaluation of his conversational language impossible, he frequently spoke in (unintelligible) phrases and sentences. In addition, his intelligence was assessed by our school psychologist and was found to be within normal limits. After careful consideration, I finally diagnosed Sean's problem as a severe articulation disorder of no known cause. A summary of the articulation errors I found is given in Table 1.1.

Sean was enrolled in therapy immediately. I designed a therapy plan based on criteria I had learned in my training. In considering what sound to treat first, I weighed many factors. For example, I compared his chronological age with the age he was expected to have mastered many of his error sounds. I then examined those developmentally appropriate phonemes a step further. I considered which of them he could repeat correctly after I showed him a somewhat exaggerated model of correct production. Both of these considerations,

TABLE 1.1
Sean's Articulation Errors

Substitutions
Initial: b/f, b/v, t/θ, d/ð, d/s, t/ʃ, d/tʃ, d/dʒ, d/k, d/g, p/sp, t/sk, d/st, d/kr, t/tr, t/kl, p/fl
Medial: b/v, s/θ, d/ð, d/s, d/z, t/ʃ, t/tʃ, d/dʒ
Final: ʔ/t, s/ʃ

Omissions
Initial: /z, h/
Medial: none
Final: /p, b, t, d, k, g, f, v, θ, ð, ʒ, tʃ, dʒ/

Distortions
Initial: /r/
Medial: /r/
Final: /ɚ/

---

developmental age and *stimulability*, are important in devising a plan of treatment. After looking at these two factors and many others, I decided on a therapy plan. My plan was to teach the /k/ sound first. When that sound was corrected, I would move on to the /g/. When it was corrected, I would teach the /f/, and so on until Sean could say all of his error sounds correctly in conversational speech.

Notice that I made up a plan that entailed teaching one sound at a time. At the time Sean was my client, almost all clinicians taught one sound at a time. Some clinicians, however, were just beginning to try out some new procedures based on principles derived from learning theory. They were writing treatment programs for speech sounds that looked a little like those written for teaching machines and, in fact, were based on them to a large extent. But still, it was one sound at a time in therapy.

In therapy with Sean, I taught him first how to become a good listener. Before I showed him how to say a target sound, I "trained his ears" to know how his target phoneme sounded. I made sure he could identify his error sound as well as isolate it from other sounds. I bombarded him with instances of his new sound so he would develop an internal auditory model of that sound. Most of all, I made sure he could tell the difference between his new sound and his error sound. All of this work was part of what we called "ear training."

Production therapy also followed traditional methods. I always spent time establishing correct production of a new sound in isolation first. I then trained Sean to say the sound right in a series of increasingly more difficult stages—in syllables, in words, in phrases, in sentences, and then in conversation. I wouldn't let him move from one stage to the next unless he could say his sound correctly and consistently in the preceding stage. All of Sean's articulation errors were essentially corrected in this manner, with the process taking approximately 2 years. I somehow managed it with the help of his parents and teacher, some natural maturation, and all the state-of-the-art training I had at my command at that time.

It was not as easy as it all may sound. There were many times when I thought what I was doing was simply too difficult for Sean. My concept and his concept of a phoneme were very different, and I had him doing some rather abstract tasks at times. I never realized how difficult it could be to listen for fine differences in speech sounds. I recall asking Sean to locate a certain speech sound embedded in the middle of a multisyllabic word and his looking at me as though I were crazy. It was a look that said, "Why am I doing this? It doesn't make any sense." He sometimes gave me that same look when I'd have him say the same set of words over and over again.

My approach to Sean's articulation problem reflected my philosophy about it at that time. I thought then that speech sound errors were phonetic in nature and so my therapy emphasized both the auditory and articulatory properties of a phoneme. Had I the opportunity to undertake the clinical management of Sean today, I would handle his case differently. My philosophy with regard to the nature of disorders like his has changed, influenced by changes in our profession over the last 15 years. We no longer consider all articulation errors phonetic in nature. Many have been shown to be predictable occurrences in a complex phonological system. Many are based on a delayed or deviant system of rules a speaker uses. Moreover, our philosophies concerning treatment have also changed. We are no longer so rigid as to teach just one sound at a time. We now look for underlying patterns or processes that may account for a larger number of errors and attempt to remediate them. For example, notice (Table 1.1) how Sean leaves off most final consonants. This is a pattern called *final consonant deletion,* and indeed, Sean used it regularly. If I had targeted that process instead of teaching one sound at a time, I might have substantially changed many error sounds at once. I didn't know that then. What I knew and did then, however, was effective, and the traditional approach is still used by many clinicians today.

The traditional approach to therapy used with Sean is explained in much more detail in chapter 5. Later chapters show how approaches to therapy have changed in the last 15 years. As you read this book, refer to the case of Sean occasionally and consider how his case might have been treated differently. We will refer to Sean several times more in this introductory chapter as we lay the foundation for the remainder of the text.

CHANGING PERSPECTIVES

Traditionally, the specific errors of speech sound production, or articulation errors, have been described as omissions, substitutions, or distortions (Milisen, 1954). A particular sound of speech such as an /s/ might be omitted, as in saying "oup" for "soup" (omission); it might be replaced by another sound, as in saying "thoup" for "soup" (substitution); or it might be produced in such a manner as to be recognized as an approximation of the correct utterance, but off-target to some degree (distortion). Table 1.1 shows Sean's errors in each category.

In traditional practice, if the cause of the defective utterance is related to a structural deformity or physical defect, the articulatory problem is classed as *organic* in nature. When structure, hearing, and all observable physical systems appear to be normal, the articulatory problem is termed *functional* in nature, and its origin attributed to faulty learning (Curtis, 1956). Most articulation disorders are considered to be of this latter type.

In recent years, the profession of speech pathology has been influenced substantially by the contributions of linguistics. For example, the name of the profession has been changed from speech pathology to speech-language pathology. The influence of linguistic conceptions is also apparent in relation to disorders of articulation, which are now analyzed in terms of underlying principles or rules that govern speech production.

The description of these principles or rules is part of *phonology*, the study of the sound system of language. This field is concerned with the underlying system that governs the use of speech sounds (segments) and of stress, intonation, and pausing (suprasegments) in the production and discrimination of meaningful utterances. From the linguistic point of view (Compton, 1970; Pollack & Rees, 1972; Ingram, 1976), errors of speech sound production are phonological in nature and can be shown to be systematic in pattern based on a relatively few underlying phonological principles. Sean omitted nearly all final consonants, reflecting a rule in his personal phonological system that is different from the rules of normal speakers. This concept is elaborated in a number of later chapters.

While a phonological perspective of speech production is extremely helpful, it is also important to consider speech production as motor behavior. Speech sounds are uttered through the movement of the tongue, lips, and other parts of the articulatory mechanism. This aspect of articulation is an important consideration when treating organic disorders, as described in chapter 10. In the case of Sean, an organic disorder was one possibility that the clinician ruled out in the assessment process.

Thus, when considering deviant articulation, it appears useful to account for both phonological and articulatory aspects of speech production. Although there is some ambiguity in terminology for describing different facets of communication (Ferguson & Yeni-Komshian, 1980), for the moment it appears possible to consider the actual mouthing or production of speech sounds as "articulation" and the rule system governing their correct use as "phonology."

In addition to the trend toward a more linguistically oriented conception of speech disorders, there has been a growing acknowledgment that speech and language are part of a larger system of human behavior called *communication*, and that speech and language disorders may profitably be classified and treated as disorders of communication. One of the areas that has contributed to this broader communication approach to speech and language problems is pragmatics, a field that goes beyond linguistics and focuses on the intentions, use, and effects of communication (Morris, 1938, 1946; Rees, 1978; Lucas, 1980; Prutting, 1982). Pragmatics requires that human communication be considered in terms of the total communicative situation in which communicative interactions take place, not just the lexical meaning of words (semantics) and surely not just the structural features of verbal utterances (syntax). Chapter 8 explains articulation therapy within the overall communication framework.

THE COMMUNICATION SYSTEM

Although this book focuses on articulation, it is important to consider the entire communication system. In the case of Sean, treatment focused on the speech sounds themselves. Little attention was given to those sounds as part of a larger system of communication. Consider, however, what happens when two people talk to each other. As they talk, there is an unceasing flow of information between them. The one who is actually talking at any particular moment is not the only one sending messages. The listener is also sending messages through posture, facial expressions, gestures, and other communicative signs. Further, the communicative interchange is not strictly back and forth. The two persons do not only take turns sending and receiving; they are, in fact, sending and receiving simultaneously and constantly, and both are influenced by the complex of verbal and nonverbal signs that constitute the pragmatic context of communicative acts (Morris, 1946; Rees, 1978).

Even though two people in communication are sending and receiving messages simultaneously and constantly, it is impossible to analyze and discuss all aspects of their communication at once. Therefore, analysis must proceed at a slower pace, treating each element in turn. There are two main divisions of the communicative system: expression and reception.

Reception is one half of the communication process and includes the following components: (a) sensation, which occurs at the level of the sense organs, which are the periphery of the receptive system; (b) perception, which is the input processing of information in the communication system; (c) conceptualization, or the association of meaning with signs or symbols (words, gestures, etc.); and (d) cognition, which includes thinking, reasoning, problem solving and similar forms of behavior. Chapter 9 discusses the relationship between the auditory components of reception and articulatory learning.

The other half of the two-part system is expression, including (a) ideation, or creative cognition, which is the generation of thoughts, ideas, or concepts by cognitive processes; (b) codification, which is the process of putting a thought, feeling, or idea into a conventional code; (c) code retrieval, or selection of the appropriate code from previous experience to express the message; (d) neuro-motor patterning, or coordination of motor nerves to bring about muscle action; and (e) production, which requires a complex and harmonious blending of the actions of several muscle groups.

Other factors influence both reception and expression of speech. They include (a) affect and motivation, (b) attention, (c) feedback, (d) memory, and (e) communicative relationships.

These elements are not separate and distinct entities, but in large measure are so interrelated as to be inseparable in the practical sense. Together they form a system. The use of the term *system* implies that each element, feature, or process in the communication-learning system functions as an integral part of the whole, and the entire system is influenced by the functioning of each of its parts. If any part of the system fails, then the entire system is affected.

TREATMENT OF ARTICULATION DISORDERS

The primary focus of this text is but one aspect of the total communication process—speech production. However, all of the other facets affect and interrelate with this one, and must, therefore, be considered in any assessment or treatment program. Many areas of Sean's development, for example, were examined in assessing his disorder.

In order to remediate disordered articulation, it is necessary to understand certain background information, including the anatomy and physiology of articulation and the phonological rules of the language. This information is presented in chapter 2. In order to understand delayed and disordered articulation, one must also have information regarding normal development. Accurate assessment requires thorough knowledge of normal behavior, and remediation goals and procedures are often based on the developmental process. In chapter 3 the development of adult articulation and phonological rules by the child are described.

Chapter 4 discusses assessment. Careful assessment is a necessary prerequisite to remediation. In particular, linguistic approaches require in-depth assessment procedures to analyze patterns of error. Time spent in analysis will be reflected in more effective and efficient remediation. In addition, ongoing assessment must continue throughout therapy as the clinician evaluates progress and the effectiveness of specific procedures.

This text focuses heavily on remediation procedures. Two sections are devoted to this topic. In Part II the major types of therapy are described. They include traditional approaches, behavioral approaches, and linguistic approaches. In addition, considerations for working with specific populations are discussed.

In Part III four contemporary therapy techniques are described. Each of these chapters is written by an author who has developed and used the particular approach. Each includes the author's rationale in developing the approach, his or her own description of the procedures, and analysis of the strengths and weaknesses.

As might be expected, considerable overlap of ideas and therapy procedures is represented. On the other hand, there may be some inconsistencies or apparent contradictions. The most important idea to be drawn from the book is that no one therapy program is best or should be used with every client. A given type of disorder or a disorder resulting from a specific etiology may be more amenable to a given therapy approach. In addition, individuals may respond differently regardless of identifiable symptoms or causes. This kind of information can be obtained only through thorough evaluation prior to and during therapy. Thus the clinician must have a large "bag of tricks" in the form of several overall approaches and a number of specific strategies. The purpose of Parts II and III is to provide an overview of the remediation process and specific approaches so that the clinician can choose what is best for each setting and each client. Every facet of communication must be considered in making this choice.

The choice of therapeutic approach should also be based on past experience in the field and current research findings. Shelton and McReynold's (1979) review of research on remedial practices provides an excellent update on what research has taught us about training procedures. Following are a few brief summary statements based on their chapter.

1. It is not necessary to choose one of the general approaches discussed in Part II. They are all based on sound learning principles and may supplement each other. Each style has a place and contribution.
2. Use of the new sound outside of therapy does not occur until a discriminative stimulus is established in the new situation (see chapter 6). For example, the child's mother can become a discriminative stimulus if she participates in therapy or if she reminds the child to use the new sound outside of therapy.
3. Children differ greatly in the use they make of listening as they attempt to change their articulation. In general, children presenting problems in articulation are a heterogeneous group, and training programs should consider each child's uniqueness.
4. Ability to imitate overrides other articulatory behaviors; therefore, early acquisition of imitative skill in training seems beneficial.
5. The likelihood of a language problem in children with articulation disorders increases as the severity of the misarticulations increases.

The research of Diedrich and Bangert (1980) also offers many findings of interest to clinicians. Their data, gathered over a period of 4 years, were drawn from the work of 61 speech clinicians with 1,108 children having /r/ and /s/ articulation errors. It is important to note that some conclusions may not apply to children with other types of errors or with multiple errors. Some of their conclusions are summarized here.

1. Individual differences between clinicians account for substantial proportions of variation in articulation learning.
2. Children respond to articulation therapy at different rates. One type of child starts with low articulation skills and rises rapidly to a high level. A second type of child starts low and ends the school year with a high level of ability, but does not rise as quickly as the first type of child. A third type of child begins the year with a high articulation score and finishes the year with an even higher score. A fourth type of child begins the school year with very low ability and makes little improvement.
3. Children show a pattern of immediate generalization. That is, children begin to use the new sound outside of therapy almost immediately, before clinicians expect carry-over and program it into therapy. Clinicians should plan for carry-over earlier in therapy.
4. Older children with articulatory problems do not respond more poorly to therapy, as some believe.
5. One therapy session per week seems as effective as meeting twice a week.
6. Whether children are taught in groups of two, three, or four seems to make no difference.
7. Previous therapy experience seems to make no difference in current learning.
8. Using multiple errors to predict success on learning /r/ and /s/ is not effective.

9. Types of /s/ errors are unrelated to extent of learning.
10. Training the target sound in isolation, followed by its use in initial and then mixed positions in words, phrases, and sentences is a common procedure. Under this format, many children learn; some do not.
11. If a child is 75% accurate in the use of the target phoneme in connected speech for two successive probes (1 week apart), he/she can be dismissed from therapy. Follow-up probes (checks) should be made until 95% accuracy is achieved.

These conclusions suggest that many of the things that we "believe" about articulation therapy may not be true. This means that clinicians must always be testing their assumptions about articulation disorders and the therapy process with their real clients. They must also be open to modifying their beliefs as their clients provide them with new information.

Later chapters of this book will expand on many of the ideas presented in this introduction. The purpose of all of these chapters is to help clinicians become more effective in their assessment and treatment of articulatory and phonological disorders.

REFERENCES

Compton, A. J. (1970). Generative studies of children's phonological disorders. *Journal of Speech and Hearing Disorders, 35,* 315–343.

Curtis, J. F. (1956). Disorders of articulation. In W. Johnson, S. Brown, J. Curtis, C. Edney, & J. Keaster (Eds.), *Speech handicapped school children* (rev. ed). New York: Harper & Row.

Diedrich, W. M., & Bangert, J. (1980). *Articulation learning.* Houston: College-Hill Press.

Ferguson, C. A., & Yeni-Komshian, G. H. (1980). An introduction to speech production in the child. In G. H. Yeni-Komshian, J. F. Kavanagh, & C. A. Ferguson (Eds.), *Child phonology: Vol. 1. Production.* New York: Academic Press.

Ingram, D. (1976). *Phonological disability in children.* New York: American Elsevier.

Lucas, E.V. (1980). *Semantic and pragmatic language disorders.* Rockville, MD: Aspen Systems Corporation.

Milisen, R. (1954). The disorder of articulation: A systematic clinical and experimental approach. *Journal of Speech and Hearing Disorders,* Monograph Supplement 4.

Morris, C. W. (1938). Foundations of the theory of signs. In O. Nuerath, R. Carnap, & C. W. Morris (Eds.), *International encyclopedia of unified science* (Vol. 1, No. 2). Chicago: University of Chicago Press.

Morris, C. W. (1946). *Signs, language and behavior.* Englewood Cliffs, NJ: Prentice-Hall.

Perkins, W. H. (1977). *Speech pathology: An applied behavioral science.* St. Louis: The C. V. Mosby Co.

Pollack, E., & Rees, N. S. (1972). Disorders of articulation: Some clinical applications of distinctive feature theory. *Journal of Speech and Hearing Disorders, 37,* 451–461.

Prutting, C. (1982). Pragmatics as social competence. *Journal of Speech and Hearing Disorders, 47,* 123–134.

Rees, N.S. (1978). Pragmatics of language. In R. L. Schiefelbusch (Ed.), *Bases of language intervention*. Baltimore: University Park Press.

Shelton, R. L., & McReynolds, L. V. (1979). Functional articulation disorders: Preliminaries to treatment. In N. J. Lass (Ed.), *Speech and language advances in basic research and practice* (Vol. 2). New York: Academic Press.

PART I

Prerequisites for Therapy Planning

The first section of this text presents background information regarding articulation and phonology. A clinician must have such knowledge prior to remediation for several reasons. First, it is important to understand the production of speech sounds and the rules that specify their use in language production. Without a good picture of the normal system, it is not possible to evaluate adequately one that is deviant. This information is presented in chapter 2.

Second, the clinician must be well versed in the normal development process to make judgments about adequacy of a child's skills at various ages or determine if a child's delayed production is following a normal sequence. Additionally, many principles of normal development are used in planning remediation programs. Normal development is discussed in chapter 3.

Information from these two areas is used in carrying out diagnostic procedures upon which a remediation program is based. Evaluation is important not only for planning remediation, but for assessing progress and revising goals throughout the therapy process. Assessment principles and techniques are presented in chapter 4.

2

Articulatory Phonetics and Phonology

Speech production is a vehicle for carrying language. Language is generally considered to consist of four sets of rules: the rules of pragmatics, semantics, syntax and phonology. Although these sets of rules are closely interrelated, this chapter will focus only on the last set—phonology.

Phonology is the study of linguistic rules governing the sound system of the language, including speech sounds, speech sound production, and the combination of sounds in meaningful utterances. *Phonetics* is the specific branch that deals with individual speech sounds, their production, and their representation by written symbols. *Articulation* refers to the actions of the organs of speech in producing the sounds of speech.

The first part of this chapter presents basic information on articulatory phonetics. The latter portion discusses other aspects of phonology.

THE ARTICULATORY SYSTEM

Many parts of the human body, from the pelvis to the cranium, are involved with the process of speech production (see Figure 2.1). All of these parts form a system that operates with remarkable synergy. Within this system

This chapter was written by **Nancy A. Creaghead** and **Parley W. Newman**.

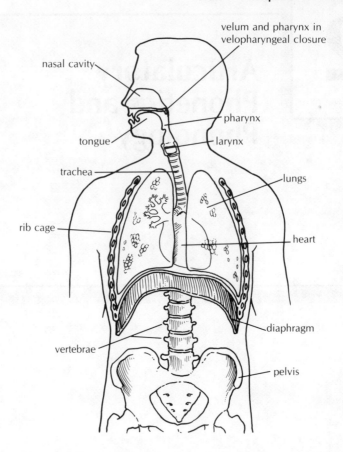

FIGURE 2.1
The articulatory system. This simplified schema of the articulatory system identifies the major anatomical parts of the system. All parts with their associated nerve and muscle tissues work in concert to produce the sounds of speech.

there are subsystems, each of which contributes to articulation. The articulatory system integrates all of the following: the breathing apparatus; the larynx, the controlling valve of airflow; the pharynx, the general passageway that connects all of the orifices and the cavities of the system; and the other parts, including the tongue, lips, teeth, mandible, hard palate, velum, oral cavity, and nasal cavity.

Traditionally, the parts of the system have been thought of in a kind of linear sequence beginning with respiration, then moving on through phonation, resonance, and articulation. Actually, all of these elements are interrelated parts of the articulatory system and must be coordinated during the process of articulation. For example, within the breathing apparatus, air pressure below the glottis (opening in the larynx) is influenced not only by expiratory muscle forces but also by resistance to the airstream at the glottis or higher in the vocal tract by constrictions formed by the tongue or lips. There is no simple relationship between muscle activity and the production of syllables.

There is changeover from one muscle group to another during different aspects of articulation. Different types of muscle activity occur prior to and following the production of syllables that are stressed or unstressed. In addition, productions of different speech sounds are accompanied by different types of breathing-muscle interplays (Draper, Ladefoged, & Whitteridge, 1959; Ladefoged, 1962). The breathing apparatus is not just a simple supplier of wind that other systems utilize. Instead, it is a dynamic, complex, interacting part of the articulatory process. Similarly, the human larynx is not simply an organ of phonation, but serves as an important and active contributor to speech articulation (Sawashima & Hirose, 1983). In the voiced-voiceless contrasts of cognate pairs such as /s/–/z/, /t/–/d/, /k/–/g/, etc., the laryngeal musculature provides the control of voicing or devoicing that is an integral part of the production of these consonants (Hirose, 1976). Coordinated actions of different combinations of laryngeal musculature activity also bring about the production of different types of stop consonants (Hirose, Lee, & Ushijima, 1974).

These findings emphasize the dynamic nature and interconnectedness of the articulatory system. The action and function of any part affects the actions and functions of the other parts, and all parts working together in different patterns produce the varieties of human noises that we call speech. The production of the sounds of speech that are the creations of this articulatory system will now be considered.

As the discussion of articulatory phonetics progresses, it is necessary to symbolize the sounds of speech. For convenience, the symbols that will be used are listed in Figure 2.2. An accompanying key word is given with each symbol so that the speech sound it represents can be identified.

VOWEL ARTICULATION

Vowels are characterized in their production by an open vocal tract (see Figure 2.3). Vowels are also termed *syllabics* because each one forms the nucleus of a syllable. Some other vowel-like sounds occasionally provide this syllable-forming function. These are /m/, /n/, and /l/. When these consonants serve as vowels, a short line is placed under them in transcription (/m̩/, /n̩/, /l̩/).

For general phonetic purposes, vowel production can be described by specifying the positions of the tongue, lips, and pharynx. Lips contribute to lengthening and shortening the vocal tract; rounding and protruding them lengthens the tract, as in the production of the high and mid back vowels, and retracting them shortens the vocal tract, as in production of the front vowels.

The tongue and pharyngeal cavity can be considered together. Although the elevating and constricting muscles of the pharynx influence the configuration of the pharyngeal cavity, its shape in vowel production is determined largely by the front-to-back placement of the tongue. When the tongue is carried forward the pharyngeal cavity enlarges. As the tongue moves toward the rear, the pharyngeal portion of the vocal tract diminishes in size. The changing shape of the vocal tract creates a variety of oral tract configurations each of which has its own resonance characteristics that result in the production of the different vowels (see Figure 2.4). The vowels of English can be categorized with regard to tongue position as follows:

Vowels (Syllabics)					
Front Vowels		*Central Vowels*		*Back Vowels*	
symbol	key word	symbol	key word	symbol	key word
i	h<u>ea</u>t	ɝ	b<u>ir</u>d	u	f<u>oo</u>d
ɪ	h<u>i</u>t	ʌ	b<u>u</u>t	ʊ	w<u>oo</u>d
e	h<u>a</u>te	ɚ	butt<u>er</u>	o	c<u>oa</u>t
ɛ	h<u>ea</u>d	ə	<u>a</u>bout	ɔ	s<u>au</u>ce
æ	h<u>a</u>d			ɑ	h<u>o</u>t

Contrastive Diphthongs		*Noncontrastive Diphthong Examples*	
symbol	key word	symbol	key word
aɪ	k<u>i</u>te	eɪ	vac<u>a</u>tion
aʊ	c<u>ow</u>	oʊ	l<u>ow</u>
ɔɪ	c<u>oi</u>l	ɪr	<u>ear</u>
ju	c<u>u</u>te	ɑr	<u>are</u>

Syllabic Consonants		
m̩ love '<u>em</u>	n̩ more '<u>n</u> more	l̩ midd<u>le</u>

Consonants (Nonsyllabics)						
Stops		*Fricatives*		*Nasals, Glides, Liquids*		
symbol	key word	symbol	key word	symbol	type	key word
p	<u>p</u>in	f	<u>f</u>ile	m	nasal	<u>c</u>ome
b	<u>b</u>id	v	<u>v</u>oice	n	nasal	<u>n</u>ice
t	<u>t</u>en	θ	<u>th</u>umb	ŋ	nasal	ri<u>ng</u>
d	<u>d</u>og	ð	<u>th</u>ose	l**	liquid	<u>l</u>et
tʃ*	<u>ch</u>ew	s	<u>s</u>ee	r	liquid	<u>r</u>ed
dʒ*	<u>j</u>ump	z	ea<u>s</u>y	j	glide	<u>y</u>es
k	<u>k</u>ic<u>k</u>	ʃ	<u>sh</u>oot	hw	glide	<u>wh</u>ite
g	<u>g</u>o	ʒ	trea<u>s</u>ure	w	glide	<u>w</u>et
ʔ	mi<u>tt</u>en	h	<u>h</u>ot			

*also termed affricates
**also termed a lateral

FIGURE 2.2
Vowel and consonant symbols.

High front vowels: /i/ /ɪ/   High back vowels: /u/ /ʊ/
Mid front vowels: /e/ /ɛ/   Mid back vowels: /o/ /ɔ/
Low front vowels: /æ/   Low back vowels: /ɑ/
   Mid central vowels: /ɝ/ /ʌ/ /ɚ/ /ə/

  Vowel production is also considered on a tense-lax dimension. Vowels with
more extreme tongue adjustments and longer duration are termed *tense* vowels.
In general, tense vowels can appear in open syllables, as in *sew, sue, sir, see,* and
say and in closed syllables such as *cope, coop, curt, keep,* and *cape.* The shorter
vowels, which appear in closed syllables, but not in open syllables, are called *lax*

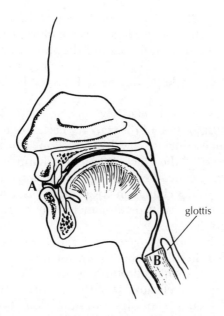

FIGURE 2.3
The vocal tract. The curved line from A to B travels through the vocal tract. Its length indicates the front-to-back boundaries of the tract. Velopharyngeal closure is shown also. The area of the glottis is indicated. The glottis is the chink between the vocal folds.

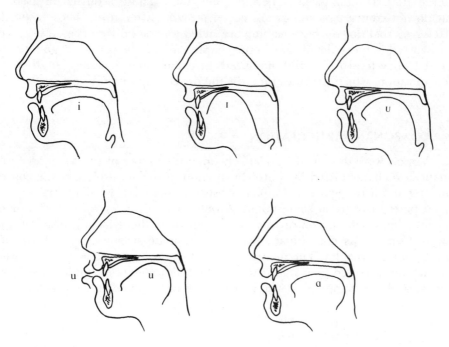

FIGURE 2.4
Approximate positions of the tongue and lips in producing the vowels /i/, /ɪ/, /u/, /ʊ/, and /ɑ/. Other vowel positions lie between and among these.

17

vowels. Closed syllables with lax vowels are *bit, bet, but*, and *book*. These syllables (vowels) are produced with relatively less extreme movements. Tense-lax differences can be felt to some degree by placing the thumb and forefinger on the undersurface of the lower jaw and while pressing up and in, feeling the different muscle tensions while producing /i/ followed by /ɪ/, /e/ followed by /ɛ/, and so forth.

The vocal tract assumes a relatively specific shape for each vowel, and there is a different configuration of the tract for each. Sometimes the configuration of the tract changes during vowel production, which in turn alters the resonating characteristic of the tract. When this happens, a modification in resonance occurs, with a concurrent change in the quality of the vowel. This shifting of resonance and the change in vowel quality is termed *diphthongization*. Thus, in a single syllable pulse two resonances may occur, one blending into another, creating a diphthong.

Some vowels can be diphthongized without changing the meaning of the word they form, while other diphthongs contrast specific meanings. The combined vowel elements in a single diphthong are indicated by the way diphthongs are symbolized phonetically. Diphthongs that contrast meaning are: /aɪ/, /aʊ/, /ju/, and /ɔɪ/. Examples of dipthongs that do not contrast meaning are /eɪ/ and /oʊ/. For instance, the word *cake* when spoken is perceived as *cake* whether it is uttered as [kek] with a pure vowel [e] or pronounced [keɪk] with a diphthongized [eɪ]. With the contrastive diphthongs, however, the vowel /ɔ/ has an entirely different meaning from its diphthong /ɔɪ/. The word *tall* might be uttered [tɔl]. Dipthongized it becomes *toil* [tɔɪl]. Those acoustic differences that do not contrast meanings are called *phonetic* differences. Those acoustic differences that do contrast meaning are called *phonemic* differences. These will be discussed in more detail later in the chapter. When the vowels /e/ and /o/ are stressed, they tend to be diphthongized. Stressing them includes lengthening their duration, which provides time for the diphthongization to occur.

CONSONANT ARTICULATION

Vowels were described as relatively open-tract types of productions. Consonants are characterized by more constriction in the vocal tract. Some consonants temporarily require a complete closure of the tract, while others require only a partial closure at some point. Vowels are the carriers of syllables or in fact are the syllables; consonants are attached to the syllabic pulses of the vowels. Consonants may initiate syllables, terminate syllables, or both initiate and terminate syllables. The manner in which consonants are joined to vowels is sometimes referred to as *syllable shape*. The following are examples of syllable shapes. In these examples, V stands for vowel and C stands for consonant.

V shape:	oh	E
VC shape:	oat	eat
CV shape:	toe	tea
CVC shape:	tote	beat
CCVC shape:	float	clean

CCVCC shape:	cloaks	pleats
CCCVCC shape:	strokes	streets
CVCCCC shape:	sixths	
CCCVCCC shape:	sprints	

Note in these examples of different syllable shapes how consonants can cluster against a vowel. There is one vowel for each syllable, but there may be none or several consonants clustered in a syllable.

Some consonants are characterized by vibration of the vocal folds, while others are activated by the breath stream only; on this basis, consonants are classified as voiced or voiceless. There is great economy in the system with this voiceless-voicing contrast. The output of the system in consonant production is nearly doubled by the addition of the voicing contrast. From /p, f, θ, t, s, ʃ, tʃ, k/ the following are derived by the addition of voice: /b, v, ð, d, z, ʒ, dʒ, g/. In general, the voiceless consonants are uttered with greater physiological force than the voiced.

Consonants are named and described by the nature of the constriction of the vocal tract and also by the location of this constriction. Both contribute to type and quality. The nature of the constriction is referred to as *manner of production*, and the location of the constriction is referred to as *place of articulation*. All consonants are classified in terms of manner and place.

The places of constriction and actual contact points are identified in Figure 2.5. In general, these places are the lips (bilabial), lower lip and upper front teeth (labiodental), tip of tongue and teeth (linguadental), tongue and

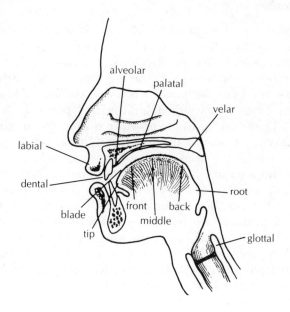

FIGURE 2.5
Places of constriction or contact in articulation: labial, dental, alveolar, palatal, velar and glottal. Also indicated are the areas of the tongue used in articulatory contacts: tip, blade, front, middle, back, and root.

alveolar ridge (lingua-alveolar or just alveolar), tongue and hard palate (linguapalatal or just palatal), tongue and velum (linguavelar or just velar), and glottis (glottal). For some sounds, the tongue comes into contact with the corresponding structure, actually blocking the vocal tract. For other consonants, it moves close to the part so that there is a narrowing of the tract. Both of these conditions have been referred to as constrictions in the vocal tract that make up consonant production.

The manner of production reflects the nature of the constriction. If the tract is temporarily closed off, the sound is a *stop,* indicating the temporary stoppage of sound production. Sometimes the release from the stoppage is forceful in nature, and the stop might be referred to as a *stop-plosive.* Another manner of production results from a very narrow constriction that sets up a friction type of noise. Sounds produced in this manner are termed *fricatives.* In a few cases sounds are formed as stops followed by a fricative release. These sounds are called *affricates.* Another type of sound is produced when the velum drops, coupling the nasal pharynx with the vocal tract and producing nasal resonance. These sounds, produced by the opening of the velopharyngeal port, are termed *nasals.* Some consonants are produced primarily by a movement of the tongue from one area of the oral cavity to another. Sounds produced by this transitional motion are *glides.* A narrowed tongue permitting air to pass around its sides produces a *lateral.* The consonants are depicted by manner and place of production in Table 2.1.

Stops or Plosives

In the production of stops, the oral cavity is sealed at some point. This closure for stops creates within the oral cavity a rapid growth of air pressure, which is suddenly released with the opening of the closure. There is an audible burst of air, a transient. However, in running speech, the word-final stops are often unreleased. For example, in the word *pop,* speakers release the first /p/, and the aspirate escape of air is heard, but the final /p/ may be held without the aspirate release. The build-up of air pressure during the articulation of stops requires velopharyngeal closure during their normal production so that air does not escape through the nose.

Each of the stops occurs in a cognate pair. That is, there is a voiced and a voiceless counterpart for every English stop. The relative timing of the initiation or cessation of voicing during the transition between stop and vowel is the characteristic that distinguishes between the voiced and voiceless stops. This time element is referred to as *voice onset time* (VOT) or *voice termination time* (VTT). In English, a second characteristic differentiates voiced and voiceless stops in the initial position of syllables: voiceless stops are characterized by a greater degree of aspiration than those that are voiced.

/p/ **and** /b/.   Except for the voicing component, /p/ and /b/ are formed in the same manner. The breath stream is impounded by closure of the lips. Air pressure builds up behind the seal during a moment of hold, which is followed by the release of the pressure with the parting of the lips.

TABLE 2.1

Classification of Consonants by Manner and Place of Production

Manner of Articulation	Place of Articulation													
	Bilabial		Labial-Dental		Lingua-Dental		Lingua-Alveolar		Palatal		Velar		Glottal	
	−	+	−	+	−	+	−	+	−	+	−	+	−	+
Stop	p	b					t	d			k	g		
Fricative			f	v	θ	ð	s	z	ʃ	ʒ			h	
Affricate							tʃ	dʒ						
Nasal		m						n				ŋ		
Glide	hw	w								r, j				
Lateral								l						

− absence of voicing
+ presence of voicing

/t/ **and** /d/.   Except for the voicing difference, /t/ and /d/ are formed in the same manner. In forming these sounds, the tongue tip and blade are in contact with the alveolar ridge behind the upper front teeth, with the sides of the tongue in contact with the upper teeth and gums, forming an airtight seal. As with all plosives, breath pressure is built up within the oral cavity, then released as the tongue moves toward the next sound.

/k/ **and** /g/.   Again, except for the voicing distinction, these two sounds are produced in the same manner. The back of the tongue is placed in contact with the velum. Breath pressure is built up behind this closure and then released as the tongue moves toward the next sound to be articulated.

Fricatives

A variety of noises can be produced in the vocal tract by sending the voiced or voiceless breath stream through different constrictions formed in the tract. The flow of air must be sufficiently strong and the constriction sufficiently narrow to create friction noise or aperiodic sound. Because fricatives are pressure consonants, they require a firm velopharyngeal closure. Except for /h/, all fricatives have voice-voiceless cognate pairs.

/f/ **and** /v/.   Except for the voicing distinction, /f/ and /v/ are formed in the same way. The inner border of the lower lip is raised to a close approximation with the cutting edge of the upper front teeth. The breath stream passes through this light contact, creating a disturbance in the air stream that produces the friction noise characteristic of sounds of this class.

/θ/ **and** /ð/.   Except for the voicing distinction, /θ/ and /ð/ are formed in the same fashion. They are produced by placing the flattened tip of the tongue on, or very close to, the cutting edge of the upper front teeth. The airstream is directed through the thin but broad space between the tongue and teeth. The lower teeth probably are in contact with the undersurface of the tongue. These two sounds are the weakest of the fricatives.

/s/ **and** /z/.   Except for the voice-voiceless distinction, /s/ and /z/ are formed the same way. The sides of the tongue are in contact with the teeth and gums. The blade of the tongue is near but not touching the alveolar ridge. There is a narrow groove in the midline of the tongue through which the breath stream passes. The /s/ and /z/ have been called narrow-channel fricatives. This position creates turbulence in the airstream, producing the fricative quality of these sounds. The /s/ is often spoken of as a high-frequency sound. This is because there is little energy in the /s/ below 4000 Hz. There are two prominent bands of energy in the /s/, one at about 6000 Hz and the other at approximately 8000 Hz.

/ʃ/ **and** /ʒ/.   Except for the voice-voiceless distinction, the /ʃ/ and /ʒ/ are formed in the same way. The sides of the tongue are in contact with the upper teeth and gums. The tip and blade of the tongue are raised toward, but do not touch, the alveolar ridge and front part of the palate. With the tongue in this position, the breath stream is directed against the hard palate and the alveolar ridge. The channel in the midline of the tongue is broad compared with /s/ and /z/. The /ʃ/ and /ʒ/ are broad-channel fricatives. A large portion of the body of the tongue is arched toward the palate in the production of this pair of fricatives. Also, there tends to be an everting or protrusion of the lips with their production. The special hissing quality of the /s, z/ and /ʃ, ʒ/ has earned them a subtitle among the fricatives. They are also called *sibilants*.

/h/.   The last of the fricatives to be described is /h/. It is voiceless, and the source of the turbulence which creates its fricative nature is sometimes attributed to a glottal constriction. However, the glottal constriction, if it exists, is very slight. Perhaps the more accurate way to describe the /h/ is to say that it is a voiceless onset of the following vowel.

Affricates

There are two affricates, which are a cognate pair. These sounds combine plosive and fricative characteristics.

/tʃ/ **and** /dʒ/.   Except for the voicing distinction, these sounds are produced in similar fashion. They are formed by placing the blade and body of the tongue in broadly distributed contact with the hard palate, often including the alveolar ridge. The sides of the tongue are in contact with the upper teeth and gums. Air pressure is built up behind the tongue, followed by an affricate release as the tongue quickly drops and shapes itself as in production of /ʃ/ or /ʒ/.

Nasals

Most of the sounds of English are produced in a two-part tract consisting of the pharyngeal and oral cavities, extending from the lips down to the glottis. There are three exceptions: /m/, /n/, and /ŋ/. These three sounds are produced with the addition of the nasal pharynx, which is coupled to the vocal tract by the lowering of the velum. The absence of the velopharyngeal closure during the production of the nasals, in effect, lengthens the vocal tract. This lengthening changes the resonance characteristic by adding low-frequency components, which creates the nasal quality of the sound. The passage of sound through the convoluted nasal cavity also absorbs sound energy, weakening the amount of emitted energy.

/m/.   In producing /m/, the lips are closed and the voiced sound travels through a tract including both oral and nasal pharyngeal resonators. The tongue position is of no consequence. It usually assumes the shape for the following vowel.

/n/.   To produce /n/, the tip and blade of the tongue are placed on the alveolar ridge with the sides of the tongue in contact with the upper teeth and gums so that air cannot escape through the oral cavity. With the tongue in this position voice is produced.

/ŋ/.   The /ŋ/ is produced by bringing the body of the tongue into contact with the lowered soft palate. With the tongue in this position, voiced sound is produced and is resonated primarily in the pharyngeal cavities, including the nasal pharynx. Little oral cavity resonance is possible, for it is blocked off by the tongue.

Semivowels, Glides, and Liquids

Glides are sometimes called semivowels because, like vowels, they are resonant phenomena, very similar to diphthongs. In fact, if /w/ and /j/ are spoken slowly, they sound like diphthongs. In the production of glides, the vocal tract is open as for vowels. Yet glides are considered consonants because, like consonants, they serve in initiating vowels or diphthongs. The term *semivowels* includes both the glides /j/ and /w/ and the liquids /l/ and /r/. Velopharyngeal closure accompanies the articulation of these sounds of speech. Their individual production characteristics will now be described.

/j/.   The /j/ is initiated with voicing and an on-glide with the front part of the tongue raised toward the anterior part of the hard palate in the approximate position of the /i/ and /ɪ/ vowels. The glide is made as the tongue moves to the position for the following vowel of the word being spoken. Resonance change is the most distinctive characteristic of this sound.

/w/ **and** /hw/.   The chief distinction between /w/ and /hw/ is presence or absence of voicing. The /w/ is articulated primarily by rounding the lips. Production of /w/ creates the most extreme position of all the lip-rounding productions. The lips are puckered to almost a point of closure, very similar to their position when whistling. In this position, voicing occurs, and the lips move quickly to the subsequent vowel position, thus producing the glide. Again, resonance change is the distinguishing characteristic of /w/. In General American speech the use of /hw/ is disappearing. It is being replaced by /w/.

/l/.   The /l/ is produced with the tip of the tongue pressed against the alveolar ridge. The tongue is narrowed so that its sides do not touch the teeth toward the rear of the mouth. In this position there are apertures on each side of the tongue which influence the resonance characteristic of the oral cavity, creating the unique quality of /l/. The tongue basically has two settings in /l/ production. In a less narrowed condition it produces the /l/ heard in words such as *let* and *love*. With a more narrowed position, it produces the variation heard in words such as *ball* and *pill*, and vowel utterances such as in *turtle*. The /l/ is a liquid, and because of the resonance chambers at the sides, it is sometimes termed the *lateral*.

/r/.   The /r/ is termed a liquid, and it is also a glide. When it serves as an on-glide, initiating a vowel, the tongue moves from the /ɝ/ position (see Figure 2.6) to that of the subsequent vowel. If /r/ terminates a syllable as an off-glide, the tongue moves from a vowel position to or toward the /ɝ/ position. The essence of the sound is movement either toward or away from the /ɝ/.

Figure 2.6 illustrates the bunched tongue positions used in producing /ɝ/. The variety of tongue shapes used in producing an /ɝ/ without specific contact points in the oral cavity make it difficult to describe. The lack of articulatory points of contact and the three-chamber resonance cavities that the tongue and pharynx create perhaps account for the difficulty children have in mastering this sound in speech. The drawings in Figure 2.6 are adapted from an X-ray study of DeLattre and Freeman (1968). In the literature on /r/ productions, the retroflex tongue position is often described. In this position the tip of the tongue is turned back. However, the presence of the retroflex position was not supported by the X-ray data of DeLattre and Freeman. The tongue position for /ɝ/ can best be described as bunched with three resonance chambers, one in front of the tongue, a second directly behind the tongue, and the third in the region of the laryngeal pharynx. Ladefoged (1975) uses the term *rhotacization* to describe the quality of r-coloring. This term includes both retroflex and bunched tongue positions.

DYNAMICS OF SPEECH PRODUCTION

In the discussion thus far, speech sounds have been identified and described. It is now appropriate to consider them in the context of conversational or

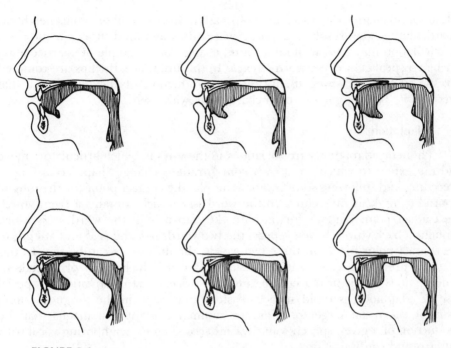

FIGURE 2.6
Representative shapes of the tongue in productions of the /ɝ/ in the word *curb*
by General American speakers. Note the three resonance chambers, one in
front of the tongue, a second directly behind the tongue, and a third in the
laryngeal pharynx. (*Source:* "A Dialect Study of American R's by X-ray Motion
Pictures" by P. DeLattre and D.C. Freeman, 1968, *Linguistics, 44,* p. 41.
Copyright 1968 by *Linguistics*. Adapted by permission.)

connected or running speech. The words printed on this page are made up of
letters of the alphabet, and it is reasonable to think of the sounds of speech as
being joined in a similar manner. However, this comparison between connected
speech and words on a page is very misleading, for in reality speech is a
continuously changing physiological and acoustic stream produced by the articulatory system. Speech sounds that we have discussed are segments, but speech
is not segmented. It is a flow of syllable pulses with the articulators in constant
motion except when the flow stops for pauses. The genuine dynamic connection between the sounds of speech can be considered in light of their influence
upon each other. They affect each other and alter each other. There are three
aspects of sound influence: coarticulation, adaptation, and assimilation.

Coarticulation

One type of phonetic influence that occurs in connected speech is
coarticulation. Strictly speaking, coarticulation means that two articulators are
moving simultaneously to produce two different phones. This creates adaptation,
in which an articulator modifies its movements due to the influence of a
preceding or following phone. It also creates assimilation, in which there is an

actual sound change due to a feature spreading from one phone to its neighbor. Coarticulation may result in a smear of features as found in assimilation, yet coarticulation may exist without a sound change. An example of coarticulation is when a speaker says the word *through.* In this utterance, the lips are rounded for the upcoming vowel /u/ during the production of the /θr/ cluster that precedes it. The tongue can even coarticulate with itself.

Adaptation

Phonetic adaptations are variations in the ways in which articulators move and the extent to which vocal tract configurations change shape according to preceding and following sounds. For example, the contact point for the tongue in producing /k/ is the velum. In the word *seek,* which contains a front vowel, the contact point is more forward for /k/ than it is in the word *book,* which contains a back vowel. If one repeats the two words *seek* and *book* and attends to the contact point for /k/ in these two words, the difference can be felt. In this case the preceding vowel influences the place in which /k/ is produced. In general, no sound is produced the same way twice, due to adaptation. A special case of adaptation is rapid speech. Faster rates result in the tongue's falling short of the usual target position. In summary, adaptation means that the production of a given speech sound varies according to neighboring vocal tract patterns and configurations.

Assimilation

If changes in a given sound are extensive enough, the sound may actually take on audible characteristics of its neighbor. These modifications in the way a phone (speech sound) sounds are called *assimilation* and will be discussed later in the chapter.

Conclusion.   Coarticulation, adaptation, and assimilation are pervasive in connected speech. These processes make speech production efficient. The activities of the articulatory system are not restricted to producing one sound at a time and producing sounds in sequence; rather, movements are overlapping, and preparations for several sounds are going on simultaneously. Sounds are not produced as beads on a string with one following another, but instead phones overlap and flow into each other in a continuously changing stream of sound.

PHONOLOGICAL RULES

Phonological rules describe the sound system of a language. Some of these rules tend to be universal across languages, partly because the available set of rules is bound by the articulatory mechanism and the perceptual limitations of human beings. Other rules vary among languages. For example, all languages have a set of both vowels and consonants, but some languages have very few different sounds while others have a larger set. English, for example, has approximately 17 vowels, while other languages like Eskimo and some dialects of Arabic have only 3—/i/, /ɑ/, and /u/ (Schane, 1973). Phonological rules describe the following parameters of a language: (a) the phonemes of the language, (b) the allophones of the phonemes and the conditions for appearance of the allophones, and (c) the allowable word positions and combinations of these phonemes.

The Phoneme

The phoneme is the smallest unit of sound that is capable of affecting meaning in a language. The concept of the phoneme is an idealized notion about what constitutes the discrete spoken units of the language. Any individual who is a native speaker of a given language intuitively knows the phonemes of his language. He needs no course in linguistics to know the difference between two words that differ by only one phoneme. Further, meaning is not necessary, because if a native speaker of English heard the syllables *peeb* and *beeb*, which have no meaning, he would report that they differ by the first sound. They have the potential for being different words. They might be used as names for a pet or a new detergent. Each language has a set of phonemes which are combined to form all of the words of the language. The phoneme set of all languages consists of both vowels and consonants. The number of different phonemes in a language is always balanced by two opposite forces.

1. A larger number of phonemes provides more flexibility in forming new words without making words longer. For example, if our language had only two phonemes, /p/ and /o/, we could have the words /o/, /po/, /op/, and /pop/, and then the only way to make new words would be to add syllables: /popo/, /opop/, /opopo/, /popop/, /opopop/, /popopop/, /popopopo/, etc. Very quickly, such strings of syllables would be beyond our memory capacity.

2. On the other hand, having fewer phonemes in the language places less burden on our articulatory and perceptual capabilities. If our only phonemes are /p/ and /o/, we have great latitude in production of both with the assurance that the listener will not confuse them. We could pronounce /p/ as /b/, or even as /t/, /k/, /f/, etc., and the listener would still assume the sound to be /p/ because there are no other consonant choices. In the same way, /o/ could be pronounced as a wide range of vowels with no concern for confusion. With fewer phonemes there is also less burden on the listener because he does not have to listen so carefully to be sure he heard the correct sound. If a language has two different phonemes, like /s/ and /ʃ/, that are similar except for place of articulation, then the speaker must be careful to achieve correct tongue placement so that the listener does not confuse such words as *see* and *she*. Likewise, the listener must be more alert and often make use of context to detect the difference.

The smallest phoneme set that has been found is 5 phonemes. English has 46, which ranks with other languages having large numbers of them. The considerations just discussed influence learning the sound system of a language and affect intelligibility of children with defective articulation.

The Allophone

A phoneme is a class or category of speech sounds that have the same role in contrasting meaning. More simply expressed, a phoneme is a family or group of sounds that are perceived as belonging to the same category. A phone is the actual speech sound uttered. Each spoken phone is classified as belonging to a particular phoneme according to its effect on meaning.

An allophone is an articulatory gesture that is a variant of a phoneme category within the language. For example, in English, the voiceless plosives have aspirated and unaspirated allophones which are determined by word position. At the beginning of a word /p/, /t/, and /k/ are aspirated; at the end they are not. Therefore, although aspirated and unaspirated variants are different phones, they are not different phonemes because the difference does not change the meaning of the word. It is possible that a language could have two different words, /pil/ and /p^{h}il/ (with an aspirated /p/). In that case, /p/ and /p^h/ would be two phonemes. In English, [p] and [p^h] are allophones. Note that slashes are used to enclose phonemes. This is called *broad phonetic transcription*. Brackets are used to enclose allophones. When allophones are transcribed, it is called *close phonetic transcription*. From the above example, it can be seen that the specific language being discussed may determine whether slashes or brackets are appropriate to enclose a given phone. Diacritical markings may be used to define allophones in close transcription. Examples of diacritical markings include "~" to denote nasality, as in [kæ̃n], or "ㅓ" to denote a lateralized production, as in a lateral lisp, e.g., [sɪt].

Two observations can help us determine whether two phones are phonemes or allophones in a language:

1. If we can find two words in the language that differ only in regard to the two phones, then we have two phonemes. In English, /pæt/ and /bæt/ are different words, and therefore /p/ and /b/ are phonemes. These two words, which differ by only one phoneme, are called a *minimal pair*. However, [hæt^h] and [hæt] are not different words. Therefore, this pair gives no evidence that [t^h] and [t] are phonemes.

2. If the two phones always appear in complementary distribution (i.e., never appear in the same context in a word), they are not classified as different phonemes. In English, [p^h] appears only in the syllable-initiating position ([p^{h}æt]); [p] appears only in syllable-final position ([hop]), or as the second member of a consonant cluster ([spɪn]). Thus although these /p/s are produced differently and sound different, they all belong to the same phoneme category.

All of the various allophones are the direct result of the environment, or phonetic context, of the phoneme. In other words, we can say that allophones are the result of context-sensitive rules. In the above example, the use of [p] or [p^h] is determined by the surrounding sounds—i.e., whether the /p/ is preceded or followed by a vowel, a consonant or nothing. Context-sensitive rules describe the allophonic modifications that speakers make in rapid speech. Many of these modifications have become part of the standard production of individual words. Context-sensitive rules will be described under "Phonological Processes."

Rules for Sound Combinations

Phonological rules also describe the allowable syllable structures and sound combinations of a given language. All natural languages contain vowels and consonants and allow them to combine with one another in certain ways. Consonant-vowel (CV as in *go*), vowel-consonant (VC as in *up*), or consonant-vowel-consonant (CVC as *cat*) syllable structures are very common across languages. In English, there are no restrictions on which vowels may occur with which consonants. All possible combinations of single vowels and single consonants are allowable.

Earlier in the chapter a variety of syllable shapes was shown. There are in English, as well as in other languages, restrictions regarding the combination of consonants with one another. These limitations determine allowable syllable structures. In English, in addition to the CV structure, it is possible to have CCV (*true*) and CCCV (*strew*), but not CCCCV. A consonant or consonant cluster may close the syllable, as in CCCVC (*strike*). In addition to the VC syllable, we can have VCC (*nats*) and VCCC (*arms*), but not VCCCC. There are altogether 16 allowable syllable structures in English, including V (*a*). The largest possible syllable structure is CCCVCCC (*strands*–/strændz/).

There are also rules specifying which consonants may be combined with one another and in what order. At the beginning of English words, we can use the consonant clusters /st/ (*stick*), /sp/ (*spoon*), /sk/ (*skate*), /sl/ (*slip*), and /sw/ (*swim*), but not /sr/, /sʃ/, /sθ/, etc. We can further have /str/ (*strike*), /spr/ (*spring*), /skr/ (*scream*), but not /slr/ or /swr/. In addition, we can say /br/ (*break*), /bl/ (*blue*), /gr/ (*great*), /gl/ (*glue*), /tr/ (*tree*), /dr/ (*drink*), but not /tl/, or /dl/. Similar but not identical rules exist for the final word position. These rules are not the same for other languages.

Morphophonemics

Earlier, the phoneme was described as the smallest unit of sound that is capable of affecting meaning. A morpheme, on the other hand, is the smallest unit of meaning. How are they different? /p/ and /b/ are phonemes. They do not mean anything by themselves. However, in the minimal pair /pæt/ and /bæt/ the meaning of the word depends on which of the two is present. /s/ is also a phoneme. The sequence /sæt/ has a different meaning than /pæt/ or /bæt/. But /s/ is also a morpheme. When attached to a word, it can carry other meanings: plural, or possession. In the same way *ed* (pronounced /t/, /d/, or /əd/) is a morpheme, meaning past, as are *un* meaning "not," *pre* meaning "before," etc. These are bound morphemes, which means that they must be attached to another morpheme. Free morphemes such as *dog, window, truth, go, pretty,* and so forth have meaning by themselves. Thus words are also morphemes, but what is seen as a single word may be made up of more than one morpheme as in *undeniable,* which is three morphemes, each adding to the meaning of the whole.

Morphophonemic rules govern the production of sounds in combinations of morphemes. It may be said that they relate phonological rules and syntactic rules. For example, a morphophonemic rule specifies how the past tense marker will be produced when it is attached to a specific word. It may be pronounced as /t/ (*walked*), /d/ (*played*), or /əd/ (*skated*), depending on the phonetic context. Morphophonemic rules will be discussed further under "Assimilation" and "Writing Rules."

DISTINCTIVE FEATURES

One goal of linguistics is to describe a language using the smallest number of different rules which can account for all of the possible combinations and sequences that can be generated. One attempt to describe the set of phonemes in a language is the theory of distinctive features. A distinctive feature is an articulatory or acoustic parameter whose presence or absence defines a phoneme. Most distinctive feature systems are binary systems that describe each phoneme by the presence or absence of a set of features. Some phonemes, such as /p/ and /b/, differ by the presence or absence of only one feature. These two phonemes share an identical set of features with the exception of voicing. /p/ is voiceless, while /b/ is voiced.

/p/	/b/
+ stop	+ stop
+ anterior	+ anterior
− coronal	− coronal
+ consonant	+ consonant
− voice	+ voice

On the other hand, the phonemes /u/ and /p/ have no + features in common.

/u/	/p/
+ vocalic	− vocalic
− consonantal	+ consonantal
− anterior	+ anterior
+ back	− back
+ coronal	− coronal
+ sonorant	− sonorant
+ rounded	+ stop
+ voiced	− voiced

Several different feature systems exist. Chomsky and Halle (1968) proposed a set of binary features which could describe all English phonemes, including both vowels and consonants. The features that they proposed are defined in Table 2.2. Table 2.3 shows a feature matrix for the vowels and consonants of English based on the Chomsky and Halle system. Other feature systems have been proposed and used by various researchers (Jakobson, Fant, & Halle, 1952; Miller & Nicely, 1955; Singh & Black, 1966; Singh & Polen, 1972; Singh & Singh, 1972). It is important to be aware of and understand these feature systems because some research on articulation disorders and distinctive feature therapy approaches has been based on them.

At least some of the feature distinctions have proved to be quite relevant in describing children's patterns of errors. It should be remembered, however,

TABLE 2.2
Definition of Features Used by Chomsky and Halle (1968)

Consonantal	sounds that have a marked constriction in the vocal tract
Vocalic	voiced sounds that do not have a marked constriction in the vocal tract
Sonorant	sounds that allow the air stream to pass unimpeded through the oral or nasal cavity
Interrupted	sounds in which the air stream is completely blocked at some point during production
Strident	sounds in which noise is produced by forcing the air stream through a small opening
High	sounds made with the tongue elevated
Low	sounds made with the tongue lowered
Back	sounds made with the tongue retracted
Anterior	sounds in which the point of constriction is anterior to the point for production of /ʃ/
Coronal	sounds in which the tongue blade is raised
Rounded	sounds in which the lips are rounded
Distributed	sounds in which the constriction extends over a long part of the vocal tract
Lateral	sounds in which the midline is constricted so that the air escapes laterally
Nasal	sounds in which the air passes through the nasal cavity
Voiced	sounds in which the vocal folds vibrate

that linguistic terminology is often devised to describe the language itself, not the production of the language or the producer (Walsh, 1974). In actual practice, a system based on the traditional parameters of manner, place and voicing may be more useful. The use of traditional terminology will not produce a purely binary system which can describe every sound with the same small set of features; however, it may better describe what the speaker of English does with his mouth. Manner, place, and voicing characteristics were described earlier in the chapter and categorized in Table 2.1. This table can be used to determine the type of articulation error in terms of natural features. One can see, for example, that a substitution of /p/ for /b/ (written p/b) constitutes a voicing error; the substitution t/k indicates a place error toward the front of the mouth; a t/s substitution reveals an error of manner.

Markedness Theory

Markedness theory is an attempt to account for finer details of relative articulatory and perceptual complexity within a distinctive feature system. The theory is that the presence of certain features makes a sound more difficult to produce or more difficult to discriminate from other sounds. Usually the plus value of the feature is the marked value and presumably makes the sound more difficult. In general, a sound with more plus features is considered to be more marked and thus more difficult to produce than a sound with fewer plus features. Toombs, Singh and Hayden (1981) give the following criteria for determining the unmarked member of a consonant pair. The unmarked phoneme is the one which (a) requires less articulatory effort, (b) is less complex acoustically, (c) is less ambiguous perceptually, (d) is acquired earlier in normal

TABLE 2.3
Distinctive Feature Composition of English Segments

	ɨ	ī	ū	ē	ō	ǣ	ā	æ̃	ɔ̃	i	u	e	ʌ	o	æ	ɔ	y	w	ɛ	r
vocalic	+	+	+	+	+	+	+	+	+	+	+	+	+	+	+	+	–	–	–	+
consonantal	–	–	–	–	–	–	–	–	–	–	–	–	–	–	–	–	–	–	–	+
high	+	+	+	–	–	–	–	–	–	+	+	–	–	–	–	–	+	+	–	–
back	+	–	+	–	+	–	+	–	+	–	+	–	+	+	–	+	–	+	+	–
low	–	–	–	–	–	+	+	+	+	–	–	–	–	–	+	+	–	–	–	–
anterior	–	–	–	–	–	–	–	–	–	–	–	–	–	–	–	–	–	–	–	–
coronal	–	–	–	–	–	–	–	–	–	–	–	–	–	–	–	–	–	–	–	+
round	–	–	+	–	+	–	–	+	+	–	+	–	–	+	–	+	–	+	–	
tense	+	+	+	+	+	+	+	+	+	–	–	–	–	–	–	–	–	–	–	–
voice																				+
continuant																				+
nasal																				–
strident																				–

Note: č = /tʃ/, ǰ = /dʒ/, š = /ʃ/, ž = /ʒ/.
Source: From *The Sound Pattern of English* by N. Chomsky and M. Halle, 1968, New York: Harper & Row. Copyright © 1982 by Harper & Row. Reprinted by permission.

development, and (e) occurs more often in the phoneme inventories of natural languages.

Table 2.4 from Toombs et al. (1981) shows the marked and unmarked values for English consonants based on Singh and Singh's (1972) feature system. From this table, it can be seen that the voiced member of a voice-voiceless cognate pair is the marked member because voicing must be coordinated with the other required articulatory gestures. Comparing /t/ and /k/, it can be seen that /k/ is more marked because "back" is the marked value for the front-back feature. In later chapters, it will be seen that /t/ is a common substitution for /k/ in normal speech development and in children with articulation disorders. Other phoneme pairs can be examined in the same way to determine the more marked member of the pair. It should be noted, however, that markedness theory is a tentative hypothesis regarding a very complex issue, and its validity in explaining articulatory phenomena has not been proven (Grunwell, 1982).

The use of distinctive features for articulation therapy will be discussed in chapters 7 and 14.

PHONOLOGICAL PROCESSES

Phonological processes are modifications of speech sound production away from the standard adult production in isolation. In general, processes simplify sound productions. Some processes occur in normal adult speech. They are considered acceptable and do not interfere with intelligibility, as in assimilation of one phoneme to an adjacent phoneme in rapid speech. The nasalization of vowels that precede nasal consonants is an example ([kæ̃n]). Nasalization may occur when the velopharyngeal port is opened in preparation for the succeeding nasal sound so that the vowel also sounds nasal. Phonology

TABLE 2.3 *(continued)*

l	p	b	f	v	m	t	d	θ	ð	n	s	z	c	č	j	š	ž	k	g	x	ŋ	h	kʷ	gʷ	xʷ
+	−	−	−	−	−	−	−	−	−	−	−	−	−	−	−	−	−	−	−	−	−	−	−	−	−
+	+	+	+	+	+	+	+	+	+	+	+	+	+	+	+	+	+	+	+	+	+	−	+	+	+
−	−	−	−	−	−	−	−	−	−	−	−	−	+	+	+	+	+	+	+	+	−	+	+	+
−	−	−	−	−	−	−	−	−	−	−	−	−	−	−	−	−	−	+	+	+	+	−	+	+	+
−	−	−	−	−	−	−	−	−	−	−	−	−	−	−	−	−	−	−	−	−	+	−	−	−
+	+	+	+	+	+	+	+	+	+	+	+	+	+	+	−	−	−	−	−	−	−	−	−	−	−
+	−	−	−	−	−	−	+	+	+	+	+	+	+	+	+	+	+	−	−	−	−	−	−	−	−
																		−	−	−			+	+	+
+	−	+	−	+	+	−	+	−	+	+	−	+	−	−	+	−	+	−	+	−	+	−	+	−	−
+	−	−	+	+	−	−	−	+	+	−	+	+	−	−	−	+	+	−	−	+	−	+	−	−	+
−	−	−	−	−	+	−	−	−	−	−	+	−	−	−	−	−	−	−	−	+	−	−	−	−	−
−	−	−	+	+	−	−	−	−	−	−	−	+	+	+	+	+	+	+	−	−	−	−	−	−	−

TABLE 2.4
Markedness Values for Specific Phonemes

	Nasal-ity	Labial-ity	Voic-ing	Sono-rancy	Sibi-lancy	Contin-uancy	Front/Back
p	U	U	U	U	U	U	U
b	U	U	M	U	U	U	U
t	U	M	U	U	U	U	U
d	U	M	M	U	U	U	U
k	U	M	U	U	U	U	M
g	U	M	M	U	U	U	M
f	U	U	U	U	U	M	U
v	U	U	M	U	U	M	U
θ	U	M	U	U	U	M	U
ð	U	M	M	U	U	M	U
s	U	M	U	U	M	M	U
z	U	M	M	U	M	M	U
ʃ	U	M	U	U	M	M	M
tʃ	U	M	U	U	M	U	M
dʒ	U	M	M	U	M	U	M
w	U	U	(U)	M	U	(U)	U (flexible)
r	U	U	(U)	M	U	(U)	U
l	U	M	(U)	M	U	(U)	U
j	U	M	(U)	M	U	(U)	M
m	M	U	(U)	(U)	U	(U)	U
n	M	M	(U)	(U)	U	(U)	U
ŋ	M	M	(U)	(U)	U	(U)	M

Source: "Markedness of Features in the Articulatory Substitutions of Children" by M.S. Toombs, S. Singh, and M. E. Hayden, 1981, *Journal of Speech and Hearing Disorders, 46,* p. 186. Copyright 1982 by the American Speech-Language-Hearing Association, Rockville, Maryland. Reprinted by permission.

includes the study of sound changes as they occur in the sequencing of ongoing speech. Phonological rules are an attempt to specify these changes. For example, the sentence *Did you eat yet?* is likely to be pronounced [dʒitjɛt] in rapid speech. The rules for this production can be specified and are predictable in other similar sequences of sounds.

The term *phonological process* generally refers to a pattern of sound change that affects a class of sounds or the overall structure of words or syllables. Nasalization of vowels, for example, is a process that generally affects all vowels in the context of nasals. A phonological rule can be written to express this same information. A phonological rule is "the (more or less formal) statement of a process" (Edwards & Shriberg, 1983, p. 91). Stampe (1969), who developed a model of "natural phonology," makes a stronger distinction. He says that processes are natural in the sense that they are innate and based on the physical characteristics of the human speech capacity. Rules, on the other hand, are not innate, but are the arbitrary characteristics of a language which must be learned. In some cases, natural processes and the rules of a language may be in opposition to each other. For this reason, simplification processes, discussed in the next section, may occur.

Researchers have used the term *natural processes* to describe those which occur developmentally in normal children, which seem to occur across languages, and which can be seen in historical language change (Stampe, 1969; Edwards & Shriberg, 1983). These same processes frequently persist in the speech of children with articulation disorders. Shriberg and Kwiatkowski (1980) include the following in their list of natural processes: (a) final consonant deletion (*cat* – /kæ/), (b) velar fronting (*came* – /tem/), (c) stopping (*see* – /ti/), (d) palatal fronting (*she* – /si/), (e) liquid simplification (*rope* – /wop/), (f) assimilation (*dog* – /gɔg/), (g) cluster reduction (*please* – /piz/), (h) unstressed syllable deletion (*potato* – /teto/).

Simplification Processes

In rapid conversation, speakers tend to simplify sound sequences, either by omitting phonemes or by making adjacent phonemes more similar. Some of these changes may vary from speaker to speaker or from dialect to dialect. Some occur fairly consistently across speakers of a language. In time, these become part of the standard pronunciation of words. These simplification processes cause pronunciation of the words of the language to change over time.

Simplification occurs because of the natural constraints imposed by the articulators. These constraints help in determining the allowable sound combinations in the language. Difficult sequences are less likely to be part of the language. For example, it would be difficult to have an initial cluster consisting of /zs/ because the speaker would have to be very careful to begin with voicing, turn off the voicing for /s/, and begin voicing again for the vowel. It is extremely likely that the /s/ part of the cluster would become voiced, thus reducing the cluster to the single phoneme /z/. The degree of difficulty in production of two adjacent phonemes is determined by the features which differentiate the phonemes and the kind of movement or change the articulators must make between them. Simplifications which occur in the language over time result in spellings which do not reflect the way that the word is pronounced. Following are some specific types of simplification processes.

Omission.   The word *known* demonstrates the disparity between spelling and pronunciation that can occur over time. This word was probably once pronounced with both a /k/ sound and a /w/. These two phonemes were omitted over time because the word was easier to pronounce without them and because their absence did not cause that word to be confused with another. There are many English words with so-called silent letters which reflect this pattern of change: *sign, thumb, walk, sing.*

Assimilation.   The word *sing* listed above illustrates both omission of a phoneme and assimilation between two phonemes. Although /g/ has been omitted, its influence is seen in the preceding nasal sound. The final consonant in *sing* is not /n/, but /ŋ/—a combination of the manner of production for /n/ and the place of production for /g/. Assimilation occurs when a phoneme is changed to more nearly match another phoneme. In other words, a feature of one phone may carry over into an adjacent phone. In the example just given, the place of articulation of the lost plosive influences the nasal sound. One of the most common forms of assimilation in English is the assimilation of nasality to surrounding non-nasal sounds—that is, the nasal sound influences a neigh-boring vowel. Pronounce *cat* and *can*. The vowels are the same in respect to the shape of the oral cavity, but they sound different because of the nasality assimi-lated to the /æ/ in *can*.

Further examples of assimilation processes are shown in the past tense and plural markers for English verbs and nouns.

walked	/t/	hats	/s/
dragged	/d/	dogs	/z/
bedded	/əd/	dresses	/əz/
		ditches	/əz/
		dishes	/əz/
		judges	/əz/

Can you figure out the rule? When the final phoneme is voiceless, a /t/ is added for the past tense and an /s/ for the plural. These are voiceless sounds. When the final sound is voiced, the voiced /d/ or /z/ is added. When the final phoneme is the same as the marker to be added, a vowel is inserted. In the case of the plural, this rule extends to all /s/-like sounds or sibilants.

The above are examples of voicing assimilation. As revealed in *sing*, assimilation also occurs in place of articulation. The following set of words provides another example:

imperfect	intolerable	inconceivable
improper	indiscrete	incongruous
imbalance	innumerable	incorrect
immovable	insensitive	inglorious

In the first column, the prefix is spelled and pronounced with an /m/ to match the bilabial sound at the beginning of the root word. In the second column, the /n/ matches the lingua-alveolar position of /t/, /d/, /n/, and /s/. In the final column, the prefix is spelled the same as in the second. However, many of us produce an /ŋ/ in these words, especially in rapid speech.

The examples of past tense and plural marker suffixes and the prefix meaning "not" illustrate morphophonemic rules. As discussed earlier, these rules govern the production of sequences of morphemes. They may be based on assimilation.

Carry-over of a feature from one sound to the next is called left-to-right or progressive assimilation. English past tense and plural markers illustrate this type of assimilation. Nasal assimilation, as in the word *can* ([kǣn]), is an example of right-to-left or regressive assimilation.

Assimilation, then, may occur at the single-word level; spelling will only sometimes reflect it. However, it occurs even more frequently in rapid speech and may extend across word boundaries. Unacceptable assimilation and other simplification rules may occur in the speech of individuals with articulation problems.

Vowel Reduction.   A third type of simplification is vowel reduction. There is a tendency in English and other languages for unstressed vowels to become lax and centralized, thus moving toward the schwa (/ə/, the mid central vowel). Once again, spelling may reflect the original vowel as in the following words:

beautiful	button
about	butter
calorie	collar
describe	parlor

Note the variety of different vowel spellings that are pronounced as /ə/ or /ɚ/ in the unstressed syllables. This illustrates the tendency for all vowels to become schwa when unstressed. In some cases, vowel reduction may be less complete. Sometimes the vowel may become lax, but retain the tongue position so that /i/ becomes /ɪ/ (*receive*); /u/ becomes /ʊ/ (*petulant*); /e/ becomes /ɛ/ (*vacation*).

Syllable Reduction.   When vowel reduction is carried even further, the vowel may be lost entirely and consequently the syllable will disappear. Pronouncing the word *probably* as /prɔblɪ/ (*probly*) is an example of syllable reduction. Words with double vowels such as *lead, motion, receive* may have originally been pronounced with the two adjoining vowels as separate syllables.

WRITING RULES

Linguists use a formal notation system for writing the rules that we have discussed in this chapter. The goal in writing a linguistic rule is to make it as general as possible so that it will cover the largest number of actual utterances while excluding those cases that do not fit the rule. The phonological rule specifies the phoneme or class of phonemes to be used and describes the context in which the phoneme or class will appear. The following rules describe the use of plural endings in English discussed in an earlier section.

1.
$$\text{PLURAL} \longrightarrow \begin{bmatrix} + \text{ sibilant} \\ + \text{ anterior} \\ - \text{ voice} \end{bmatrix} \Big/ \# \underline{\quad\quad}$$

2.
$$\emptyset \longrightarrow \begin{bmatrix} + \text{ vocalic} \\ - \text{ high} \\ - \text{ low} \\ - \text{ front} \\ - \text{ back} \end{bmatrix} \Big/ + \text{sibilant} \underline{\quad\quad} \begin{bmatrix} + \text{ sibilant} \\ + \text{ anterior} \\ - \text{ voice} \end{bmatrix}$$

3.
$$\begin{bmatrix} + \text{ sibilant} \\ + \text{ anterior} \\ - \text{ voice} \end{bmatrix} \longrightarrow + \text{ voice} \Big/ \begin{bmatrix} - \text{ sibilant} \\ + \text{ voice} \end{bmatrix} \underline{\quad\quad}$$

These three rules say that the plural marker becomes /s/, /z/, or /əz/ depending on the phoneme before it. The arrow means "becomes," the slash means "in the context of," # indicates the end of the word, and the blank indicates the position in the word of the element on the far left. In this case, the plural markers follow the context phoneme, and three rules are needed to describe what happens. The first rule generates the plural marker. As stated in this rule, the underlying form of the plural marker is assumed to be /s/. Rule 2 inserts the schwa when the final sound in the word is a sibilant. Rule 3 changes /s/ to /z/ when the previous phoneme is voiced. These rules must be ordered as shown here. If Rules 2 and 3 were reversed, the plural marker on *dress* would remain /s/, then it would be changed to /əs/, and finally the second rule would have to apply again to form /əz/.

The following rule describes nasalization of vowels preceding nasal consonants:

4.
$$+ \text{ vowel} \longrightarrow + \text{ nasal} \Big/ \underline{\quad\quad} \begin{bmatrix} + \text{ consonant} \\ + \text{ nasal} \end{bmatrix}$$

This rule says that sounds with the feature +vowel take on the additional feature +nasal when followed by sounds with the features +consonant and +nasal. The following rule could also be written, but it is so specific that it would not provide an adequate generalization of what happens in the language.

5. æ $\longrightarrow$ æ̃ $\Big/ \underline{\quad\quad}$ n

The assimilation rule for the set of words with the prefix *in-* or *im-* is as follows:

6.
$$\begin{bmatrix} + \text{ consonant} \\ + \text{ nasal} \end{bmatrix} \longrightarrow \begin{bmatrix} \alpha \text{ anterior} \\ \beta \text{ coronal} \end{bmatrix} \Big/ \underline{\hspace{2cm}} \begin{bmatrix} - \text{ sonorant} \\ \alpha \text{ anterior} \\ \beta \text{ coronal} \end{bmatrix}$$

(Schane, 1973)

This rule specifies that the nasal sound acquires the features + or – anterior and + or – coronal depending on the presence of those features in the following sound; i.e., if the following sound is +anterior, the nasal will be +anterior. The α and β represent this dependent relationship.

Devising formal rules implies the concepts of "underlying phonological representation" and "surface or derived representation" (Schane, 1973). The form to the left of the arrow is the *underlying form* in that it is not actually produced. The form that is derived by application of the rule (the form to the right of the arrow) is actually produced and is called the *surface form.*

The concept of underlying representation can also be applied to the difference between phonemes and allophones. Remember that phonemes are the family of sounds which listeners perceive as belonging to the same category. The allophone is the sound that is actually produced. A rule such as Rule 4 converts the phonemic or underlying representation (e.g., /æ/) into the phonetic or surface representation ([æ̃]). In Rule 6, we do not even know what the underlying representation is! The surface form is [ɪm], [ɪn], or [ɪŋ], but which of the three is the underlying form? For cases such as this, linguists hypothesize an abstract underlying form. It may or may not be possible to determine what the underlying form actually is. Attempts are based on such factors as ability to predict all surface forms, simplicity of the solution, plausibility, spelling and historical sound change (Edwards & Shriberg, 1983; Schane, 1973). In the above example, /ɪn/ is generally considered to be the underlying form.

This type of investigative work to uncover underlying forms may be necessary in working with children with articulation problems, as will be seen in chapter 4.

SUMMARY

Information regarding the production of speech sounds and the organization of the speaker's language is imperative for the clinician who attempts to modify individual articulation errors and/or incorrect articulatory patterns. This chapter has described the production of each of the vowels and consonants of English in regard to place and manner of articulation and voicing. When these sounds are combined in running speech, their production is modified through the effects of coarticulation, adaptation, and assimilation.

Phonological rules specify the phonemes of the language and their combination into meaningful words. A distinctive feature system is one way of describing individual sounds. Changes that occur in running speech, in child language, in disordered articulation, or in the language over time can be described by phonological processes or assimilation rules. Linguists use a formal notation for writing these rules.

Information about the production of speech sounds, English phonology, and terminology for describing the rules is a necessary basis for understanding the material in later chapters.

REFERENCES

Chomsky, N., & Halle, M. (1968). *The sound pattern of English.* New York: Harper and Row.

DeLattre, P., & Freeman, D. C. (1968). A dialect study of American R's by X-ray motion pictures. *Linguistics, 44,* 29–68.

Draper, M. H., Ladefoged, P., & Whitteridge, D. (1959). Respiratory muscles in speech. *Journal of Speech and Hearing Research, 2,* 16–27.

Edwards, M. L., & Shriberg, L. D. (1983). *Phonology: Applications in communicative disorders.* San Diego: College Hill Press.

Grunwell, P. (1982). *Clinical phonology.* Rockville, Maryland: Aspen Systems Corporation.

Hirose, H. (1976). Posterior cricoarytenoid as a speech muscle. *Annals of Otology, Rhinology and Laryngology, 85,* 334–342.

Hirose, H., Lee, C. Y., & Ushijima, T. (1974). Laryngeal control in Korean stop production. *Journal of Phonetics, 2,* 145–152.

Jakobson, R., Fant, G., & Halle, M. (1952). *Preliminaries to speech analysis.* Cambridge, Mass.: MIT Press.

Ladefoged, P. (1975). *A course in phonetics.* New York: Harcourt Brace Jovanovich, Inc.

Ladefoged, P. (1962). Sub-glottal activity during speech. In A. Sovijarvi & P. Aalto (Eds.), *Proceedings of the Fourth International Congress of Phonetic Sciences, Helsinki 1961.* The Hague: Mouton & Company.

Miller, G., & Nicely, P. (1955). An analysis of perceptual confusions among some English consonants. *Journal of the Acoustical Society of America, 27,* 338–352.

Sawashima, M., & Hirose, H. (1983). Laryngeal gestures in speech production. In P. F. MacNeilage (Ed.), *The production of speech.* New York: Springer-Verlag.

Schane, S. (1973). *Generative phonology.* Englewood Cliffs, New Jersey: Prentice-Hall Inc.

Shriberg, L., & Kwiatkowski, J. (1980). *Natural process analysis.* New York: John Wiley and Sons.

Singh, S., & Black, J. (1966). Study of twenty-six intervocalic consonants as spoken and recognized by four language groups. *Journal of the Acoustical Society of America, 39,* 312–387.

Singh, S., & Polen, S. (1972). Use of a distinctive feature model in speech pathology. *Acta Symbolica, 3,* 17–25.

Singh, S., & Singh, K. (1972). A self-generating distinctive feature model for diagnosis, prognosis, and therapy. *Acta Symbolica, 3,* 89–99.

Stampe, D. (1969). The acquisition of phonetic representation. In R. I. Binnick, A. Davison, G. M. Greene, & J. L. Morgan (Eds.), *Papers from the Fifth Regional Meeting, Chicago Linguistic Society.* Chicago: Chicago Linguistic Society.

Toombs, M. S., Singh, S., & Hayden, M. E. (1981). Markedness of features in the articulatory substitutions of children. *Journal of Speech and Hearing Disorders, 46,* 184–191.

Walsh, H. (1974). On certain practical inadequacies of distinctive feature systems. *Journal of Speech and Hearing Disorders, 39,* 32–43.

Phonological Development

How is it possible that children learn language so quickly? They are born without any knowledge of their language and without the ability to produce sounds other than crying, much less the phonemes or words of the language. Yet by the time they are 1 year old, they have learned enough to produce words, and by the age of 4, they are able to speak essentially like adults. The amount to be learned is huge, and the learning process is fascinating.

THE OVERALL SEQUENCE OF ACQUISITION

For most children, the acquisition of the sounds of their language takes place during the first 4 years. By age 4 children know a great deal about the phonological system of the language, with later development to occur primarily in the areas of morphophonology of complex word forms and metalinguistic knowledge (Ingram, 1976). Some children produce nearly all phonemes correctly in sentences by 2½ to 3 years, while others continue to have a few phonetic errors at age 6. Most children can be understood by strangers by 3½ years or earlier and exhibit adult-like articulation by 5 years.

This chapter was written by **Nancy A. Creaghead**.

At birth, the infant's only vocalization is crying. During the first year, children move through several stages while developing the ability to produce a variety of speech sounds. At this time their productions are limited to nonmeaningful cooing and babbling sounds, but they are surrounded by the meaningful speech of others. Hearing the language around them and practicing sounds prepare them for speech production. At 1 year, at least a few sounds are used in sequences which are consistent enough to be identified as words. During the next 3 years, the child's repertoire of sounds expands and correct production is stabilized. In addition, the child learns the rules for combining these sounds into the words of the language.

Ingram (1976) has identified six stages of phonological development. He relates these stages to Piaget's (1962) stages of cognitive development and describes what happens phonologically at each cognitive stage. These stages are outlined below:

Piaget's Period of Sensorimotor Development

Ingram identifies two stages of phonological acquisition during this period.

Birth to about 10 or 12 months.   During this stage, the child communicates through crying and gestures. Certain prerequisites for speech are also developing— speech perception, babbling or sound play, and the ability to imitate speech sounds.

12 to 18 months.   The child develops a small vocabulary of perhaps 50 single words. Ingram notes that there is a qualitative difference between the phonology of these first words and those that occur after 18 months.

Piaget's Period of Concrete Operations

This cognitive period lasts from about 18 months to 12 years. The first substage, preconceptual thought, coincides with the next stage of phonological development.

18 months to 4 years.   During this time the child acquires most of the sounds of the language and learns to combine them into simple morphemes or words. Those simplifying phonological processes which characterize the child's earliest productions are gradually eliminated so that new classes of sounds emerge.

4 to 7 years.   During Piaget's intuitional substage, the phonetic inventory is completed, and the child begins to use more complex words that are derived from root words (e.g., *sign–signature*).

7 to 12 years.   During Piaget's concrete operations substage, the child refines his knowledge of the morphophonemic rules of the language—e.g., the rules of tense markers and plurals and other derivational rules such as those that make nouns from adjectives (*able–ability*), nouns from verbs (*solve–solution*), and adjectives from nouns (*care–careful*). Ingram indicates that development during this period may be related to learning to read.

Period of Formal Operations

12 to 16 years.   The advanced development of metalinguistic understanding allows the child to make conscious judgments about the phonological system, i.e., what the sounds of the language are and how they can be combined. Ingram states that this ability may be important in learning to spell.

Ingram proposes these as tentative stages and suggests research to determine their validity in describing phonological development.

THEORIES OF PHONOLOGICAL DEVELOPMENT

Over the years a number of theories have been set forth to explain how children learn the sound system of their language. No one theory has been accepted as a complete account; the complexity of the system to be learned and of the organism learning it suggests that any one theory may be too simplistic as an explanation.

Some researchers have been interested in describing and explaining the process of phonological development in children, while others have directed their attention to developing theories. In order to understand the development of the theories, it is important to consider how the supporting data have been obtained.

Some of the research has been in the form of diary studies. Most often researchers have recorded the developing speech of their own children over a given period of time (Braine, 1974; Burling, 1959; Carlson & Anisfield, 1969; Leopold, 1947; Velten, 1943). The resulting data have been described and analyzed with regard to apparent regularities or inconsistencies in development. Some of the early diary studies have provided a wealth of data that subsequent researchers have reexamined for further interpretation, for evaluation of specific theories (Moskowitz, 1970), or for comparison with other data (Edwards & Shriberg, 1983; Ferguson & Farwell, 1975).

Large-scale cross-sectional studies of speech sound development have been an important source of normative data on which clinicians have based their decisions about adequacy of articulation in individual children. The studies of Poole (1934), Templin (1957), and Wellman, Case, Mengurt, and Bradbury (1931) have been the standards for comparison. Recently, however, new studies (Prather, Hedrick, & Kern, 1975; Arlt & Goodban, 1976) have found generally younger ages for development, suggesting the possibility of discrepancies in the earlier studies or changes in the rate of development in today's children. These studies will be described in greater detail later in the chapter.

Other research has been directed toward examining the developing sound production (Gruber, 1973; Irwin & Chen, 1946; Irwin, 1947a, 1947b, 1947c, 1948a, 1948b, 1948c, 1951, 1952; Maskavinic, Cairns, Butterfield, & Weamer, 1981; Nakazima, 1975; Oller, Wieman, Doyle & Ross, 1975; Tonkova-Yampol'skaya, 1973) and speech perception (Cutting & Eimas, 1975; Eilers, 1977; Eilers, Gavin, & Wilson, 1979; Eilers & Minifie, 1975; Eilers, Wilson, & Moore, 1977; Kuhl, 1977; Miller & Morse, 1976; Williams & Golenski, 1979) of infants and the speech sound development of one or a group of children (Blasdell & Jensen, 1970; Dyson & Paden, 1983; Ferguson & Farwell, 1975; Ingram,

Christensen, Veach, & Webster, 1980; Macken, 1980, Weir, 1966; Winitz, 1969). Many studies have examined other specific facets of speech acquisition.

While some researchers have concentrated on describing the developmental process, others have attempted to formulate theories to explain how and/or why children learn to speak their language. Ferguson and Garnica (1975) divided the proposed theories into four groups: (a) behavioral theory, as illustrated by Mowrer (1952) and Olmsted (1971); (b) structuralist theory, as proposed by Jakobson (1968) and Moskowitz (1970);(c) natural phonology theory, exemplified by Stampe (1969); and (d) prosodic theory, as suggested by Waterson (1971). A fifth division is the interactionist-discovery theory of Kiparsky and Menn (1977). Although new theoretical information has become available (Edwards & Shriberg, 1983; Vihman, 1981; Yeni-Komshian, Kavanaugh, & Ferguson, 1980), these general divisions still hold.

Behavioral theories postulate that language is learned in response to the environment through the child's imitation of adult speech and reinforcement of his attempts. Mowrer (1952) proposed what he called the *autism theory of speech acquisition.* He suggested that children initially associate the speech of their caretaker with satisfying events like feeding and holding. The speech of the caretaker thus becomes a secondary reinforcer, and subsequently so do the child's own vocalizations. As a result of emotional attachment to the caretaker, children continue to attempt to imitate the adult's vocalizations and shape their productions toward the adult model as a result of the reinforcement provided. Mowrer proposed this theory based on his observations of myna birds. It agrees with the concepts of learning theory and consequently has been widely accepted because it is in accord with explanations of the learning of other skills. Ferguson and Garnica (1975) point out that there is no experimental evidence to support this theory and that language learning may be different from other human behaviors.

The structuralist theory (Jakobson, 1968) holds that children are born with the ability to develop language and that phonological development and other aspects of language acquisition follow a universal order. Jakobson contends that there is a general order of sound development, although the exact age of acquisition may vary from child to child. He proposed that children develop their sound system by learning oppositions or contrasts of decreasing magnitude. These oppositions are expressed in terms of distinctive features (see chapter 2). The first contrast that children learn is between vowels and consonants, hence they will be likely to have a vowel and a consonant in their earliest phonetic repertoire. The consonants begin to differentiate first, with a manner distinction between oral and nasal sounds. In regard to place, a labial sound like /b/ or /m/ is likely to appear in opposition to a dental sound like /d/ or /n/. Children are then likely to develop two or three very different vowels which form the bare essentials of the vowel triangle, such as a high front vowel like /i/, a high back vowel like /u/ and a low mid vowel like /ɑ/. The vowels will continue to differentiate in this manner until all vowels in the language have been acquired.

This universal order determines that certain groups of sounds will appear before others. For example, Jakobson states that the presence of alveolar and palatal sounds implies the presence of dental sounds. Likewise, the presence of

TABLE 3.1
Possible Order of Development of Early Distinctive-Feature Contrasts in Repertoire of Hypothetical Child

First Division			
Vowel		Consonant	
/ɑ/		/b/	
Second Division			
	Oral		Nasal
	/b/		/m/
Third Division			
High front	High back		
/i/	/u/		
Low mid			
/ɑ/			
Fourth Division			
Labial	Dental	Labial	Dental
/b/	/d/	/m/	/n/
Fifth Division			
Stop	Fricative		
/d/	/s/		

fricatives implies stops. A given fricative will not be used until the homorganic (same place of articulation) stop has been acquired (Ingram, 1976). Based on these principles, Table 3.1 shows an outline of the possible early contrasts for a hypothetical child. It is not suggested that every or even most children will follow this exact order of sound acquisition.

Jakobson saw this progression as beginning with the onset of meaningful speech. According to his theory, babbling is not continuous with phonemic development. During babbling the child utters a wide variety of sounds, many of which do not appear in early meaningful speech and must be learned or relearned as speech develops.

Other researchers who have adopted Jakobson's theories see more continuity between babbling and meaningful speech (Moskowitz, 1970). Moskowitz extended Jakobson's theory, but focused on the syllable as the earliest learned unit: first CV, then VC, and finally V. According to Moskowitz, children first analyze whole syllables, then phonemes. Moskowitz states that a theory of development must include both segments (individual sounds) and distinctive features. Either alone is not sufficient. Although there may be a universal set of rules that are available to children, each child uses a slightly different subset.

Stampe's (1969) natural theory of phonological development is based on the premise that the normally developing child attempts to reproduce the adult model, but because of immature motor abilities, the productions are simplified. The child's productions differ from the adult model as a result of the innate system of phonological processes that the child brings to the language-learning task. The development of adult phonology involves progressive elimination of these processes.

In general, processes simplify sound productions and produce a reduced set of phonemes. In Stampe's words, "A phonological process merges a potential phonological opposition into that member of the opposition which least tries the restrictions of the human capacity" (p. 443). The presence of a given process may cause one sound or set of sounds to be produced like another. For example, a common process in child language is stopping of stridents, which will cause sounds like /s/ and /z/ to be produced as [t] and [d] (*see*–[ti]; *zoo*–[du]). The process of fronting may cause /k/ and /g/ to be produced as [t] and [d] (*cat*–[tæt]; *go*–[do]). Thus six potential phonemes have been reduced to two.

Children's earliest productions will reflect the innate phonological system which demonstrates the full range of processes. As they move toward the adult system, children use three types of resolutions to create contrasts: (a) suppression of a process so that it becomes optional and finally nonexistent, (b) limitation of the contexts to which the process applies, and (c) ordering of the application of processes. For example, if the child demonstrates final consonant deletion and stopping, final consonant deletion must be eliminated in order for stopping to occur in the final position (Braine, 1974; Stampe, 1969). As the child eliminates processes, the set of phonemes will expand.

Stampe (1969) suggests that this theory of natural processes explains the phenomena that Jakobson (1971) described. However, Locke (1980) disagrees with this explanation and maintains that categorizing sounds by either distinctive features or phonological processes may mask some information that can be obtained by examining individual segments.

The prosodic theory (Waterson, 1971) holds that children initially perceive adult speech in terms of whole units rather than individual phonemes, and that they attempt to produce an overall schema of what they hear rather than a sequence of individual sounds. Ferguson (1978) agrees that the total word is the important unit in the child's early learning of phonology. According to Waterson, the earliest learned sounds are based on the input that the child receives. They will be those most frequent in adult speech or clearest to the child because of repetition, strong accent, etc. In support of this theory, Blasdell and Jensen (1970) found that 2½- to 3-year-old children imitated nonsense syllables with primary stress and those in the final position of words more often than other syllables.

Waterson outlined five basic structure types used by young children in their first words. In each case certain prominent features characterize the utterance. The five types described by their notable features are (a) labial structures, (b) continuant structures, (c) sibilant structures, (d) stop structures, and (e) nasal structures. The adult word that the child is attempting to produce will contain some of the features that the child uses, but the sets of features will not be identical. Those features that the child latches on to are determined by the factors mentioned previously (most frequent, clearest) and by the child's perceptual and production capacities.

According to this theory, there is no set order of development. Children may vary with regard to both sequence and rate of development. One advantage of the theory, as Ferguson (1978) notes, is that it accounts for irregularities in development, which theories based on segments and rules fail to do. Both Ferguson (1978) and Weir (1966) have noted the role of intonation patterns in speech development, which provides indirect support for Waterson's theory.

Kiparsky and Menn (1977) and Menn (1976, 1980) propose an interactionist-discovery theory wherein the child is an active learner who attempts to discover the structure of the adult phonological system by organizing it into manageable pieces. Like Waterson, Kiparsky and Menn suggest that children learn to produce whole words before they learn individual phonemes and phonological rules. Beginning speakers will learn a few specific words or a few types of word patterns, and from those, generalize the rules of adult speakers. Since children are creative learners, they may develop their own strategies along the way. For example, children may stick with certain familiar forms and learn new words that fit those forms. They may learn words that do not fit their current rule system, but not be ready to generalize rules from the new word to other words. Since the rules are not innate, through the process of trial and error, children may develop their own temporary rules which do not fit the adult system.

Like Waterson's, this theory accounts for individual differences. It also accounts for certain strategies or phenomena which have been observed in individual children, such as progressive idioms or advanced forms (Moskowitz, 1973), overgeneralization, and selection or avoidance of sounds and words (Edwards & Schriberg, 1983).

THE FIRST YEAR

A major portion of the acquisition of the phonological system of the language occurs during the first year. At birth, reflexive crying is the only type of sound that infants emit. The sounds of crying are primarily nasalized vowels—sounds made with the velopharyngeal port open. Within the first few months, however, children begin to gain control over the vocal mechanism. Sounds continue to be reflexive, but they become more varied.

Oller (1976) has outlined the parameters of vocal and articulatory control that children must gain before learning speech. They include:

1. Control of phonation or voice and the vocal mechanism—Children must learn to turn voicing on and off at will.

2. Control of extremes and variations in pitch—Children first learn to make the distinction between very high sounds and very low sounds. Gradually they learn to make finer pitch variations, which are necessary for intonation patterns.

3. Control of extremes and variations in volume—As with pitch, children initially gain voluntary control over extremes in volume. Growth in volume control allows them to distinguish not only between yelling and speaking softly, but also among the fine variations needed for word and sentence stress and for adjusting volume to different listeners and speaking situations.

4. Control of resonance—Children do not make use of the full resonant characteristics of the vocal tract in their earliest utterances. They must learn to achieve the oral resonance required for appropri-

ate voice quality and to vary the resonance characteristics for different speech needs.

5. Control of the timing aspects of alternating resonance and constriction—Children's earliest alternations between open and closed positions of the vocal tract develop into vowels and consonants. To
produce syllables, they must develop the ability to make very rapid,
very fine alternations.

During the first year, children move through stages of phonological
development which are focused toward attainment of these five competencies.
Oller (1976) has outlined the following stages of acquisition:

0–1 month.   Quasi-resonated nucleus stage. In this stage, children are
able to produce oral sounds, but these sounds are only partially resonated
because they do not open their mouths, direct the position of their tongues
or sustain the sounds. In this stage, they make large gains in the control of
voice, but resonance is minimal.

2–3 months.   Goo stage. In this stage, vocalizations have greater resonance.
They continue to be primarily vowel-like sounds, but some constrictions or
consonant- like sounds may be introduced. Constrictions (pre- consonants) and
resonances (pre-vowels) may alternate, but they do not occur in a unit as in a
syllable.

4–6 months.   Coo stage. Alternations of resonances and constrictions
appear during this stage. These alternations will later become CV or VC
syllables. Vocalizations are more fully resonated, but they are not yet distin-
guishable as specific vowels. In the same way, specific consonants will not
generally be identified. However, greater variety in constriction types occurs.
During this stage, almost total constrictions which resemble /k/ or /g/, /p/ or /b/
may be heard. These will become stops. Raspberries appear, precursors of
fricative sounds. Experimentation with pitch and volume extremes also occurs
here. Screams and growls exemplify the extremes of pitch, while yelling and
very soft vocalizations demonstrate extremes of volume.

7–10 months.   Reduplicated babbling stage. An important step toward
the production of words and sentences is the ability to combine syllables. This
skill usually appears first in the form of exactly duplicated CV combinations
such as *baba, dada*, etc. This demonstrates a giant step in the ability to alternate
constrictions and resonances. During this stage, more definable consonant and
vowel sounds appear.

11–14 months.   Jargon stage. Jargon demonstrates the child's acquisition
of fine variations in pitch and volume, combined with lack of words. The child
appears to be using real sentences because the intonation (pitch) patterns and
stress (loudness and timing) are well established and like those of adults.
However, the child does not yet know very many of the words or grammatical
rules of the language.

During the last stage, the first real words appear. When children use their first meaningful words, they must have sufficient control over the articulatory mechanism to produce at least two sounds in a consistent manner. In order for the adults in the environment to recognize the words, they must be produced in a similar fashion on several occasions. It is at this point that children begin to acquire the phonemes of the language. Once the child has developed a small set of phonemes, this set will continue to expand, production of these sounds will become more consistent, and control over pitch and volume will become more refined.

Babbling

It has been theorized by a number of researchers that infant babbling is random in the sense that the child produces the full range of possible human speech sounds (Jakobson, 1971; Mowrer, 1952; Velten, 1943). Between the ages of about 4 months and 10 months, the infant produces a wide variety of sounds, some of which may be recognized as resembling English phonemes, and others of which may be phonemes in other languages, but not in English. Deaf and hearing children seem to begin babbling at about the same age, and their early babbling is similar. This observation lends support to the notion that initially babbling is at least partly reinforced by tactile and kinesthetic sensation in the child's mouth. Children may babble because it feels good or interesting to them. It is further theorized that this vocal play provides practice in speech sound production.

At approximately 8 months, the child begins to imitate the vocal play of adults. At this time mother can say "mama" to the child and he or she may repeat "mama". Children are also likely to repeat their own CV sequences. It is likely that babbling is now more directly under auditory control. Now the child may babble in response to an auditory stimulus and may continue because of the sound. Gradually the phonemes used by the adults in the child's environment will become more prevalent in the child's speech, and those not used in the their language will drop out. At about this time, deaf children may fall behind hearing children in their amount of babbling.

Although children may vary greatly in their choice of babbled sounds, some generalizations can be suggested. Irwin and Chen (1946) and Irwin (1947a, 1947b, 1947c, 1948a, 1948b, 1948c, 1951, 1952) reported the results obtained from records transcribed in IPA from 95 infants recorded at 1-month intervals from 0 to 2½ years. They did not distinguish between meaningful and nonmeaningful utterances in their analysis. Irwin (1952) reported that the infants had seven phoneme types at 1 month. Irwin and Chen (1946) observed that vowels were five times more frequent than consonants at birth and that they continued to be more frequent during the first 30 months. Irwin (1948a) reported that at 2 months the most frequent vowels were /ɛ/, /ɪ/, /ʌ/. The relative percentage of these decreased with age, while the percentage of /i/, /e/, and /æ/ increased. Back vowels (/ɑ/, /ɔ/, /o/, /ʊ/, /u/) began to appear at 5 to 6 months. Irwin concluded that the newborn's vowel repertoire is not like that of an adult. It begins to move toward the adult model after 5 to 6 months, but continued development occurs after 30 months.

An analysis of 18 infants showed 2 different consonants used in the initial position at 1 month (Irwin, 1951) and 11 consonants in that position at 2½ years. In regard to manner of articulation, Irwin (1947a) found that the youngest infants had only plosives, /k/, /g/, /ʔ/ (glottal stop), and a fricative, /h/. Both /h/ and /ʔ/ (glottal stop) dropped out as other plosives came in. Nasals and other plosives and glides came in at 5 to 6 months, semivowels and fricatives at 9 to 10 months. Glides and semivowels constituted a small percent of phonemes throughout the period studied. In examining sounds with respect to place of articulation, Irwin (1947b) found that during the first 2 months, velars and glottals accounted for over 90% of all consonants. At 9 to 10 months, they accounted for over 50%. Postdentals and labials became prominent by the end of the first year. Nakazima (1975) noted that American and Japanese children are similar in their early use of vowels and consonants.

In summary, many children seem to have front vowels and back consonants among their earliest productions. Sounds resembling /k/ and /g/ may appear very early. Often, however, these sounds drop out as the child moves toward reduplicated and imitative babbling, and a preference develops for /b/, /p/, /m/ and then /d/ and /n/. It seems likely that the preference for /p/ and /m/ as initial phonemes for the words "mother" and "father" in many languages reflects the child's early productive capabilities ("father"—*pop, papa, père, padre*; "mother"—*mama, mom, mère, madre*). Other early family names which may reflect this phenomenon include *nana, dada, baby*.

Oller et al. (1975) examined the babbling of 5 children between the ages of 6 months and 13 months in order to evaluate the theory that speech sound selection in infant babbling is random. They found that the infants showed the same speech sound preferences that are found in the meaningful speech of young children. Babbling reflected substitution and deletion processes well documented in the meaningful speech of normal and delayed children (Dyson & Paden, 1983; Hodson & Paden, 1983; Ingram, 1976; Jakobson, 1971; Shriberg & Kwiatkowski, 1980). The infants tended to use single consonants rather than consonant clusters (cluster reduction) and more initial consonants than final consonants (final consonant deletion). They used initial stops more frequently than fricatives and affricates (stopping), final fricatives more often than stops (spirantization), glides more than liquids (gliding), and front sounds more than back sounds (fronting). Oller et al. attributed these common phoneme preferences to the human phonological capacity.

Jargon

Jargon is defined as non-meaningful sequences of phonemes having intonation and stress patterns that sound appropriate for meaningful speech. The child exhibiting jargon sounds as though he is saying something meaningful, but it cannot be understood. Jargon develops out of babbling at about 10 months and continues after the child begins to use meaningful words. Some children produce a great deal of jargon, which may be interspersed with meaningful words. They seem to be using a gestalt strategy for producing large chunks of speech, but they do not have the meaningful words or the syntactic structure to produce sentences. Other children use very little jargon. These children tend to use single words or perhaps combinations of a few words to get their point across until they are able to put meaningful words into sentences.

Babbling and jargon can be viewed as the child's pre-speech sound practice. Children produce babbling and jargon not only in interactions with adults but also when they are alone, in bed or playing with toys. There is evidence that children may continue such practice after the development of meaningful speech (Jakobson, 1971; Weir, 1962). Weir observed the vocal play of her three children when alone in their cribs and with a sibling. Sometimes they practiced newly acquired sounds in different contexts; sometimes they practiced variable productions of a sound. While some sequences reflected articulatory practice, others seemed to be syntactic practice.

Pre-Word Transitional Forms

Children do not make a clear-cut leap from nonmeaningful jargon to meaningful words. Several authors (Halliday, 1975; Ferguson, 1978; Lund & Duchan, 1983) have noted the presence of *vocables* or *transitional forms*, which are defined as utterances produced with a phonetically consistent form (PCF) in a given context. However, these forms do not qualify as true words because they are not based on adult words. In addition, they are not generalized, but are tied to the specific context and often accompanied by a consistent gesture.

Ferguson (1978) listed four phonetic forms that are frequently used in addition to nonspeech sounds such as clicks. The phonetic types are "(1) single or repeated vowel, (2) syllabic nasal, (3) syllabic fricative, and (4) single or repeated CV syllable, in which the C is a stop or nasal" (p. 280).

THE DEVELOPMENT OF MEANINGFUL SPEECH

There are two ways of examining sound development beyond babbling and jargon. One is to look at the child's phonetic repertoire, i.e., the different phones produced in attempts to communicate. The other is to examine the development of phonemes—phones used contrastively in words so that we can say they have achieved phonemic status. For example, look at the following samples from three different children:

Sample A		Sample B		Sample C	
dog	[dɑ]	bottle	[bɑ]	dog	[dɑ]
	[tɑ]	baby	[bebi]	talk	[tɑ]
Daddy	[dæ]		[pepi]	door	[do]
coat	[do]	book	[pʊ]	toe	[to]
go	[to]	puppy	[pʌpi]	give	[dɪ]
two	[du]	put	[bʊ]	tickle	[tɪ]
	[tu]				

In Sample A both [t] and [d] are included in the phonetic repertoire, but they do not appear to be different phonemes because they are used interchangeably for any lingual stop. Sample B illustrates that although the child can produce

[p] and [b], they are not used consistently as two different phonemes. In some words, [b] is replaced by [p]; in others [p] is replaced by [b]. For some words, the child uses both sounds at different times. In addition, the samples do not include any minimal pairs in which the phones are used contrastively as they are in Sample C, where clear minimal pair contrasts demonstrate the phonemic value of /t/ and /d/. Unfortunately, real children do not produce samples as clear as this example, and it is often difficult to determine whether very young children are using sounds contrastively.

By the time children produce their first words, they have acquired a small set of sounds that can be recognized by the listener. Some of the words they use, however, will include phonemes they have not mastered and more sophisticated syllable structures than they are ready to produce.

It has been observed that the progression to adult-like speech production does not always follow a straight line (Dyson & Paden, 1983; Edwards, 1979; Ingram et al., 1980; Ferguson & Farwell, 1975). Individual children may use sounds correctly for a period of time and then regress to incorrect production, or may alternate between correct and incorrect production at a given point in time (Ingram et al., 1980). They may try out different strategies for sound production (Dyson & Paden, 1983), which may result in the use of certain processes at different points in development.

Moskowitz (1973) and Ferguson and Farwell (1975) have noted the presence of *progressive idioms*, which are defined as words which have advanced pronunciation beyond the child's current phonological system. At the same time, the child may have *regressive idioms*, where the pronunciation remains static despite the fact that the child's system has changed. These regressive idioms are likely to be often-used words or names of familiar people or pets. For example, a child whose sister's name is Cindy might call her [dɪnɪ] due to the processes, prevocalic voicing and cluster reduction. After the child is able to produce /s/ and /nd/, he may still call her *Dinnie* because to him that has become her name. Children may also tend to use words that contain their acquired sounds and avoid those that they cannot pronounce correctly (Ferguson & Farwell, 1975; Macken, 1980).

Information about the variable progression to adult speech can be gained only by observing individual children at frequent intervals over a period of time. Cross-sectional studies like those to be described next will often mask such phenomena.

A further issue in examining speech sound development is that adults may not always perceive the changes that occur in child speech, so that gradual progress goes unnoticed. For example, Macken (1980) and Macken and Barton (1980) noted that children may make changes in distinctive features that do not fit the adult's categorical analysis. A child might acquire the correct voice onset time for prevocalic voiceless stops, but since the adult's system also requires aspiration, the sound continues to be perceived as voiced.

Acquisition of Speech Sounds

The general sequence and approximate ages of consonant acquisition in meaningful words has been documented by several latitudinal studies. Table

TABLE 3.2
Age Levels for Phoneme Development According to Five Studies

	Wellman (1931)	Poole (1934)	Templin (1957)	Sander (1972)	Prather (1975)
m	3	3½	3	before 2	2
n	3	4½	3	before 2	2
h	3	3½	3	before 2	2
p	4	3½	3	before 2	2
f	3	5½	3	3	2–4
w	3	3½	3	before 2	2–8
b	3	3½	4	before 2	2–8
ŋ		4½	3	2	2
j	4	4½	3½	3	2–4
k	4	4½	4	2	2–4
g	4	4½	4	2	2–4
l	4	6½	6	3	3–4
d	5	4½	4	2	2–4
t	5	4½	6	2	2–8
s	5	7½	4½	3	3
r	5	7½	4	3	3–4
tʃ	5		4½	4	3–8
v	5	6½	6	4	4
z	5	7½	7	4	4
ʒ	6	6½	7	6	4
θ		7½	6	5	4
dʒ			7	4	4
ʃ		6½	4½	4	3–8
ð		6½	7	5	4

3.2 shows a comparison of the data obtained by Poole (1934), Templin (1957), and Wellman, Case, Mengurt, and Bradbury (1931). These researchers asked children to name pictures or objects, answer questions or repeat words. The studies varied in the number of children tested, the ages included, the type of stimuli, the number of sounds tested, and the criterion for mastery. These factors are outlined in Table 3.3.

From Table 3.2 it can be seen that the exact ages and overall sequence of mastery vary among the studies, but only slightly, despite some differences in methodology and criteria. The discrepancy between Poole and the other two studies for /f/, /r/, and /s/ may be attributed to the more stringent criterion used by Poole. In general, it can be seen that nasal sounds are mastered early, along with stops and glides. Fricatives, affricates, and liquids tend to develop later.

Sander (1972) reinterpreted the data of Wellman et al. and Templin based on a criterion of 51% accuracy in two out of three positions. This means that 51% of the children tested at a given age level produced the sound correctly in at least two positions. He called this *the age of customary production* and compared it with the age at which 90% of the children produced the sound in at least two positions. Sander argued that the stricter criteria used by the previous researchers revealed the upper age limits for correct production,

TABLE 3.3
Subjects, Stimuli, and Criteria for Mastery Used in Cross-Sectional Studies of Speech Sound
Development

	n	Ages	Stimuli	Number of Sounds	Criterion
Wellman et al.	204	2–6	pictures questions	133	75% 3 positions
Poole	140	2.6–8.5	pictures objects questions	23	100% 3 positions
Templin	480	3–8	pictures	176	75%
Prather	147	2–4	pictures		75% 2 positions

whereas the majority of children may produce the sounds correctly at an earlier age. Figure 3.1 shows the age range from the point of 51% mastery to the point of 90%. This graph shows great variability in the length of time required for acqusition by different children.

Prather, Hedrick, and Kern (1975) obtained data on 147 children for phoneme productions in the initial and final positions of words using the 75% criterion. They found earlier ages of acquisition than the previous researchers (Table 3.2), a fact which may be attributed to their inclusion of only two word positions for each consonant. When comparing the findings of Prather et al. with those of Sander, which were based on the early studies (Table 3.2), it can be seen that Sander's lower or 50% age limits correspond to the Prather et al. data, especially for the early-developing sounds. The upper or 90% age limits (for the early studies) tend to be much later than for the Prather et al. data.

Arlt and Goodban (1976) also found that previously established norms were inconsistent with the articulation abilities that they found in 240 children between 3 and 6. Nearly half of the phonemes tested in this investigation were produced correctly by 75% of the children from 6 months to 4½ years earlier than the Templin (1957) norms, while the other half were produced at about the same age. One third of the phonemes appeared at least 1 year earlier than would be expected from the established norms. Some sounds, including /s, z, tʃ, l, v/, were produced from 2 to 4½ years earlier than previously reported. Phonemes which were produced at the same age as the established norms included /m, n, h, ŋ, b, w/.

These studies of consonant development have shown that there is a general sequence of acquisition which can be used to help determine the adequacy of articulation development of a given child. While there will be individual variation in specific age of acquisition and in the exact sequence of phoneme development, some generalizations can be made. It can be expected that phonemes such as /p/, /b/, /m/, /w/, /t/, /d/, /n/, /k/, /g/, /h/ will be developed early—before 3 years. In addition, preschoolers younger than 4 years will not be expected to have acquired /θ/, /ð/, /z/, /v/, /ʃ/, /ʒ/, /tʃ/, /dʒ/ (Sander, 1972). Beyond these generalizations, decisions regarding articulatory adequacy will be based on number of sounds acquired and overall intelligibility.

Age Level

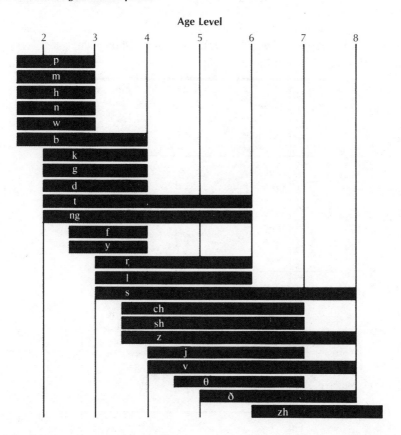

FIGURE 3.1

Average age estimates and upper age limits of customary consonant production. The solid bar corresponding to each sound starts at the median age of customary articulation; it stops at an age level at which 90% of all children are customarily producing the sound (From Templin, 1957; Wellman et al., 1931). *(Source: "When Are Speech Sounds Learned?" by E. K. Sander, 1972, Journal of Speech and Hearing Disorders, 37, p. 62. Copyright 1972 by the American Speech-Language-Hearing Association, Rockville, Maryland. Reprinted by permission.)*

Grunwell (1982) presented this developmental data in another form. She outlined seven stages in the development of phonology and specified the sounds that might be expected at each stage. Table 3.4 shows the suggested phonological system of the child at each stage with sounds grouped according to manner of articulation and labial or lingual placement.

It cannot be stressed too strongly that developmental norms must be interpreted with caution. The norms are averages based on evaluation of large numbers of children and as such do not reflect the performance of any given child. As Jakobson (1971) noted, the general sequence of acquisition is more stable across children than is the timetable; however, both may vary. Some children have nearly adult articulation by 2 years, while others, still within normal limits, continue to make a few errors at 5 years.

TABLE 3.4
Profile of Phonological Development: Phonological System

Stage (age)	Manner	Labial	Lingual
Stage I (0;9–1;6)	Nasal		
	Plosive		
	Fricative		
	Approximant		
Stage II (1;6–2;0)		m	n
		p b	t d
		w	
Stage III (2;0–2;6)		m	n (ŋ)
		p b	t d (k g)
		w	h
Stage IV (2;6–3;0)		m	n ŋ
		p b	t d k g
		f	s
Stage V (3;0–3;6)		w	(l) j h
Stage VI (3;6–4;0) / (4;0–4;6)		m	n ŋ
		p b	t d tʃ dʒ k g
		f v	s z ʃ
		w	l (r) j h
Stage VII (4;6<)		m	n ŋ
		p b	t d tʃ dʒ k g
		f v θ ð	s z ʃ ʒ
		w	l r j h

Source: Clinical Phonology (p. 98) by P. Grunwell, 1982, Rockville, MD: Aspen Systems Corporation. Copyright 1982 by Aspen Systems Corporation. Reprinted with permission of Aspen Systems Corporation.

Acquisition of Distinctive Features

Menyuk (1968) examined consonant development of children from a distinctive-feature viewpoint based on the Jakobson, Fant and Halle (1963) system. Using spontaneous speech samples, she analyzed the use of the following features by preschool children: gravity, diffuseness, voicing, continuancy, stridency, nasality. She determined the percentage of sounds containing each feature which were used correctly at age levels between 2½ and 5 years for American children and 1 and 3 years for Japanese children. The order of mastery of the features for both American and Japanese children was: nasal, grave, voiced, diffuse, continuant, strident.

Menyuk suggested that the + nasal and + voiced features may be acquired early because of their "on-off" nature—the velopharyngeal port is either open or closed for nasal and non-nasal sounds; the vocal folds either vibrate or they do not for voiced and voiceless sounds. In contrast, degree of stridency is on a continuum—/θ/ has a small degree of stridency, but is not considered to be a strident sound; /f/ contains more stridency, and is considered to be + for that feature. Another early-learned feature, + grave, carries a maximum distinction between the + and – contrasts. Those consonants which are + grave (e.g., /b/, /g/) are produced at either the front or the back of the oral cavity. This line of reasoning has also been used to account for the early appearance of these sounds in babbling.

Menyuk observed that the sequence of acquisition of the features did not correspond directly with their frequency of occurrence in adult speech, with the order of maintenance in adults' perceptual confusions, or with the order of maintenance in substitutions made by normally developing children or children with articulation problems. Maintenance of a feature means that the feature is present in both sounds when one sound is substituted for another in perception or production. It was found that the features + nasal and + voiced were well maintained in each case. This observation lends support to Menyuk's argument regarding the on-off nature of these features.

Prather et al. subjected their data from 147 children to the feature analysis used by Menyuk. As in their comparison with the Sander data, they found a similar sequence of acquisition with earlier age levels. Unlike Menyuk, Prather et al. also examined the – value of the features and found their order of acquisition to be close but not identical to the reverse order of the + features. The rank order for the three analyses is shown in Table 3.5.

Weiner and Bernthal (1976) examined the acquisition of the following features by 250 2- through 6-year-old children:

TABLE 3.5
Rank Order of Feature Acquisition Found by Menyuk (1968)
and by Prather, Hedrick, and Kern (1975)

Menyuk	Prather et al.	Prather et al.
+ nasal	+ nasal	– continuant
+ grave	+ grave	– strident
+ voice	+ diffuse	– diffuse
+ diffuse	+ voice	– voice
+ strident	+ continuant	– nasal
+ continuant	+ strident	– grave

anterior	coronal	nasal
high	low	lateral
back	distributed	delayed release
continuant	voice	

They found that the features most frequently in error during production of fricative sounds were –anterior, +coronal, +high, –distributed, +continuant and +voice. In producing stops, children had the highest number of errors on –anterior, +high, +voice, and +delayed release. There were very few errors for the features +nasal and –continuant at any age. By 5 years only +coronal, –distributed and +voice exceeded an error rate of 5%. The results for four of the eleven features agreed with the predictions of markedness theory (see Chapter 2).

Singh (1976) applied distinctive feature analysis to a number of developmental studies (Wellman et al., 1931; Poole, 1934; Irwin, 1947; Templin, 1957; Nakazima, 1962; Snow, 1963; Bricker, 1967; Messer, 1967; Menyuk, 1968; Menyuk & Anderson, 1969; Cairns & Williams, 1972; Prather et al., 1975). These conclusions were noteworthy: (a) Based on Irwin's (1947) data, the child's priority of features is very different at 1 month from the adult's but moves between 1 and 30 months toward approximation of the adult system, and (b) examination of a variety of studies with different purposes reveals similar results regarding the role of distinctive features in speech sound acquisition.

Phonological Process Analysis of Developing Speech

As noted earlier, Stampe (1969) proposed that learning the sound system of a language involves suppressing a number of innate simplifying processes. As these processes are eliminated, the child develops an increased number of contrasts in his speech and eventually acquires the full set of sounds of the adult model. A number of authors have described the phonological processes which characterize child speech.

Ingram (1976) collected data on early child phonology from a variety of sources, including both English-speaking children and children learning other languages. He identified the probable phonetic repertoire and the processes that are common in the first words of children.

Ingram (1976) holds that the child's variations from the adult model do not depend entirely on underdeveloped articulatory skills, but also result from faulty perception of the adult model. For example, the child who consistently fails to use final consonants may be able to make sense only of the CV part of the word at that point in time. The final consonant may be perceived only as meaningless noise.

Oller (1976) indicated that the child learns pitch and volume variations by beginning at the extremes and gradually refining the smaller variations. Jakobson (1968) suggested the same process in the learning of individual phonemes. Examining the data of 4 children who had vocabularies of about 50 words, Ingram (1976) found the following common inventory of sounds:

Consonants			*Vowels*	
p	t		i	u
b	d			ɑ
f	s	h		

An individual child would not be likely to have all of the above sounds in his first words, but his set would be likely to be chosen from among them. The sounds which a given child might use would probably be maximally different from one another. This is seen most clearly in the vowel set shown above. The three vowels, high front, high back, and low mid, are extremely distinct. Following this line of reasoning, we might expect a hypothetical child to have /b/ and /h/ as his two-consonant repertoire. In fact, not all children follow the theoretical model exactly, but all do tend to use quite distinct sounds as their early phonemes.

Ingram (1976) discussed the processes which characterize the speech of children from 1 year, 6 months to 4 years. Table 3.6 summarizes the processes, provides an example of each, and suggests ages at which children are likely to use them for those cases where Ingram provides this information.

As noted in Table 3.6, certain processes are more common in normal child speech than others. Grunwell (1982) listed the following processes as being the most common in normal development: weak syllable deletion, final consonant deletion, reduplication, consonant harmony (assimilation), cluster reduction, stopping, fronting, gliding, and context-sensitive voicing. She also proposed ages at which these processes might be expected to occur and to be eliminated. Table 3.7 summarizes this information.

Dyson and Paden (1983) examined the elimination of five phonological processes by 40 two-year-old children. On eight occasions at 3-week intervals, they elicited 36 words to provide opportunity for the five processes to occur. At the first testing, the processes were ordered as follows in regard to frequency of occurrence: gliding, cluster reduction, fronting, stopping, and final consonant deletion. At the last testing 7 months later, the order remained the same. Final consonant deletion was almost completely eliminated; fronting and stopping were infrequent; gliding and cluster reduction, on the other hand, were still common.

Phonological processes do not always occur in isolation. It is not uncommon for two or more processes to co-occur in children's speech. The following productions are examples of such co-occurrence:

[bæt]   *bag*   fronting and final consonant devoicing
[taɪd] *slide* cluster reduction and stopping

When processes co-occur, it becomes more difficult to determine the relationship between the realized form and the target form. What may look like random substitution is likely to be the result of the application of several processes.

The processes most common in normal children are those that are also most frequently seen at later ages in children with disordered articulation.

TABLE 3.6
Summary of Phonological Processes Described by Ingram (1976)

Syllable Structure Processes

Final consonant deletion ([kæ] for *cat*). Usually eliminated by 3 years.
Unstressed syllable deletion ([nænə] for *banana*). Usually eliminated by 4 years.
Syllable reduplication ([bɑbɑ] for *bottle*). Most common in the phonology of the first 50 words.
Cluster reduction, including deletion of the entire cluster ([ɪnk] for *drink*), reduction to one member ([dɪnk]), or substitution for one member, ([dwɪnk]). May last for a long time during the acquisition stages.

Assimilatory Processes

Contiguous assimilation between consonants:
    Labial assimilation ([fwi] for *tree*). Probably eliminated by 4 years.
    Final consonant devoicing ([dɔk] for *dog*). Eliminated by 2 years.
Contiguous assimilation between a consonant and a vowel:
    Alveolars become velars when adjacent to back vowel ([ku] for *to*).
    Prevocalic voicing ([dæt] for *cat*). May last for only several months.
    Vowel lengthening before voiced consonant ([bæ:] for *bad*).
    Vowel nasalization ([grĩ] for *green*). Very common.
Noncontiguous assimilation between consonants:
    Back assimilation ([gɔg] for *dog*).
    Labial assimilation ([bɑp] for *stop*).
    Nasalization ([nʌ̃nə] for *another*). Not a common process.
Noncontiguous assimilation between vowels:
    Progressive assimilation ([æbæ] for *apple*).
    Regressive assimilation ([bibi] for *baby*).

Substitution Processes

Those affecting obstruents:
    Stopping of fricatives and affricates (t/s). May persist over several years.
    Fronting of palatals and velars (t/k). Most common before 3½ years.
Those affecting nasals:
    Fronting (n/ŋ). Occurs with fronting of other velars.
    Denasalization (b/m). Not a strong process.
Those affecting liquids:
    Stopping (d/r). Probably very early in development.
    Gliding (w/r). May last for some time.
    Liquid replacement (l/r). May occur late in development.
Those affecting glides:
    Frication (z/j). Not a common process.
Those affecting syllabic liquids and nasals:
    Vocalization (ə/ɚ). Very common process.
Those affecting vowels:
    Neutralization (/ə/ substituted for any vowel).
Deletion: can affect any segment. Earliest process available to child. It must be eliminated before others can occur.

TABLE 3.7

Chronology of Phonological Processes

	2;0–2;6	2;6–3;0	3;0–3;6	3;6–4;0	4;0–4;6	4;6–5;0	5;0—
Weak Syllable Deletion							
Final Consonant Deletion							
Reduplication							
Consonant Harmony							
Cluster Reduction (Initial) obstruent + approximant /s/ + consonant							
Stopping /f/							
/v/							
/θ/ →[f] /θ/							
/ð/→ [d] or [v] /ð/							
/s/							
/z/							
Fronting '[s] type' /ʃ/							
Fronting [ts, dz] /tʃ, dʒ/							
Fronting /k, g, ŋ/							
Gliding /r/ → [w]							
Context-Sensitive Voicing							

Source: Clinicial Phonology (p. 183) by P. Grunwell, 1982, Rockville, MD: Aspen Systems Corporation. Copyright 1982 by Aspen Systems Corporation. Reprinted with permission of Aspen Systems Corporation.

SPEECH PERCEPTION

A great deal of research has recently been directed toward determining the infant's capacity for discriminating between the perceptual features that distinguish phonemes. Analysis of the responses of infants is difficult, but researchers have attempted to determine differential responses by analyzing sucking rate, heart rate, and head orientation. One typical method is to repeat the same phoneme over and over while the child sucks on an electronically wired nipple, has his heart rate measured, or gazes at a toy. The child's sucking rate or heart rate during the constant condition is measured. It is then determined if a change in response occurs when a novel stimulus is presented. For the head turn response, the child is conditioned to look at a toy when one of the phonemes is heard. Using these methods, researchers have suggested that infants as young as 1 month are able to distinguish between /p/ and /b/, which differ only in the voicing feature (Cutting & Eimas, 1975).

Cutting and Eimas further found that 1- and 4-month-old infants perceived the difference between /p/ and /b/ on the basis of voice onset time at the same critical boundaries as did adults. Eilers and Minifie (1975) found that infants aged 4 through 17 weeks varied their sucking rate to indicate discrimination between /sɑ/ and /vɑ/ and between /sɑ/ and /ʃɑ/, but not between /sɑ/ and /zɑ/. Eilers, Wilson and Moore (1977) found that their youngest infants (1 month) discriminated between /vɑ/ and /sɑ/ and between /sɑ/ and /ʃɑ/; their 6- to 8-month group discriminated between /sɑ/ and /zɑ/. Their oldest group (12 to 14 months) did not discriminate between /θɑ/ and /fɑ/. Eilers et al. also found that 1- to 3-month-old infants were able to discriminate voiced versus voiceless consonants in the final position of syllables when given the full set of clues that are used in production of English words, i.e., lengthening of vowels before final voiced plosives and fricatives. These syllable contrasts are /ɑt/ versus /ɑːd/ and /ɑs/ versus /ɑːz/ (where ":" denotes vowel lengthening). Overall, they found developmental changes for certain speech contrasts. Other studies (Eilers, 1977; Kuhl, 1977, 1979; Miller & Morse, 1976) have confirmed that infants at 1 month are able to perceive certain speech contrasts and that others develop during the first year.

Research examining the perceptual abilities of children older than 12 months has indicated that speech sound discrimination abilities continue to develop during the preschool years (Barton, 1976; Edwards, 1974; Garnica, 1973; Shvachkin, 1973; Templin, 1957). Some authors have suggested a universal order of the acquisition of phonemes and phonemic distinctions (Garnica, 1973; Shvachkin, 1973), while others have questioned a strict or even general order and have noted the importance of such factors as the meaningfulness of the material, familiarity with the words, attention, and production abilities (Barton, 1976, 1980; Edwards, 1974; Strange & Broen, 1980).

Zlatkin and Koenigsknecht (1976) examined the continuing development of perception and its relationship to production in 2- and 6-year-olds. Ten children in each of these age groups and 20 adults read word pairs or named picture pairs such as *peas–bees, time–dime, coat–goat.* Using spectrographic analysis, Zlatkin and Koenigsknecht examined the distinction between voiced and voiceless consonants as measured by voice onset time. They found significant differences between the productions of 2- and 6-year-olds, but all subjects' data fell into similar regions. The adults' productions were more consistent than those of children. Another finding was that the subjects' productions tended to agree with their perceptual responses regarding the critical voice onset time for distinguishing between voiced and voiceless consonants. However, the 2-year-olds were not able to discriminate their own productions when they were played back to them, whereas the 6-year-olds were. In general, perceptual ability preceded production.

Graham and House (1971) studied the role of distinctive features in 3- to

4½-year-old girls' ability to discriminate among pairs of consonants. They found that in general pairs that differ by a greater number of features were more easily discriminated. The highest number of errors occurred on pairs that differed by only one feature. In addition, the high-error contrasts often reflected common substitutions. The children's performance was similar in kind to that of adults; they simply made more errors.

Strange and Broen (1980) examined the ability of 3-year-old children to discriminate among /w/, /l/, and /r/ in meaningful word pairs. They found that in a very structured task the children were able to discriminate among these consonants, which share most of the same features (approximant consonants). Further, they found that there was a relationship between perception and production in that the children who did not produce these sounds correctly made more errors in discrimination. However, all of the children had better than chance performance.

This research raises certain questions regarding the nature of speech sound discrimination. First, is there an inborn human ability to identify certain contrasts which speakers then use in language, or do children learn the contrasts that they hear around them? On the one hand, the ability of the youngest infants to make certain discriminations argues in favor of an innate device. There is, however, contradictory evidence. Eilers, Gavin and Wilson (1979) tested 6- to 8-month-old infants from English-speaking homes and from Spanish-speaking homes. In English the difference between voiced and voiceless consonants is cued by the amount of voice onset lag time (voicing is started after the initiating of the articulation of the consonant), whereas in Spanish voice onset lead time (voicing begins before the initiation of the articulation of the consonant) is crucial. Both groups of infants were able to distinguish pairs of consonants by lag time, but only the Spanish children made the distinction on the basis of lead time. This and other data suggest that certain perceptual distinctions (such as discriminating voice-voiceless on the basis of voice onset lag time) may be innate. Other distinctions (such as discriminating on the basis of voice onset lead time as in Spanish) may be learned.

Kuhl (1980) suggests that we do not have sufficient evidence to answer this question regarding innateness. However, Aslin and Pisoni (1980) propose a compromise view called *the atunement theory*. This theory holds that infants are capable of making at least some phonetic-contrast discriminations at birth, but this ability is not fully developed. Early experience is needed to sharpen discrimination abilities. Thus, because experience does play a role, children are likely to become more attuned to contrasts important in the language they hear around them.

A second question that is important to the speech-language pathologist is the following: What is the relationship between perception and production or, more importantly, what is the role of perception in determining articulation errors and in mediating their correction? Graham and House (1971) observed that their preschool subjects tended to make discrimination errors that were similar to common substitutions. Strange and Broen (1980) found that 3-year-olds who misarticulated /l/ and /r/ had higher error rates on the discrimination task than those with correct articulation. However, the developmental data does not provide a clear answer to the perception/production question. Further information can be gained from studies involving children with articulation problems (see chapter 9).

SUMMARY

Analysis of the developing speech of normal children suggests that learning the phonological system of a language is a rule-governed process. In order to describe the acquisition process, researchers have collected data on the speech sound production of large numbers of children at a given age, or they have examined the development of one or a few children over time. Based on these data, differing theories have been proposed regarding the nature of the rules and learning strategies. These theories can be divided into the following groups: behavioral theory, structuralist theory, natural phonology theory, prosodic theory, and interactionist-discovery theory.

Children tend to follow the same general sequence of development despite the fact that ages for acquisition vary greatly. A great deal of important learning in regard to speech perception and the basics of speech production occurs during the first year of life, before the child begins to produce intelligible speech. We expect children to say their first consistent words at about 1 year, to be intelligible by 3 years, and to have near-perfect articulation by the time they begin school.

The development of meaningful speech and the errors that children make can be described in relationship to speech sound segments, distinctive features or phonological processes. More often than not, children with disordered articulation will demonstrate the same kinds of errors as younger normal children. Their speech production can be described in the same ways. Therefore, information about normal development is imperative for designing effective remediation procedures.

REFERENCES

Arlt, P. B., & Goodban, M. T. (1976). A comparative study of articulation acquisition as based on a study of 240 normals, aged three to six. *Language, Speech and Hearing Services in Schools, 7,* 173–180.

Aslin, R. N., & Pisoni, D. B. (1980). Some developmental processes in speech perception. In G. H. Yeni-Komshian, J. F. Kavanagh, & C. A. Ferguson (Eds), *Child phonology: Vol. II. Perception.* New York: Academic Press.

Barton, D. P. (1976). *The role of perception in the acquisition of phonology.* Unpublished doctoral dissertation, University of London.

Barton, D. (1980). Phonemic perception in children. In G. H. Yeni-Komshian, J. F. Kavanagh, & C .A. Ferguson (Eds.), *Child Phonology: Vol. II. Perception.* New York: Academic Press.

Blasdell, R., & Jensen, P. (1970). Stress and word position as determinants of imitation in first-language learners. *Journal of Speech and Hearing Research, 13,* 193–202.

Braine, M. D. S. (1974). On what might constitute learnable phonology. *Language, 50,* 270–299.

Bricker, W. A. (1967). Errors in echoic behavior of pre-school children. *Journal of Speech and Hearing Research, 7,* 67–76.

Burling, R. (1959). Language development of a Garo and English-speaking child. *Word,* *15,* 45–68.

Cairns, H. S., & Williams, F. (1972). An analysis of the substitution errors of a group of standard English-speaking children. *Journal of Speech and Hearing Research, 15,* 811–820.

Carlson, P., & Anisfield, M. (1969). Some observations on the linguistic competence of a 2-year old child. *Child Development, 40,* 569–575.

Cutting, J. E., & Eimas, P. D. (1975). Phonetic feature analyzers and the processing of speech in infants. In J. F. Kavanaugh & J. E Cutting (Eds.), *The role of speech in language.* Cambridge: M.I.T. Press.

Dyson, A., & Paden, E. (1983). Some phonological acquisition strategies by two-year olds. *Journal of Childhood Communication Disorders, 7,* 6–18.

Edwards, M. L. (1974). Perception and production in child phonology: The testing of four hypotheses. *Journal of Child Language, 1,* 205–219.

Edwards, M. L. (1979). Phonological processes in fricative acquisition. *Papers and Reports on Child Language Development, 17,* 98–105.

Edwards, M. L., & Shriberg, L. D. (1983). *Phonology: Applications in communicative disorders.* San Diego: College Hill Press, Inc.

Eilers, R. E. (1977). Context sensitive perception of naturally produced stop and fricative consonants by infants. *Journal of the Acoustical Society of America, 61,* 1321–1336.

Eilers, R. E., Gavin, W., & Wilson, W. R. (1979). Linguistic experience and phonemic perception in infancy. *Child Development, 50,* 14–18.

Eilers. R. E., & Minifie, F. D. (1975). Fricative discrimination in early infancy. *Journal of Speech and Hearing Research, 18,* 158–167.

Eilers. R. E., Wilson, W. R., & Moore, J. M. (1977). Developmental changes in speech discrimination in infants. *Journal of Speech and Hearing Research, 20,* 766–780.

Ferguson, C.A. (1978). Learning to pronounce: The earliest stages of phonological development in the child. In F. D. Minifie & L. L. Lloyd (Eds.), *Communicative and cognitive abilities: Early behavioral assessment.* Baltimore: University Park Press.

Ferguson, C. A., & Farwell, C. B. (1975). Words and sounds in early language acquisition. *Language, 51,* 419–439.

Ferguson, C.A., & Garnica, O. K. (1975). Theories of phonological development. In E. H. Lenneberg & E. Lenneberg (Eds.), *Foundations of language development.* New York: Academic Press.

Garnica, O. K. (1973). The development of phonemic perception. In T. Moore (Ed.), *Cognitive development and the acquisition of language.* New York: Academic Press.

Graham, L. W., & House, A. S. (1971). Phonological oppositions in children: A perceptual study. *Journal of the Acoustical Society of America, 49,* 559–566.

Gruber, J. S. (1973). Playing with distinctive features in babbling of infants. In C. A. Ferguson & D. I. Slobin (Eds.), *Studies of child language development.* New York: Holt, Rinehart and Winston.

Grunwell, P. (1982). *Clinical phonology.* Rockville, Maryland: Aspen Systems.

Halliday, M. (1975). *Learning how to mean: Explorations in the development of language.* London: Edward Arnold.

Hodson, B. W., & Paden, E. P. (1983). *Targeting intelligible speech.* San Diego: College Hill Press.

Ingram, D. (1976). *Phonological disability in children.* New York: American Elsevier.

Ingram, D., Christensen, L., Veach, S., & Webster, B. (1980). The acquisition of word-initial fricatives and affricates in English by children between 2 and 6 years. In G. H. Yeni-Komshian, J. F. Kavanaugh, & C. Ferguson (Eds.), *Child phonology: Vol. I. Production.* New York: Academic Press.

Irwin, O. C., & Chen, H. P. (1946). Infant speech: Vowel and consonant frequency. *Journal of Speech Disorders, 11,* 123–125.

Irwin, O. C. (1947a). Infant speech: Consonant sounds according to manner of articulation. *Journal of Speech Disorders, 12,* 402–404.

Irwin, O. C. (1947b). Infant speech: Consonant sounds according to place of articulation. *Journal of Speech Disorders, 12 ,* 397–401.

Irwin, O. C. (1947c). Infant speech: The problem of variability. *Journal of Speech Disorders, 12,* 173–176.

Irwin, O. C. (1948a). Infant speech: Development of vowel sounds. *Journal of Speech and Hearing Disorders, 13,* 31–34.

Irwin, O. C. (1948b). Infant speech: The effect of family occupational status and of age on use of sound types. *Journal of Speech and Hearing Disorders, 13,* 224–226,

Irwin, O. C. (1948c). Infant speech: The effect of family occupational status and of age on sound frequency. *Journal of Speech and Hearing Disorders, 13,* 320–323.

Irwin, O. C. (1951). Infant speech: Consonantal position. *Journal of Speech and Hearing Disorders, 16,* 159–161.

Irwin, O. C. (1952). Speech development in the young child: Some factors related to the speech development of the infant and young child. *Journal of Speech and Hearing Disorders, 17,* 269–279.

Jakobson, R. (1968). *Child language, aphasia and phonological universals.* The Hague: Mouton.

Jakobson, R. (1971). *Studies on child language and aphasia.* The Hague: Mouton.

Jakobson, R., Fant, G., & Halle, M. (1963). *Preliminaries to speech analysis: The distinctive features and their correlates.* Cambridge, Mass.: MIT Press.

Kiparsky, P., & Menn, L. (1977). On the acqusition of phonology. In J. Macnamara, (Ed.), *Language learning and thought.* New York: Holt, Rinehart and Winston.

Kuhl, P. K. (1977). Speech perception in early infancy and perceptual constancy for the vowel categories /a/ and /ɔ/ [Abstract]. *Journal of the Acoustical Society of America, 61* (Suppl. 1), 539.

Kuhl, P. (1979). The perception of speech in early infancy. In M. Lass (Ed.), *Speech and language: Advances in basic research and practice* (Vol. I). New York: Academic Press.

Kuhl, P. K. (1980). Perceptual constancy for speech-sound categories in early infancy. In G. H. Yeni-Komshian, J. F. Kavanagh, & C. A. Ferguson (Eds.), *Child phonology: Vol. II. Perception.* New York: Academic Press.

Leopold, W. (1947). *Speech development of a bilingual child: A linguist's record.* Evanston, Ill.: Northwestern University Press.

Locke, J. L. (1980). Prediction of child speech errors: Implications for a theory of acquisition. In G. H. Yeni-Komshian, J. F. Kavanaugh, & C. A. Ferguson (Eds.), *Child phonology: Vol. I. Production.* New York: Academic Press.

Lund, N. J., & Duchan, J. F. (1983). *Assessing children's language in naturalistic contexts.* Englewood Cliffs, N.J.: Prentice-Hall, Inc.

Macken, M. A. (1980). Aspects of the acquisition of stop consonants: A cross-linguistic perspective. In G. H. Yeni-Komshian, J. F. Kavanaugh, & C. A. Ferguson (Eds.), *Child phonology: Vol. I. Production.* New York: Academic Press.

Macken, M. A., & Barton, D. P. (1980). A longitudinal study of the acquisition of the voicing contrast in American-English word-initial stops, as measured by voice onset time. *Journal of Child Language, 7,* 41–74.

Maskavinic, A. S., Cairns, G. F., Butterfield, E. C., & Weamer, D. K. (1981). Longitudinal observations of individual infants' vocalizations. *Journal of Speech and Hearing Disorders, 46,* 267–273.

Menn, L. (1976). Evidence for an interactionist-discovery theory of child phonology. *Papers and Reports on Child Language Development,* Stanford University, *12,* 169–177.

Menn, L. (1980). Phonological theory and child phonology. In G. H. Yeni-Komshian, J.

F. Kavanaugh, & C. A. Ferguson (Eds.), *Child phonology: Vol. I. Production.* New York: Academic Press.

Menyuk, P. (1968). The role of distinctive features in children's acquisition of phonology. *Journal of Speech and Hearing Research, 11*, 138–146.

Menyuk, P., & Anderson, S. (1969). Children's identification and reproduction of /w/, /r/, /l/. *Journal of Speech and Hearing Disorders, 12*, 39–52.

Messer, S. (1967). Implicit phonology in children. *Journal of Verbal Learning and Verbal Behavior, 6*, 609–613.

Miller, C. L., & Morse, P. A. (1976). The "heart" of categorical speech discrimination in young infants. *Journal of Speech and Hearing Research, 19*, 578–589.

Moskowitz, A. I. (1970). The two-year-old stage in the acquisition of English phonology. *Language, 46*, 420–441.

Moskowitz, A. I. (1973). Acquisition of phonology and syntax: A preliminary study. In G. Hinitikka, J. Moravcsik, & P. Suppes (Eds.), *Approaches to natural language.* Dordrecht, Holland: Reidel Publishing Co.

Mowrer, O. H. (1952). Speech development in the young: The autism theory of speech development and some clinical applications. *Journal of Speech and Hearing Disorders, 17*, 263–268.

Nakazima, S. A. (1962). A comparative study of the speech developments of Japanese and American English in childhood. *Studies in Phonology, 2*, 17.

Nakazima, S. (1975). Phonemicization and symbolization in language development. In E. H. Lenneberg & E. Lenneberg (Eds.), *Foundations of language development.* New York: Academic Press.

Oller, D. K. (1976, November). *Analysis of infant vocalizations: A linguistic and speech scientific perspective.* Miniseminar presented at the American Speech-Language-Hearing Association Annual Convention, Houston.

Oller, D. K., Wieman, L. A., Doyle, W. J., & Ross, C. (1975). Infant babbling and speech. *Journal of Child Language, 2*, 1–11.

Olmsted, D. (1971). *Out of the mouth of babes.* The Hague: Mouton.

Piaget, J. (1962). *Play, dreams, and imitation in childhood.* New York: Norton.

Poole, E. (1934). Genetic development of articulation of consonant sounds in speech. *Elementary English Review, 11*, 159–161.

Prather, E., Hedrick, D., & Kern, C. (1975). Articulation development in children aged two to four years. *Journal of Speech and Hearing Research, 40*, 179–191.

Sander, E. (1972). When are speech sounds learned? *Journal of Speech and Hearing Disorders, 37*, 55–63.

Shvachkin, N. K. (1973). The development of phonemic speech perception in early childhood. In C. A. Ferguson & D. I. Slobin (Eds.), *Studies of child language development.* New York: Holt, Rinehart and Winston.

Shriberg, L., & Kwiatkowski, J. (1980). *Natural process analysis.* New York: John Wiley.

Singh, S. (1976). *Distinctive features: Theory and validation.* Baltimore: University Park Press.

Snow, K. (1963). A detailed analysis of the articulation responses of normal first grade children. *Journal of Speech and Hearing Disorders, 6*, 277–290.

Stampe, D. (1969). The acquisition of phonetic representation. In R. I. Binnick, A. Davison, G. M. Greene, & J. L. Morgan (Eds.), *Papers from the Fifth Regional Meeting, Chicago Linguistic Society.* Chicago: Chicago Linguistic Society.

Strange, W., & Broen, P.A. (1980), Perception and production of approximant consonants by 3-year-olds: A first study. In G. H. Yeni-Komshian, J. F. Kavanaugh, & C. A. Ferguson (Eds.), *Child phonology: Vol. II. Perception.* New York: Academic Press.

Templin. M. (1957). *Certain language skills in children: Their development and interrelationships.* Institute of Child Welfare, Monograph 26. Minneapolis: The University of Minnesota Press.

Tonkova-Yampol'skaya, R.V. (1973). Development of speech intonation in infants dur-
    ing the first two years of life. In C. A. Ferguson & D. I. Slobin (Eds.), *Studies of child
    language development.* New York: Holt, Rinehart and Winston.

Velten, H. (1943). The growth of phonemic and lexical patterns in infant language.
    Language, 19, 281–292.

Vihman, M. (1981). Phonology and the development of the lexicon: Evidence from
    children's errors. *Journal of Child Language, 8,* 239–264.

Waterson, N. (1971). Child phonology: A prosodic view. *Journal of Linguistics, 7,* 179–211.

Weiner, F., & Bernthal, J. (1976). Acquisition of phonetic features in children 2–6 years
    old. In S. Singh, (Ed.), *Distinctive feature theory and validation.* Baltimore: University
    Park Press.

Weir, R. H. (1962). *Language in the crib.* The Hague: Mouton.

Weir, R. H. (1966). Some questions on the child's learning of phonology. In F. Smith &
    G. Miller (Eds.), *The genesis of language: A psycholinguistic approach.* Cambridge,
    Mass.: MIT Press.

Wellman, B., Case, I., Mengurt, I., & Bradbury. D. (1931). Speech sounds of young
    children. *University of Iowa Studies in Child Welfare, 5.*

Williams, L., & Golenski, J. (1979). Infant behavioral state and speech sound discrimination.
    Child Development, 50, 1243–1246.

Winitz, H. (1969). *Articulatory acquisition and behavior.* Englewood Cliffs. N.J.: Prentice-
    Hall, Inc.

Yeni-Komshian, G., Kavanaugh, J., & Ferguson, C. (Eds.). (1980). *Child phonology: Vol. 1.
    Production.* New York: Academic Press.

Zlatkin, M. A., & Koenigsknecht, R. A. (1976). Development of the voicing contrast: A
    comparison of voice onset time in stop perception and production. *Journal of Speech
    and Hearing Research, 19,* 93–111.

Assessment of Articulatory Disorders

In an articulatory or phonological assessment, a clinician's task is to evaluate the nature of the disorder by sampling the speech, analyzing it, and specifying its characteristics to provide a base for therapeutic intervention. The purpose of this chapter is to explain how to carry out this evaluation. Although many of our assessment procedures have been used for years, many others are new. The first section of this chapter explains traditional assessment procedures used in any articulatory evaluation. In the second section, a discussion of more recent linguistic rule-based procedures is presented. Knowledge of both is important in appraising the wide variety of articulatory and phonological disorders a speech-language pathologist will encounter.

TRADITIONAL METHODS OF ASSESSMENT

Obtaining Samples of Speech

Screening Tests. Screening tests identify persons whose speech may need correction. They are commonly used in public schools and may also be

---

This chapter was written by **Nancy A. Creaghead** and **Parley W. Newman**.

used as part of entrance procedures in colleges and universities. When people do not pass a screening examination, they are referred for a more formal appraisal.

Screening examinations are relatively brief and simple. They usually consist of an inquiry of name, and a simple question or two to elicit a brief sample of conversational speech. Then the person being tested might be asked to repeat a few words or sentences that contain examples of the speech sounds most frequently misarticulated. Alternatively, test sentences might be constructed so that in one or two sentences, all of the consonant sounds of the language are included. A few screening tests for articulation are available commercially; they can be obtained from sources given in Appendix 4.1.

Picture Inventories.   For many years, speech clinicians have used pictures to obtain samples of speech from children. In general, a child names a picture of an object or event. The word spoken contains a speech sound that the examiner wishes to hear the child produce, providing the opportunity to assess the child's production of that particular sound. In a typical inventory, there are sufficient pictures so that a production of each speech sound is obtained in the initial, medial, and final positions of words. Another possibility is to ask a child simply to repeat words after the clinician. This would seem to be more efficient than having the subject name pictures on cards, but research findings suggest that the results are not the same. Although the evidence is a bit equivocal and differences are not large, it appears that if the child names pictures, the responses will be more representative of typical performance than will utterances obtained through imitation (Templin, 1947; Snow & Milisen, 1954; Carter & Buck, 1958; Ham, 1958; Siegel, Winitz, & Conkey, 1963; Smith & Ainsworth, 1967; Kresheck & Socolofsky, 1972; Paynter & Bumpas, 1977). Another reason for using picture cards is motivation. In general, children seem to enjoy naming pictures more than repeating words after the examiner.

There are many picture inventory articulation tests on the market; sources are provided in the appendix to this chapter. A clinician may also choose to make a personal set of pictures. Making up one's own set of test cards takes a little time in the beginning, but it provides opportunities for creativity and flexibility. A personal set of cards can be added to, subtracted from, or modified as needs or assessment approaches dictate. For example, the clinician may wish to supplement the main inventory with additional pictures representing the most commonly misarticulated sounds. Or additional cards may be constructed that show pictures whose names contain certain consonant clusters. If a particular stimulus item is not reliable in obtaining the desired response, then a different stimulus card can be substituted readily. In addition, there may be some words particularly suited to a specific locale. Finally, as current events, television shows, and moving pictures create new characters that capture the public imagination, a personal set of articulation cards can be adapted to heighten their interest value.

There are, however, certain disadvantages to consider in constructing one's own test. These include (a) the time required, (b) the potential lack of uniformity of the pictures, (c) the limits of the clinician's knowledge regarding test construction methods, and (d) the difficulty in obtaining a varied population for standardization.

For those who are interested in making a personal picture inventory, it might be helpful to describe it in more detail. A test card should be of convenient size, 3 by 5 inches or 5 by 7 inches. It should contain a few pictures whose names include the phoneme under test. Test words must be appropriate to the vocabulary level of preschool children. It is often convenient to have three pictures on a card: one representing the test phoneme in the initial position of a word, one in the medial position, and one in the final position. For example, three pictures on one card designed to elicit the /s/ might be *sun* (initial), *pencil* (medial), *house* (final). On the back of the card the following information might be provided to aid test presentation and recording of data: (a) the number of the card corresponding to the item number of the test record blank, (b) the symbol of the phoneme under test, and (c) the test words, and perhaps a sentence to foster elicitation of each word. For example, for the test word *sun*, the question might be: What rises in the sky each morning and makes the night go away? With this information on the back of the card, the clinician need not see the face of the card, which is toward the child, yet all information is available to facilitate administration and recording of information. The sequence of the picture cards should correspond to the listing of items on the recording blank. Recording blanks may be obtained commercially or can be developed by the individual as well. Figure 4.1 gives an example of the front and back of a stimulus card.

Figure 4.2 is an example of a recording form. It is taken from a commercially available articulation test called the T-MAC Test of Minimal Articulation Competence (Secord, 1981b). Note the following information on the recording form:

1.   a number to correspond with the appropriate test card
2.   the symbol representing each phoneme tested
3.   the test words representing the phoneme in the initial (pre), medial (inter), and final (post) positions of the test word. The terms prevocalic, intervocalic, and postvocalic refer to the relationship of the consonant to the vowel in the syllable, i.e., whether the consonant precedes the vowel, occurs between two vowels, or follows the vowel.
4.   the last column in each set headed "Stim." This is an abbreviation of the word *stimulability*, which will be explained later.

Note also that in a few cases the full complement of initial, medial, and final test words is missing. These absences reflect instances in English in which some phonemes do not occur in certain positions of words. For example, in item 8, /h/ does not appear in the final position, and in item 12, /w/ does not occur in the final position.

There are varied sources of pictures. They may be cut out of magazines and pasted on cards, or may be drawn if the clinician has an artistic bent. Pictures should be in color, and if the clinician draws or paints them, they should be of consistent style. It is helpful to laminate the cards so that children can handle them without fear of damage. Actual items like a button or coin

Front of picture-naming card

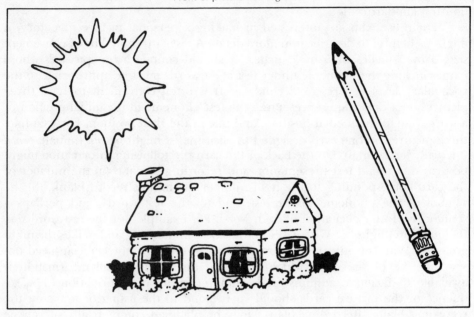

Back of picture-naming card for examiner's use

12.   /s/

   sun

   pencil

   house

Sun: What rises in the sky each morning and makes the night go away?

Pencil: What do we write with?

House: What do we call a place where people live?

FIGURE 4.1
Front and back sides of articulation test card.

make the cards somewhat difficult to handle. The more of these there are and the bulkier they are, the more unwieldy the set becomes.

Sometimes children do not respond to a picture by saying the word it

Consonants

Card	Phoneme	Pre	Inter	Post	Stim.
1	p	pie	apple	cup	
	b	boat	baby	bathtub	
2	t	table	letter	hat	
	d	door	ladder	bed	
3	k	cat	turkey	book	
	g	gun	wagon	egg	
4	s	sun	glasses	bus	
	z	zipper	scissors	nose	
5	ʃ	shoe	dishes	fish	
	ʒ		television	garage	
6	θ	thumb	toothache	teeth	
	ð	that	feather	smooth	

Card	Phoneme	Pre	Inter	Post	Stim.
7	f	fire	elephant	knife	
	v	vest	shovel	five	
8	h	house	treehouse		
9	tʃ	chair	matches	watch	
	dʒ	giraffe	pajamas	cage	
10	m	monkey	hammer	comb	
	n	nail	banana	bone	
11	ŋ		hanger	ring	
12	w	water	flower		
	j	yo-yo	yo-yo		
13	l	lamp	balloon	ball	
	r	rabbit	carrot		

Comments:

FIGURE 4.2

Example of recording form for an articulation test. (*Source: T-MAC: Test of Minimal Articulation Competence* (p. 2) by Wayne Secord, 1981, Columbus: Charles E. Merrill Publishing Co. Copyright © 1981 by Bell & Howell Company. Reprinted by permission.)

was intended to elicit. If the clinician then names the picture for the child, this accurate production may elicit a better than usual performance from the child. Therefore, it is wise to have prompts available for all test words in order to avoid giving the child a model to imitate. The clinician might say, "Can you give me another name for the picture?" Or the examiner might name the picture, and then say something in addition to diminish the influence of the spoken cue. For example, refer to the picture card shown in Figure 4.1. Suppose the child names the test word, *house,* as "home." The examiner is listening for the production of /s/ in the final position, and the word *home* does not satisfy the test requirement. So another name for the picture is requested. If the child says "house," then the objective is achieved. But if the child demurs or cannot think of another word, the clinician might say, "You are right. People live in homes. A place where people live is also called a *house.* Now can you tell me another word for *home?*" Weiner (1979) calls the interjection of an utterance following the test word *delayed imitation*. This approach is suggested because it is reasonable to assume that the intervening words will weaken the influence of cues provided in the model. However, we do not have research evidence to support this assumption.

Other Tests. Other methods may be used for obtaining samples of speech. For example, for older children and adults who read, lists of sentences to be read aloud are often provided. Many clinicians contend that the use of pictures with these individuals is somewhat demeaning. As with the picture articulation test, a clinician can prepare a set of such sentences or they may be obtained commercially. A number of the articulation tests at the end of this chapter contain sentence tests in addition to their picture-naming tests.

In general, sentence tests consist of a list of sentences, each of which is designed to elicit several examples of the same phoneme. The sentences are numbered to correspond to the recording blank. As far as is possible, each sentence is created so test words provide the opportunity for the phoneme under test to appear in the initial, medial and final positions of words.

Other procedures to obtain samples of speech are discussed later in this chapter. These other methods, in some cases, may be more valid than picture-naming procedures. Nevertheless, picture-naming tests have clinical utility, are widely used, and probably will continue to be used for the foreseeable future. Some of their limitations will be considered later in the chapter.

Recording Responses

Several times, thus far, reference has been made to recording responses on a recording blank. What does the examiner record on these blanks? There is considerable variety in recording methods, but the following description represents common techniques. If the child produces the phoneme correctly, a check or plus mark might be made on the recording sheet. However, any type of mark might be misinterpreted later when reviewing the recording form, so the best procedure to denote a correct response is to leave the item blank. Refer again to Figure 4.2, and note there is a separate blank for the phoneme under test in the initial, medial, and final position of words. Thus an entry is made for the manner in which the phoneme is produced in at least three positions, except when the language does not allow a particular sound in a particular word position.

There are three general ways in which a speech sound is produced in error: (a) distortion, (b) substitution, and (c) omission. These types of errors are presented in this particular order to represent degrees of severity (Milisen, 1954; VanRiper & Irwin, 1958; Jordan, 1960). Distortions, which are considered the least severe type of misarticulation, offer the most difficulty in recording if the examiner is attempting to be precise. At the simplest level, the examiner could simply make some type of notation such as a capital D to indicate the error was one of distortion. That is, the sound was not omitted, neither was another sound substituted in its place, but to some degree it was produced in an unusual manner. Milisen (1954) attempted more precision in recording the nature of distortion errors by using a rating scale. A rating of 3 was given to a production interpreted to be so severe that it would attract the attention of most lay persons and frequently would make the sound difficult to recognize. A rating of 2 was given to a phoneme production mildly distorted to the degree that it would attract the attention of many lay persons, but would not make it difficult to recognize. He gave a rating of 1 to normal production.

A more precise way of considering distortions is to regard them not as distortions at all but as substitutions. That is, the so-called distorted sound actually represents a substitution of a non-English sound (Van Riper & Irwin, 1958; Van Riper, 1972; Winitz, 1975). For example, one type of lisp is referred to as a *lateral lisp*. It is produced with the tongue in position to produce an /l/, but no voicing occurs, and air is blown out of the mouth. The result is a "slushy" /s/, which might be considered a distortion of the /s/, but in some ways is like a substitution of a devoiced /l/ for an /s/. Another example is the substitution ts/tʃ, as in [tser] for *chair*. This substitution, which is often recorded as a distortion, is actually another affricate that occurs in other languages (e.g., German), but not in English.

Narrow phonetic transcription can usually indicate the manner and place of a sound substitution that might be recorded as a distortion. If this type of recording is to be made, it is good practice to tape-record the child's responses so that utterances can be played back and studied more carefully. Thus, the difference between a substitution and a distortion is frequently based upon the transcription skills of the examiner. Does it really matter whether or not an error is recorded as a substitution or a distortion? The answer depends upon what is done with the information. If a distinctive feature analysis is going to be made, the features present in the substituted sound can contribute to the data of the analysis. Distinctive feature analysis is discussed later in this chapter and in chapter 14. If the error production is simply identified and the clinician plans to correct the individual phoneme, then perhaps it does not matter how the error is classified.

The preceding discussion of distortions required using the term *substitution*. However, by tradition, a *substitution* consists of replacing the intended, correct phoneme with another one from the language. Examples are common. For instance, /θ/ may be substituted for /s/ as in *think* for *sink*, /f/ for /θ/ as in *baftub* for *bathtub*, /w/ for /r/ as in *wabbit* for *rabbit*, and so forth. On the recording blank of the articulation test, common practice is simply to write in the blank the sound substituted for the target phoneme. When a recording blank is not being used, the examples just discussed are commonly written θ/s, (substitution of /θ/ for /s/); f/θ (substitution of /f/ for /θ/); and w/r (substitution of /w/ for /r/).

Omissions are recorded with a minus sign (−) or a zero in the appropriate record blank. If a zero is used, a slash should be placed in it so that it is not confused with /o/. The notation would look like this: Ø. Actually, this notation is very similar to a phonetic symbol, but its use is rare and does not create problems.

Omissions are not as simple as they first appear. Just as a so-called distortion is in reality a substitution, many omissions may also be substitutions of a more subtle nature. As Van Riper and Irwin (1958) point out, some omissions, when examined closely, are actually unvoiced articulatory gestures lacking the breath or voice of the correct sound or a substituted sound.

Weismer, Dinnsen, and Elbert (1981) analyzed the acoustic signal of three children who omitted final stops. Two of the three children produced longer vowel durations that were reliably sensitive to the voicing characteristic of the omitted final stop. Smit and Bernthal (1983) also found that "syllable reducers," children who reduced CCV or CVC syllables to CV syllables (reduction of the consonant cluster or omission of the final consonant), tended to use longer vowels on average. There were some ambiguities in the data, but in some instances the syllable reducers had significantly larger vowel duration ratios between minimal pairs with final voiced and voiceless obstruents (*bead–beet*). Again, this revealed evidence of the voicing characteristic of some word-final obstruents. Some of the syllable reducers demonstrated a second kind of contrast in production by using a glottal stop for a final voiceless target (/biʔ/for *beet*) and a vowel glide into the last word of the carrier phrase (/bij/ for *bead* before *away*). These data clearly imply that in many instances the "omission" is actually represented by some feature or articulatory gesture. As Elbert and McReynolds (1978) and Bankson and Bernthal (1982a) put it, some children "mark" the so-called omitted sounds in their productions.

There is another type of articulation error: addition. Additions are seen much less frequently than the other error types in functional articulation disorders. An example might be the child who says [stərit] for *street*. This type of addition error is called an *intrusive schwa*. This error may occur as an intermediate step in learning to produce consonant blends. Additions are more common in individuals who exhibit the articulation disorder known as *apraxia of speech* (described in chapter 10).

Testing for Stimulability

A logical first step in the evaluation of the articulation test results is to test for stimulability. Curtis (1956, p. 115) includes this as the last step of the articulation test. The purpose of the test of stimulability is to determine how readily a child can modify his/her errors when asked to imitate the examiner's correct production of them. The term *stimulability* was coined by Milisen (1954), who used three levels of stimulability: sound in isolation, syllable, and word. In Milisen's procedure, the clinician provided a model for the child to imitate and exaggerated the presentation to make the stimulus as vivid as possible. Milisen termed this energetic presentation *integral stimulation*.

The term *stimulation* and the procedure to test a client's ability to imitate misarticulated sounds correctly has been around for a long time (Travis, 1931; Van Riper, 1947). To make the distinction between this relatively common practice and Milisen's attempts at a more vivid form of modelling correct productions, the newer term was introduced. Basically, the procedure required the clinician to produce a sound, syllable, or word so that the child heard it, saw it, and perhaps felt it. Special effort was taken to make the focal point of the articulation as visible as possible. Each error phoneme identified in the articulation test was produced in this way by the clinician, and the child was asked to reproduce it. How well the child performed was, of course, recorded.

Diedrich (1983) describes stimulability testing as a measure of consistency, used to determine if there is consistency in a child's performance on two different speech tasks. The first task is the spontaneous response of the child to a picture stimulus. In the second task, the child imitates the speech model provided by the examiner. The child is consistent if similar errors are made in both tasks. The child is inconsistent to the degree that his productions on the two tasks vary. If the child is consistent, with similar errors in both tasks, the performance is regarded as showing low or poor stimulability. If there are marked differences in performance on the two tasks, the child is said to evidence high or good stimulability.

The concept of stimulability has two possible clinical applications. Both are based upon the assumption that high stimulability indicates readiness in the child to move in the direction of more normal speech. For therapeutic purposes, it would seem that error sounds that are highly stimulable would respond readily to instruction, giving the client feelings of success that would provide motivational impetus. A second implication of high stimulability is that the child may be on the verge of overcoming misarticulations without intervention and may only need more time. Thus, stimulability has been used both as a predictor of therapeutic responsiveness and as a predictor of growth and change through maturation.

Several investigators have reported that the ability of children ages 5 through 7 years to imitate syllables or words is related to the probability of their spontaneously correcting their misarticulations (Carter & Buck, 1958; Farquhar, 1961; Sommers, Leiss, Delp, Gerber, Smith, Revucky, Ellis, & Haley, 1967). Carter and Buck reported in a study of first-grade children that stimulability testing can be used for such predictive purposes. They suggested that first-grade children who correctly imitate nonsense syllables containing the error sounds 75% of the time (7 out of 9 times) are likely to correct those sounds themselves, and thus instruction is not recommended for such children. Kisatsky (1967), in an evaluation of the Carter-Buck prognostic tests, compared pretest to posttest gains over a 6-month period with no speech therapy between a group of kindergarten children identified as a high-stimulability group and a similar group of children identified as a low-stimulability group. Results indicated that significantly higher posttest articulation scores were obtained by the high-stimulability group, which showed 50% spontaneous correction. The low-stimulability group had only 10% spontaneous correction.

A thorough review of the literature on stimulability and its predictive value has recently been published by Diedrich (1983). He concluded that precise interpretation of information from stimulability testing is not possible for any of the usual purposes of such testing, including selecting error sounds for correction, deciding upon beginning remediation at the level of isolation, syllable, word, or phrase, and selecting children who do not need therapy from among those who do. Diedrich pointed out that there is risk in postponing treatment for a child who shows high stimulability. Because stimulability data are based upon groups of children, individual variability makes prediction uncertain for any given child. His conclusions do not imply that there is no predictive power in the results of stimulability testing. All of the studies reviewed found significant positive relationships between stimulability and maturation or responsiveness to therapy, but the strength of these relationships is not great enough for accurate predictions concerning individuals. Diedrich suggests that the best evidence to foretell articulatory performance might come from a trial period of diagnostic therapy. However, this statement is more of a hypothesis to be researched than a conclusion to be drawn.

In light of the preceding, a logical question might be: Is it worthwhile to check on the stimulability of error sounds? On the one hand, the answer can be no, for the intent of the clinician is to eliminate errors regardless of their stimulability. Also, it is interesting to note a rather surprising finding in one stimulability study (Sommers et al., 1967) that children in kindergarten and first and second grades with poor stimulability scores benefited more from therapy than those with good stimulability. Nevertheless, there is a general relationship between stimulability and speech improvement. Therefore, the clinician has some reasonable assurance that speech sounds that show high stimulability have a better chance of responding readily to therapy. The clinician might just as well capitalize on that relationship to increase the probability of early progress to motivate the child. Even though it has some limitations, stimulability has potential as a clinical tool (Kisatsky, 1967; Moore, Burke & Adams, 1976; Madison, 1979).

Oral-Facial Examination

A major aspect of any articulatory assessment is an appraisal of the structures and functions of the speech mechanism, particularly the orofacial structures. The intent is to determine whether both the movable and immovable articulators are adequate for speech production. This examination is usually performed soon after all testing of articulation has been completed. In this way, the clinician can be guided in the examination by knowledge about the number and types of speech sounds that are produced in error. For example, if an individual produces a large number of alveolar sounds incorrectly, then the examiner should test carefully all structures and functions involved in alveolar articulation.

The orofacial examination is also an important part of the differential diagnostic process. A clinician gains important information not only about the factors that may have either predisposed or precipitated the present articulatory condition but also about factors presently serving to perpetuate it. The examination often allows the clinician to determine whether a disorder is *functional* or *organic* in nature. Such determinations, although sometimes misleading, usually help the clinician develop more realistic therapy goals and plan more helpful therapy experiences.

A routine oral-facial examination usually involves examination of the following: (a) facial characteristics, (b) the teeth, (c) palatal and pharyngeal areas, and (d) the tongue.

To prepare for the exam, a clinician would obtain equipment such as a penlight or flashlight, examining gloves, and a tongue depressor. It should be noted that the oral-facial examination procedures discussed here represent a set of general procedures that an examiner might follow in a routine oral-facial exam. Naturally, what an examiner uncovers in performing the exam may require more in-depth probes of oral-mechanism functioning. For example, if routine appraisal of tongue mobility reveals sluggish side-to-side movement, then the clinician will no doubt ask the patient to perform a number of different tasks which probe tongue mobility. It is extremely important to go beyond what is "routine," departing from a set procedure, in order to secure the most accurate and detailed information possible. Further details concerning oral-mechanism examination procedures can be found in Dworkin (1978), Dworkin and Culatta (1980), Mason and Simon (1977), St. Louis and Ruscello (1981), and also in chapter 10, where articulatory considerations in organically based disorders are discussed. The oral-facial exam worksheet of Mason and Simon (1977) is included in Appendix A as one example of a useful set of examination procedures.

Oral-Facial Exam Procedures. This section describes the process of assessing the various areas involved in the oral-facial exam.

Facial Characteristics. In examining the facial areas, the clinician checks very general aspects such as the client's facial expression, his overall appearance, coloration, facial health, size and shape of the head, and overall symmetry of the head and facial structures.

The Teeth. Some individuals, especially children, have been shown to have difficulty producing or learning certain speech sounds because of factors related directly or indirectly to either the occlusal relationship of their teeth or to the teeth themselves. On the other hand, some children compensate remarkably well and show few if any adverse effects.

In examining the dentition, the clinician first makes a general assessment of the teeth, making sure to check for (a) overall dental health, (b) obvious structural deviations, (c) the presence of any dental appliance, and (d) supernumerary (extra) teeth. Although poor dental health will not directly affect speech production, the presence of structural deviations, dental prostheses or appliances, or extra teeth may interfere with articulation. After these preliminary procedures, an examiner will usually direct a client to close his or her teeth so that the back teeth come together. The purpose of this is to assess the dental occlusion. In a normal occlusion, the maxillary central incisors extend just slightly over the mandibular central incisors about one fourth of an inch. In reality, however, normality is measured by the relationship between upper and lower molars. When the lower first molars are approximately one half of a tooth ahead of the upper first molars, a normal occlusion exists. This is termed a class I normal molar occlusion. Three classes of abnormal occlusions, or *malocclusions*, are also recognized. A class I malocclusion consists of a normal molar relationship with some other minor variability in the dentition. In the class II malocclusion, the maxillary first molar is ahead of the mandibular first molar. Finally, in a class III malocclusion, the mandibular molar is located ahead of the maxillary molar by more than one half of a tooth.

Palatal and Pharyngeal Areas. Assessing the palatal and pharyngeal areas involves examining the general integrity of component structures and functions. Of primary concern here is velopharyngeal closure and whether the oral structures involved function adequately for this purpose. Areas to be examined include the hard palate, the soft palate, and the pharyngeal area.

In examining the hard palate, a clinician is concerned primarily with its structure. Hence, inspecting for clefts or other immediately apparent structural deviations is of primary importance. Some deviations of the hard palate are not so apparent. In these instances, palatal coloration often leads the examiner to suspect a structural deformity. Anomalies such as a submucous cleft often give themselves away by the presence of a blue coloration close to the midline of the palate. An examiner can also check more closely for a submucous cleft by very gently rubbing his or her finger across the hard palate to feel for soft spots. Other concerns with regard to the hard palate include the presence of palatal fistulas, which are openings in the palate often caused by insufficient healing after surgery, and, to a lesser extent, the size and height of the palatal vault, which may limit the space available for tongue movement. Many clients make compensatory movements to adjust for this, while in others this limited space can have an adverse effect.

The soft palate or *velum* should be examined first for any major abnormalities, such as the presence of clefts or scar tissue. In addition, its overall size and coloration should be checked. The velum is one of the most important articulators. Its valving action is important in the control of both the dispersion of nasal resonance and the ability to build up the intra-oral breath pressure that is so necessary in producing many consonant sounds. In order for the velum to valve the outgoing breath stream adequately, it must be of sufficient length. Its overall length, then, is one important consideration. The velum, however, is not the only structure which works to bring about velopharyngeal closure. Other structures located in the pharyngeal area are also involved.

In discussing procedures for examining the pharyngeal area, we will again concern ourselves first with the important structures. Then, we will look at some specific procedures important in examining both velar and pharyngeal function in velopharyngeal closure.

The most important structures of the pharyngeal area, including the lateral pharyngeal walls and the posterior pharyngeal wall, cannot be examined adequately via intra-oral observation. These structures, along with the velum, combine to produce the total sphincter action needed for velopharyngeal closure. Closure can be observed, however, by nasopharyngoscopy (a method of direct visualization) and by videoflouroscopy or cineradiographic studies (methods of indirect visualization).

Some general procedures that might be used in inspecting the velum and pharyngeal areas intra-orally follow:

1.   Make general observations first regarding the overall size, shape and symmetry of the velar structure. Observe the general length and mobility of the velum. Have the client prolong /ɑ/ followed by repeated interrupted but sudden bursts of /ɑ/. During phonation the velum should raise symmetrically in a superior and posterior direction. It should raise to the level of the hard palate. Here, however, the examiner is cautioned that even some normal speakers may show

little velar movement on these isolated productions. Look for reciprocal motion of the lateral and posterior pharyngeal walls during
phonation.

2. Inspect the size, symmetry, coloration, and general appearance of
    the faucial pillars, the palantine tonsils, and the uvula. Some consid-
    erations here include: (a) size of the air passage and whether any
    obstruction exists, (b) the possible presence of a bifid uvula or a
    uvula that deviates to one side, which typically indicates a paresis,
    and (c) the potential effects of the presence/absence of the tonsils in
    addition to their general appearance.
3. Check for the presence of oro-nasal fistulae.
4. Lightly touch the velum with a tongue depressor to elicit the gag
    reflex. There should be considerable movement during this reflex.
5. Look for signs of a submucous cleft in the velar area. Again, color-
    ation differences may alert the examiner.
6. Consider the general articulatory and/or resonance characteristics
    generally associated with velopharyngeal incompetence, such as: (a)
    excessive nasal resonance or hypernasal tone, (b) nasal emission of
    the breath stream, (c) weak or omitted consonants, and (d) compensa-
    tory articulation productions, e.g., glottal stops, pharyngeal fricatives,
    pharyngeal plosives, and use of nasal for oral phonemes.
7. A lack of nasal resonance on nasal consonants may indicate almost
    anything, from a structural deviation in the nasal cavity to something
    as basic as a cold.

The Tongue.   The tongue is unquestionably the most important articulator.
Its movement is necessary in practically all speech sounds. Its examination
begins in a manner consistent with earlier procedures: First the structure itself
is examined, and then its functions.

The tongue is usually checked first for the presence of obvious growths or
lesions of any kind and also for its appearance. Then, its overall size is considered.
Some tongues may appear to be either too small or too large, but in reality
there is a rather large range of normality. It is rare that a clinician actually gets
to view a congenitally small tongue (*microglossia*) or a congenitally enlarged
one (*macroglossia*). In spite of substantial variability in tongue size, some individuals can compensate very well.

A second observation that can be made is how the tongue is positioned
when it is at rest in the mouth. The examiner should note its symmetry, the
presence of any scar tissue, and whether the tongue appears to quiver or
undulate in any abnormal manner.

Next, the tongue tip should be elevated with a tongue depressor to permit
inspection of the lingual frenum. A "tied" lingual frenum can restrict tongue
movement considerably. Again, many clients compensate quite well for this so
that the actual number of individuals who are affected adversely is no doubt
much smaller than would be expected. This will come up again in discussing
the examination of tongue functioning.

Several procedures can be used to examine tongue functions. In general,
they assess the movement, mobility, and general strength of the tongue. All

three of these areas should be considered in a routine oral-facial examination. These procedures are summarized briefly below:

1. Hold the client's lower jaw down and ask him to elevate the tongue tip to the maxillary central incisors, then have him retract it backward and upward toward the alveolar ridge. This should give the clinician some idea of his upward range of movement, while also allowing observation of any effect an apparent restricted frenum might have. This would be an obviously important procedure if this individual misarticulated a number of alveolar consonants.

2. Ask the client to perform different tongue exercises, including: (a) protruding the tongue out of the mouth, upward and downward then licking his lips in a circular fashion, (b) moving the tongue up and down inside the mouth, (c) moving it from front to back at various speeds, (d) protruding it and moving it from side to side, (e) touching the tongue tip to various locations on the hard and soft palate after these areas have been stimulated by a tongue depressor, and (f) making a clicking noise with the tongue. Many of these procedures have been used by clinicians for years in order to determine if the tongue is physically capable of performing the range and speed of movements necessary for speech production.

   An examiner should consider carefully certain types of movements that are often related to organically based articulation disorders. For example, some children and adults diagnosed as developmental apraxics or as adult apraxic speakers, respectively, experience difficulty in the volitional planning of certain oral and even facial movements. Individuals with physical impairments such as these often differ substantially in their abilities to perform imitative versus volitional movements. Therefore, an examiner should consider both oral and facial movements elicited by imitative command and those called forth voluntarily (by verbal command only). These movements then must also be viewed in light of the actual movements required for speech. Much more detailed information about the nature and assessment of apraxia of speech is presented in chapter 10, along with a more in-depth presentation of oral-facial examination procedures.

3. Make a quick determination of tongue strength by holding a tongue blade vertically in front of the client's teeth and instructing him to push it away with his tongue. Alternatively, have the client close his mouth and push his tongue outward and against his cheek to make it appear as if there were a large gum ball in his mouth. The clinician then tries to push the tongue back in the client's mouth while the client attempts to resist this motion. If there is normal and sufficient tongue strength available, the client will have little difficulty with this task.

4. Finally, assess rate of movement by obtaining measures of *diadochokinetic rate*. The client is asked to repeat /pʌ/, or /pʌtʌ/, and then /pʌtʌkʌ/. Usually the clinician gives the client an opportunity to practice these

phonetic groups before actually performing the measurement. Most experienced examiners are well aware of the very shocked look you get from a client, especially a young child, when you suddenly ask him to repeat /pʌtʌkʌ/ as fast and as accurately as possible. Norms for diadochokinetic rate are presented in Appendix C. More detailed discussion of diadochokinesis is presented in chapter 10.

These are the general procedures followed in performing an oral-facial exam, but it is important to go beyond what is considered "routine" when the results merit it. No oral-facial examination should be a set of rigid procedures that prevent probes for more information. Only by getting the best and most accurate information possible can a clinician become a truly effective diagnostician.

Comparing Performance to Age Norms

In conducting the articulation assessment, each error phoneme is considered in relation to the age of the child. The previous chapter on normal development presented data on phoneme acquisition as it relates to age. In general, vowels are acquired before consonants. Normally all vowels are included in speech by the age of 3 years. Consonants take more time to be mastered. On average, the order of acquisition of consonants is something like this: 18 months–/p, m, h, n, w, b/; 2 years–/k, g, d, t, ŋ/; 30 months–/f, j/; 3 years–/r, l, s/; 42 months–/ʃ, tʃ, z/; 4 years–/dʒ, v/; 54 months–/θ/; 5 years–/ð/; 6 years–/ʒ/ (Sander, 1972). These data are summarized from chapter 3, where a more complete presentation is given.

This information should be used in making judgments about whether the child should be given more time for phoneme development to occur through maturation, or whether to intervene therapeutically. However, reason and caution should be exercised in the use of normative data. Norms are statistical averages, so that their application to the development of one child is problematic. In addition, Winitz (1975) explains that developmental tests should not be used for predictive purposes. That is, the speech clinician cannot predict, from normative data, where a given child will be in 6 months or a year in phoneme acquisition. Winitz suggests that normative data can be used for a guide in counseling parents, but if a parent is concerned about a particular child and desires professional help, then it is wise to improve the whole situation by providing the service.

Olmsted (1971) reports that the course of speech-sound development consists of a mixture of successes and errors in successive attempts to produce a given phoneme, with gradual increases in the percentage of successes and decreases in the relative number of errors, and that coexistence of success and error is the most frequent pattern of developing use of the sounds of speech. Normative data conceal this pattern as well as obscuring the fact of high individual variability in mastering the phonology of adult language.

Turton (1980) points out that there are two basic problems in the use of normative data in articulation assessment. The first is that speech sound development is not normally distributed; the second is that children cannot be placed into discrete categories. He indicates a need for better assessment procedures, more akin to those that are discussed later in this chapter. He also recommends criterion-referenced testing instead of normative-based testing. In criterion-referenced testing, the items of the test are selected from a teaching model that is determined by the goals of an instructional program. The level of performance of the person being assessed is not compared to a statistical average but rather to a predetermined performance goal (criterion). Of course, criterion-referenced testing requires knowledge on the part of the examiner of the type of behavior under study.

Contextual Testing

Contextual testing is concerned with the influence of surrounding phones on a particular phone. It is often a part of the assessment procedure. Spriestersbach and Curtis (1951) studied inconsistency in children's articulatory production of /s/ and /r/ and found that many children who misarticulated these sounds sometimes spoke them correctly in a specific context.

For example, words containing /s/ were most often produced correctly in the context /sp/, while /r/ was produced correctly more often in the context /tr/. It is well documented that adjacent sounds influence each other during speech production (Curtis & Hardy, 1959; Zehel, Shelton, Arndt, Wright, & Elbert, 1972; Gallagher & Shriner, 1975a, 1975b; Hoffman, Schuckers, & Ratusnik, 1977). Context change produces variability of speech sound production.

McDonald (1964) developed what he termed a *deep test* of articulation. Its purpose was to test each error sound in a variety of contexts to discover contexts in which the error phonemes were produced correctly. He objected to the traditional procedures of testing a sound in the initial, medial, and final position of three words. He pointed out that (a) three-position testing procedures are word oriented; however, words do not appear in speech as entities, but instead speech is composed of sequences of syllables, (b) consonants do not appear in initial, medial, and final positions in connected speech, but rather exist only as releasers and arrestors of syllables, (c) three-position testing simply provides too small a sample, preventing study of the influence of context, and (d) in speech there are four types of consonant connections: simple, double, compound, and abutting.

The simple consonant connection is the CV, VC, or CVC arrangement, as in *toe*, *pat*, and *tote*, respectively. A double consonant is one that occurs between two vowels, such as the fricative /s/ in the word *missing*, or across word boundaries, e.g., *passsome* as in *Pass some turkey please*. A double consonant, then, is one that can perform both an arresting and a releasing function in a sequential manner. The next type is the compound consonant. It occurs in a consonant cluster where two or more consonants combine to release or arrest a syllable. The /str/ in *street* and /st/ in *wrist* are examples. The fourth type of consonant combination, abutting, is the instance where two adjacent consonants are components of two different syllables, such as the /g/ and /p/ in *magpie*. The /g/ arrests the first syllable, while the /p/ releases the second. The McDonald deep test assesses numerous abutting contexts.

A three-position test offers limited opportunities (usually two or three) to study how various contexts influence production of error phonemes. The deep test, however, is composed of picture stimuli designed to examine production of one phoneme at a time in a variety of phonetic contexts. A consonant such as /s/, for example, can both release and arrest a syllable in English. It is tested systematically as an abutting releasor and arrestor in several different phonetic contexts. The McDonald deep test is referenced with the list of published articulation tests given at the end of the chapter.

Some researchers have considered even broader context than did McDonald. Zehel et al. (1972) studied the influence of broad and immediate context on /s/ production. *Immediate context* refers to those sounds immediately adjacent to the speech sound that is under study. *Broad context* refers to speech sounds that are part of the larger contextual environment. For example, note the location of the /s/ in the word *history*. Its immediate context is /ɪ/ and /t/, and the broader context includes /h/ and /r/. Zehel et al. found that although broad context had little influence on the articulation of /s/, immediate contexts were influential in some cases. Though subjects produced significantly more satisfactory /s/ phones in some immediate contexts than in others, it is difficult to generalize from these data to treatment of the individual. Zehel et al. indicate that the clinician who wishes to begin articulation training in contexts in which a sound is produced correctly must find contexts suitable for the individual. This implies that clinicians probably should develop contextual tests of the more commonly misarticulated phonemes that provide an even greater number of items than the McDonald deep test. These might consist of lists of words or phrases with a specific phoneme in a variety of contexts. These could be spoken by the clinician for the child to imitate. Any context in which the misarticulated phoneme is uttered correctly would be noted and used as a facilitative context for the initiation of therapy. Zehel et al. also conjecture that for those children who easily modify their articulations in response to stimulation (highly stimulable), context is relatively unimportant in articulation remediation. More investigations (Moore, Burke, & Adams, 1976; Elbert & McReynolds, 1978) support this conclusion.

Still other research supports the notion of facilitating contexts. Gallagher and Shriner (1975a, 1975b) studied the spontaneous speech of 3-year-old children and analyzed sound sequences for contextual variables related to correct and incorrect productions. They found that the correctness of /s/ and /z/ was not affected by the position of the sounds in words or the phonological acceptability of the sequences. However, more correct productions were observed in CCV contexts than in CV contexts. Also, /s/ and /z/ were produced correctly more often when followed by stop plosives, specifically /t/ and /k/, than when preceded by consonants or vowels. Their findings suggest that speech clinicians could increase assessment information by analyzing spontaneous speech samples using a VC_nV syllabic segmentation procedure. C_n represents any arrangement of consonants occurring between vowels. Within the consonantal portion of the syllable, contextual patterns that are systematically related to correct and incorrect productions should be identified. These contextual patterns could be incorporated into remediation.

Hoffman, Schuckers, and Ratusnik (1977) studied the influence of context on /r/ misarticulations. The specific contexts analyzed were: (a) lexically constrained /r/, e.g., He has *pr*ide; (b) nonlexically contrained /r/, e.g., The jeep ride was fun; and (c) nonlexically constrained /ɚ/, e.g., The kicker kicked the ball. The context that brought about the greatest number of accurate productions was the nonlexically constrained /ɚ/, the next most effective context in eliciting correct productions was the lexically constrained /r/, and the context that produced the least number of correct productions was the nonlexically constrained /r/. These differences were significant and provide the kind of helpful information that tests of context can be based upon. Similarly, in connection with contextual influences on /r/ productions, Curtis and Hardy (1959) found the most facilitative context to be C/r/ as in present and train. The second most facilitative context was C/ɚ/ as in water and river.

The McDonald deep test and C-PAC: Clinicial Probes of Articulation Consistency (Secord, 1981a) are the only commercially available instruments to assess use of context. The deep test is limited in the number of contexts provided. Hoffman et al. (1977) discuss some of its limitations. They note in particular its semantic and syntactic ill-formedness and recommend the use of short sentences for contextual testing because the effects of coarticulation transcend multiphonetic and lexical boundaries. Though stimulability may be more important in articulation remediation than the influence of context, there still is value in studying contextual influences. It is recommended that the testing go beyond that provided by the McDonald deep test, even though this requires the clinician to develop some contextual testing materials on his or her own.

More recently, Secord (1981a) introduced an instrument to assess the production of any phoneme in a variety of phonetic contexts. The C-PAC: Clinical Probes of Articulation Consistency provides an alternative to traditional picture-based deep testing. The C-PAC is a comprehensive set of articulation probes that can be used with subjects from preschool to adulthood. Each C-PAC probe assesses articulatory production in (a) pre- and postvocalic position of words, (b) initial, medial, final and word-boundary clusters, (c) sentences, and (d) conversation (storytelling). These probes can be used both to measure consistency and to identify contexts that can be used as beginning points in therapy. The types of phonetic contexts assessed by C-PAC are summarized in Table 4.1. A sample C-PAC probe for the /s/ phoneme is shown in Figure 4.3. The C-PAC is also referenced in Appendix 4.1.

Testing Auditory Discrimination

The ability to distinguish between speech sounds is termed *auditory discrimination*. Speech-language pathologists have been interested in this phenomenon for many years. In 1931, Travis and Rasmus published a study reporting that normal speakers were superior to people with functional articulation disorders in making discriminations between speech sounds. That study spawned many investigations of the subject. Testing speech sound discrimination ability became part of the speech clinician's assessment battery. Several tests of speech sound discrimination have been published. Three frequently used tests are the Wepman Auditory Discrimination Test (Wepman, 1973), the Templin Test of Auditory Discrimination (Templin, 1957), and the Goldman-Fristoe-Woodcock Test of Discrimination (Goldman, Fristoe, & Woodcock, 1970).

Although poor auditory discrimination has been thought to be a significant factor in functional articulation disorders and although testing auditory

TABLE 4.1
Phonetic Contexts Assessed by C-PAC Consonant Probes

Type	Definition
Prevocalic	Occurring before a vowel to release a one-syllable word
Postvocalic	Occurring after a vowel to arrest a one-syllable word
Intervocalic	Occurring between two vowels in a two-syllable word, acting to release and/or arrest the first, second, or both syllables
Initial cluster	Occurring in combination with another consonant to release a one-syllable word
Final cluster	Occurring in combination with another consonant to arrest a one-syllable word
Medial cluster	1. Preceding another consonant in the middle of a two-syllable word, acting to arrest the first syllable 2. Following another consonant in the middle of a two-syllable word, acting to release the second syllable
Word boundary cluster	1. Occurring postvocalically in a word followed by a prevocalic consonant in another word 2. Occurring prevocalically in a word preceded by a postvocalic consonant in another word

Source: C-PAC: Clinical Probes of Articulation Consistency (p. 5) by Wayne Secord, 1981, Columbus: Charles E. Merrill Publishing Co. Copyright © 1981 by Bell & Howell Company. Reprinted by permission.

discrimination ability has been given a place in assessment procedures, the empirical base for these beliefs and procedures is not strong. Powers (1957, p. 742), after reviewing the findings of research on the topic, wrote that results of studies on speech sound discrimination and its relation to articulation skill were conflicting and inconclusive. She also pointed out that the great weight of evidence was against there being a systematic inferiority in persons with functional misarticulations in ability to discriminate speech sounds. A decade later, as he viewed the general acceptance within the profession of the still-possible relation between speech sound discrimination ability and articulation disorders, Weiner (1967) conducted a critical review of the existing literature. His review concluded that auditory discrimination shows a developmental progression. The ceiling of this development seems to be reached at about the eighth year. The most important conclusion was that the evidence does support a link between auditory discrimination and articulation. This relationship holds until about 8 or 9 years of age. Beyond that age there does not seem to be a relationship. Strong positive findings are noted in groups with severe articulation disorders, but the relationship appears negligible when errors are few. Thus age seems to be the primary influence in studies on auditory discrimination, and number of sounds misarticulated seems to play a secondary but still important role.

The key issue in speech sound discrimination testing hinges on the nature of the stimulus material presented to the subject for a discriminating response. In general, there are two types of discriminative stimuli. The first of these consists of pairs of words or syllables that include a wide range of stimulus sounds. For example, in the Wepman Auditory Discrimination Test, the subject is presented with 40 pairs of similar-sounding words. Examples are *tub–tug, web–wed, lag–lack, gum–dumb, coast–toast*. The examiner utters a pair, and the client responds by saying "same" if the pair are perceived as the same, or "different"

PROBE /s/   (7)

Name: _____   Date: _____   Probe Score: [95]
                                                            Storytelling Score: _____ %

PREVOCALIC		POSTVOCALIC	
1. seen	8. soon	14. peace	21. goose
2. sit	9. soap	15. kiss	22. close
3. safe	10. saw	16. face	23. toss
4. set	11. sock	17. guess	24. dice
5. sat	12. sound	18. pass	25. mouse
6. surf	13. sign	19. purse	26. choice [26]
7. some		20. bus	

CLUSTER ANALYSIS

/p/ 27. spoon		/ʃ/ 48. horsehoe		/n/ 68. snake	
28. lips		49. fish sink		69. fence	
29. wasp		/z/ 50. bus zone		70. guess not	
30. whisper		51. Rose said		71. pencil	
31. knapsack		/f/ 52. laughs		/ŋ/ 72. going soon	
/b/ 32. houseboy		53. peaceful		/r/ 73. class ring	
33. rib soup		54. cough syrup		/l/ 74. slide	
/t/ 34. stamp		/v/ 55. nice view		75. false	
35. cats		56. love sick		76. asleep	
36. lost		/θ/ 57. loose thumb		77. also	
37. rooster		58. both sing		/w/ 78. swing	
38. outside		/ð/ 59. miss them		79. this way	
/d/ 39. face down		60. bathe softly		/j/ 80. kiss you	
40. road sign		/tʃ/ 61. gas check		/h/ 81. grasshopper	
/k/ 41. school		62. watch some		/s/ 82. pass some	
42. fix		/dʒ/ 63. yes Jim		Intervocalic	
43. task		64. large sun		83. Lassie	
44. ice skate		/m/ 65. smile		84. bicycle	
45. accept		66. bossman		85. glasses [59]	
/g/ 46. toss good		67. himself			
47. jigsaw					

SENTENCES

1. Mother asked me to play outside.
2. The mouse jumped over the fence.
3. Singing and dancing are fun.
4. He mowed the grass yesterday.
5. Sam drinks milk every day.   [10]

STORYTELLING

corr.	Sam	Lucy	street	school bus	stopped	swings	said
error							

corr.	nice	policeman	miss	listen	so	Let's	just	see
error								

corr. responses / total responses = _____ % correct

FIGURE 4.3
C-PAC probe for the /s/ phoneme. (*Source: C-PAC: Clinical Probes of Articulation Consistency* (p. 137) by Wayne Secord, 1981, Columbus: Charles E. Merrill Publishing Co. Copyright © 1981 by Bell & Howell Company. Reprinted by permission.)

if they are perceived as different. Bernthal and Bankson (1981) term this type of test a *general test of auditory discrimination*, meaning this type of test compares a wide variety of sounds. The three frequently used published tests mentioned in the first paragraph of this section are all general discrimination tests.

The second type of auditory discrimination test requires the client to make discriminations between the correct form of his error sound and other sounds, including the incorrect form. This type of test is phoneme specific and is called a *test of internal discrimination*.

The research of Aungst and Frick (1964) highlights important issues in the area of speech sound discrimination testing. They included in their design an idea expressed by Van Riper and Irwin (1958, p. 25) that perhaps a discrimination test will yet be devised which will match the speaker's own error against the correct utterance presented either simultaneously or successively. Aungst and Frick selected 27 children between 8 and 10 years of age, all of whom misarticulated the /r/. Four different tests of auditory discrimination were administered to each subject. In addition, an articulation consistency score was obtained for each subject on a deep test of articulation. Three of the discrimination tests were created especially for the study; the fourth was a traditional test of discrimination, consisting of 50 pairs of syllables to which the subject responded "same" or "different" following presentation of each syllable pair (Templin, 1957). The three new tests were constructed to determine the subject's ability to judge his or her own speech productions in these situations: (a) when compared to the audio-tape-recorded productions of another speaker, called the *Test of Comparison*; (b) immediately after his or her own production, the *Test of Instantaneous Judgment*; and (c) when self-productions were played back from a tape recording, the *Test of Delayed Judgment*.

Their results showed that the three new auditory discrimination tests were measuring the same ability. They also showed that some relationship exists between articulation ability and the ability to judge the correctness of one's own speech. Correlations among their three new tests of sound discrimination ranged between .93 and .95. However, correlations with the traditional test were low and nonsignificant, ranging from −.21 to −.26. The correlations between the three new tests and the articulation test were .69, .59, and .66, respectively. But again, the relationship between the traditional sound discrimination test and the articulation test was only −.03. The difference between the three new tests and the traditional test apparently was in the distinction between the judgments of one's own speech and the discrimination between pairs of general stimulus items spoken by someone else.

This study by Aungst and Frick has been reported in some detail because it suggests the kinds of tests that need to be developed. It seems reasonable to conclude from their results that traditional tests that are external to a client's specific misarticulations have limited utility. It appears more desirable to develop phoneme-specific tests of internal discrimination that have relevance for specific children. Aungst and Frick's internal discrimination test (the Test of Instantaneous Judgment), combined with a measure of articulatory consistency, might yield more accurate information. Unfortunately, work by other researchers has only brought about more debate.

The controversy over the efficacy of auditory discrimination testing was heightened by the 1971 work of Woolf and Pilberg. In a study similar to that of Aungst and Frick, in which children who misarticulated /r/ also served as subjects, results indicated that articulation ability is not related to speech sound discrimination skill. Interestingly, these findings are not in agreement with those of Aungst and Frick. Also, in an attempt to replicate part of the Aungst and Frick study, Shelton (1978) reported administering a similar test of delayed judgment to /r/- and /s/-misarticulating children before and after a period of "articulation change." Shelton could obtain a correlation no higher than .35

between any discrimination and articulation measures. Shelton stated his dis-
agreement with those who focus efforts on the child's self-discrimination, and
concluded that no one has yet demonstrated that discrimination measures
account for a significant percentage of articulation variance.

The preceding has explained that the efficacy of general auditory discrimination testing as a standard component of articulation assessment has not been
demonstrated. Indeed, it appears that the most fruitful type of discrimination
testing would be that of internal monitoring of error sound productions. It is
particularly important that the client be able to discriminate errors in his or her
own speech, though this skill is difficult to measure (Bernthal & Bankson,
1981). Thus, it appears that if the clinician is going to assess speech sound
discrimination ability, the nature of the testing instrument used will follow
models suggested by the work of Aungst and Frick or Woolf and Pilberg, in
which the clinician will need to create tests using the subjects' error phonemes
and correct articulatory targets as the material for discrimination testing. The
general commercial tests simply do not measure relevant skills.

Before concluding the discussion of speech sound discrimination, it seems
appropriate to suggest future directions these procedures may take. They are
perhaps suggested in a study conducted by Monnin and Huntington (1974). In
this investigation, the basic task for the children who served as subjects was to
identify phonemes, as opposed to making comparative judgments as required
in discrimination tasks. In comparing two phonemes in a discrimination task,
the child may perceive them as two allophones of the same phoneme because
the child's acceptable range for a given phoneme may be different from that of
adults. Phoneme identification, therefore, may be presumed to be more pertinent than the discrimination of allophonic or other differences. An appropriate
response to an identification task implies an appropriate selection of phoneme
categories. Conversely, an inappropriate response to an identification task
implies an inappropriate choice of phoneme categories, which may be due to
defects of discrimination or inappropriate labelling or both.

In their study, Monnin and Huntington included identification of two
types of phonemes: (a) those related to the misarticulations of the experimental
group, who misarticulated /r/, and (b) phonemes distant from /r/ in place and
manner of production. Vowel identification was also studied. Basically, the
child's task was to point to a picture of an object whose name was presented
from a tape recording. There were four sets of test words, and these were
presented under seven conditions, representing a continuum of distortion of
the speech signal ranging from no distortion in the first condition to maximum
distortion in the seventh. As expected, the more the speech signal was distorted,
the greater the number of errors made by the subjects. The experimental
group (/r/-misarticulating children) made significantly more errors in the identification tasks, and errors were specific to misarticulated phonemes, indicating a
positive relationship between production and identification ability.

Hoffman, Stager and Daniloff (1983) also studied discrimination of error-
specific contrasts. They recorded the speech of 12 children who consistently
misarticulated /r/ and 5 children who correctly articulated /r/. All of the children were asked to identify the recorded productions by pointing to pictures
that represented possible interpretations of /r/–/w/ contrasts such as "They run

the race" versus "They won the race" or "The clock is round" versus "The clock is wound." The two groups were about the same in their ability to identify /w/ productions. A similar result was obtained for perception of correctly produced /r/. However, the performance of the two groups differed when the children were asked to identify misarticulated /r/. Those who correctly articulated /r/ were only able to identify 35% of the misarticulated /r/ productions as members of the phoneme /r/. Apparently, children who do not misarticulate /r/ classify the misarticulated /r/ as a member of the /w/ phoneme class. The misarticulating children were apparently confused by error productions, assigning nearly 50% to each phoneme category. This guessing strategy did not apply to misarticulating children's intended productions of /w/. Misarticulating children identified 65% of these correctly. Essentially, these data suggest that children who misarticulate /r/ differ from those who do not only in regard to their perceptions of /r/ error productions. In particular, children who misarticulate adopt a guessing strategy that assigns approximately half of the error productions to the /w/ phoneme and half to the /r/ phoneme. An additional finding was a wide range of self-perception ability among the misarticulating children.

Results of the above two studies underline the need for more discrete types of analyses. These probably will consist of identification tasks as opposed to discrimination tasks. In addition, the stimuli used in the testing will probably be well-controlled synthetic stimuli. Tests using synthetic stimuli are yet to come from the speech science laboratories. In the meantime, the interested clinician might follow the kinds of procedures discussed by Locke (1980a, 1980b). Locke provides a thoughtful rationale for discrimination testing and explains the inadequacies of general tests of auditory discrimination. He also highlights the error potential in asking children to make same-different judgments. As Bernstein (1978) explains, young children interpret the word *different* to mean "same." As they mature, *different* comes to mean "similar," then finally, children acquire the adult meaning for the term. This is another justification for identification tasks as opposed to discrimination tasks. In Locke's procedure the child replies "yes" or "no" to a sequence of stimulus questions. For example, suppose the child substitutes /f/ for /θ/. The examiner extends a thumb or shows a picture of a thumb and asks, "Is this thumb?", "Is this /fʌm/?", or "Is this /sʌm/?" using a perceptually similar control phoneme. For each error phoneme, Locke elicits 18 yes or no responses from the child, using in the names of six objects or pictures (a) the correctly articulated target phoneme, (b) a perceptually similar control phoneme, and (c) the phoneme substituted by the child. This last part can be difficult in the case of substitutions that lie outside the perceptual boundaries of the phonological system of the examiner. The order of presentation is randomized to avoid establishing a pattern of response based upon order of presentation.

The place of auditory discrimination in management of articulation disorders will be discussed further in chapter 9.

PHONOLOGICAL ANALYSIS

Obtaining the Sample

Current linguistic approaches to analyzing children's speech and/or language are based on an examination of the child's habitual rule system as revealed by single words (Hodson, 1980; Weiner, 1979), phrases (Weiner, 1979) and/or conversation (Shriberg & Kwiatkowski, 1980; Ingram, 1981). The optimal sample should (a) reflect the child's production in actual communicative situations, (b) reveal both inconsistencies and consistent patterns, and (c) contain the full set of English phonemes. Ideally, the sample should include conversational speech.

Information regarding imitation, single-word production, and coarticulation has suggested several issues regarding the adequacy of various types of speech samples.

1. As noted earlier in this chapter, the child's imitated production may not reflect his spontaneous production.
2. The child's production of single words may not reflect his conversational production. Sounds may be produced correctly in single words but be misarticulated in conversation (Faircloth & Faircloth, 1970; Dubois & Bernthal, 1978; Johnson, Winney, & Pederson, 1980), or different processes may be exhibited in a single-word articulation test and in a spontaneous speech sample (Shriberg & Kwiatkowski, 1980).
3. The child may not produce a given phoneme the same way in all phonetic contexts. Coarticulation of the surrounding phonemes may influence production of a target phoneme (Curtis & Hardy, 1959; Hoffman, Schuckers, & Ratusnik, 1977; Johnson, Winney, & Pederson, 1980; McDonald, 1964).

With this set of considerations in mind, the clinician must determine what type of sample will be adequate to evaluate the phonological system of a given child.

One conclusion the clinician may draw is that a spontaneous sample of continuous speech should be obtained in order to tap the child's production in real communication and to provide for the influence of coarticulation. Dubois and Bernthal (1978) used three methods to obtain samples from children with articulation errors: (a) continuous speech in response to pictures, (b) modeled continuous speech in response to a story told by the examiner (with the story being modeled and told back in six parts), and (c) spontaneous picture naming. The children exhibited errors in spontaneous speech that they did not demonstrate by the other two methods. They also had errors on the modeled sample that they did not show in single words.

Hence, it appears that a single-word sample or even a modeled sample may not tap all of the child's errors. Shriberg and Kwiatkowski (1980) compared the canonical forms (word structures) of the words from five currently used articulation tests with the words found in speech samples of language-delayed children. They found a higher percentage of complex canonical forms on the articulation tests than in the delayed-speech samples. The articulation tests contain multisyllabic words like *telephone, Santa Claus,* and *Christmas tree,* whereas the children used words with only one and two syllables. They hypothesized that "for young children with delayed speech, the complexity of some articulation test items may trigger simplification processes" (p. 6). Further, they found that sounds such as fricatives, affricates and liquids, which are most likely to be in error, are often tested in the more complex canonical forms (*Christmas tree, Santa Claus*). This means that the likelihood of simplification is increased (p. 7).

Despite the importance of obtaining a spontaneous speech sample, simply allowing the child to talk may not elicit a sufficiently large variety of phonemes and contexts. Therefore, it is important to design materials that will encourage the child to produce variety. With very young children, a variety of toys with different phonemes in their names may be useful. For older children, action pictures can be used to elicit descriptions. Asking the child to tell a story is a useful way to elicit connected speech with somewhat controlled content. Of course, picture-naming is the most commonly used method for eliciting the total set of phonemes.

The ideal sample may be one that includes all of the above suggestions. A model for obtaining a well-rounded sample might consist of the following procedures.

Procedures for Preschool Children.   Part of a sample may be obtained by providing a set of toys for the child to play with and talk about. Included might be:

Doll	*Dishes*	*House*	*Garage*
hat	plate	chair	trucks
dress	cup	couch	cars
socks	fork	table	fire truck
shoes	spoon	kitchen	police car
shirt	knife	living room	dump truck
pants	pan	bedroom	bus
zipper		bed	train
		bathtub	
		rug	
		lamp	
		mother	
		father	
		baby	

With the four sets of toys, including about 35 items, nearly all phonemes can be represented in two positions. Engaging the child in play with the toys can elicit their names in conversation. It must be remembered, however, that asking the child to name the toys will not produce the desired results. This is a separate task, which can be used to elicit words not produced in conversation. However, these should then be recorded as single-word productions. With some very young or developmentally delayed children, it may be necessary to resort to imitated naming responses. Such responses should be attempted when spontaneous utterances cannot be obtained. However, it should be noted that they were imitated.

A second procedure is to ask the child to retell a story. It is possible to create stories which contain key words representing a variety of phonemes. These are available commercially or can be written by the clinician. Telling the entire story to the child and asking him to retell it may produce a more accurate picture of his spontaneous speech; however, key words may be lost by this method. In order to obtain a more accurate retelling, the clinician may want to tell the story in segments for the child to repeat. The Sounds in Sentences Subtest of the Goldman Fristoe Test of Articulation (Goldman & Fristoe, 1969) presents two stories which can be used for this purpose.

Procedures for School-aged Children.   Part of the sample may be obtained by holding a conversation about the child's interests. With some talkative children, it may be possible to hold the most natural sort of conversation—discussion of interests and experiences. Such a conversation can provide good information about the child's habitual speech patterns. However, with unintelligible children, the clinician may have greater difficulty in transcribing the sample because of the lack of context to help in determining what the child has said.

A second procedure is to ask the child to describe action pictures. As with toys, the content of the pictures should be controlled so that a variety of phonemes will be represented in the descriptions.

Third, the clinician may use standard picture-naming tests of articulation. An articulation test can be used to supplement the connected-speech data in order to assure that all phonemes are represented in the sample. Bankson and Bernthal (1983) have made a strong case for continued use of the traditional articulation test battery to identify phonological patterns that affect syllable shape or several sounds within a sound class.

Finally, the clinician can ask the child to retell a story. Stories can be used in the same way that they are used with preschool children.

Use of the above procedure should provide a sample which adequately represents the child's spontaneous speech and also yields the complete set of English phonemes. The goal should be to elicit as many phonemes as possible spontaneously, but failing in that, to elicit them through naming pictures or imitation.

Recording the Sample

Recording a sample of spontaneous speech is more complicated than recording picture-naming responses or imitations of single-word utterances. Grunwell (1982) states that the sample should "be recorded in such a way as to facilitate a detailed and comprehensive phonological analysis, whose validity can be checked by another analyst" (p. 198). The clinician needs to use more than one means of getting an accurate recording. All samples should be tape-recorded to permit repeated listenings for accurate transcription. However, even high-quality tape recordings have limitations. Two problems can occur in attempting to transcribe samples from the tape recorder: (a) Missing acoustic and visual clues may prevent accurate phonetic transcription, and (b) missing contextual clues may interfere with the examiner's comprehension of the situation and thereby prevent accurate transcription. For these reasons, it is important to record as much on-the-spot information as possible to supplement the tape recording.

It may be more convenient to reduce the spontaneous sample to a list of single words, but the words should be kept in order so that information regarding the effect of phonetic environment across word boundaries is not lost. Table 4.2 shows a possible abbreviated sample for a preschool child. The analysis of the sample will be discussed later in the chapter.

Phonetic Transcription.   The beginning clinician will need to give careful attention to the transcription of the sample. In normal communicative situations, listeners do not attend to individual phoneme production, but integrate sounds into meaningful units of words and phrases. This means that the clinician may overlook distortions of the signal, perceiving them as units that make the message meaningful. We do this frequently in noise. When a part of the message is not heard, we "fill in" what makes sense in the context.

In transcribing a client's articulation, it is important to extract meaning from partially unintelligible speech, but at the same time the clinician must attend to details of utterances. For example, it is important to avoid assuming that the client said "bed" when the actual production was [bɛ]. Careful listening and practice are necessary.

In order to be able to examine generalizations in the child's system, it is important to have a close phonetic transcription. In some cases, the client may substitute phones that are not English phonemes. These are more difficult for the English-speaking clinician to perceive and transcribe, but they may indicate important generalizations, errors, or approximations in the client's speech. Two examples will illustrate this fact. First, imagine a child who substitutes ʃ/s and ʒ/z. A broad transcription reveals /ʃ/ and /ʒ/ to be produced correctly or marked only as distorted. However, a closer transcription reveals x/ʃ and ɣ/ʒ, i.e., that velar fricatives are substituted for palatal fricatives. (See Table 4.3). We now see that all four sibilants are produced with a tongue position further back in the mouth than for normal speakers. We can make the generalization that sibilants are "backed."

As a second example, another child produces the following words: *thumb*–[fʌ̃], *ran*–[ræ̃], *ring*–[rĩ], all with nasalized vowels; *bad*–[bæː], *bed*–[bɛː], *car*–[kɑˠ], *ball*–[bɔˠ], all with lengthened vowels. The clinician might record these words as /fʌ/, /ræ/, /rɪ/, /bæ/, /bɛ/, /kɑ/, /bɔ/. This transcription would indicate that the child omits final consonants; however, a closer transcription reveals that the child is aware of final nasal sounds because the nasality is assimilated in the vowel. Awareness of final voiced stops is also revealed by the lengthening of the vowel. In the same way, the beginnings of final glides are exhibited by the addition of a brief schwa (*ball*—[bɔˠ]). These observations indicate that the child may be in a transition stage of developing final consonants. Thus it can be seen that careful observation and analysis yield much meaningful information.

The accurate application of phonological process analysis to be described later requires close attention to precise transcription. Table 4.3 provides a listing of phonetic symbols according to place and manner of articulation and additional diacritical markings for nasalization, syllable lengthening, etc. The student may not need to memorize the non-English symbols, but should use such a chart when transcribing samples.

TABLE 4.2

Abbreviated Speech Sample for a Preschool Child

Gloss	Transcription	Canonical Form	Substitutions I	F	Omissions I	F	Distortions
I. Spontaneous Speech Playing With Toys							
put	pʊ	CV				t	
the	ə	V			ð		
bed	bɛ	CV				d	
in	ĩ	V				n	
bedroom	bɛʊ	CVV			r	d,m	
mommy	mɑmɪ	CVCV					
in	ĩ	V				n	
the	ə	V			ð		
kitchen	tɪĩ	CVV	t/k		tʃ	n	
they	de	CV	d/ð				
gonna	dʌnə	CVCV	d/g				
eat	i	V				t	
II. Retelling a Story							
Jerry	dɛwɪ	CVCV	d/dʒ,w/r				
playing	peĩ	CVV	p/pl			ŋ	
with	wɪ	CV				θ	
his	hɪ	CV				z	
drum	dʌ̃	CV	d/dr			m	
his	hɪ	CV				z	
ball	bɔə	CVV		ə/l			
his	hɪ	CV				z	
wagon	wædə̃	CVCV	d/g			n	
III. Picture Naming							
lamp	wæ̃	CV	w/l			mp	
house	haʊ	CV				s	
cup	tʌ	CV	t/k			p	
wagon	wædə̃	CVCV	d/g			n	
wheel	wiˀ	CVV		ə/l			
telephone	tɛpõ	CVCV	p/f			n	
rabbit	wæbɪ	CVCV	w/r			t	
car	tɑˀ *imitated	CVV	t/k	ə/r			
chicken	tɪtɪ	CVCV	t/tʃ,t/k			n	
church	tʌˀ	CVV	t/tʃ	ʌˀ/ɝ		tʃ	
stove	do	CV	d/st			v	
airplane	eəpẽ	VVCV	p/pl	ə/r		n	
knife	naɪ	CV				f	
thumb	dʌ̃	CV	d/θ			m	
finger	pĩə	CVV	p/f	ə/ɚ	g	ŋ	
zipper	dɪpə	CVCV	d/z	ə/ɚ			
shoe	du	CV	d/ʃ				
ring	wɪ	CV	w/r			ŋ	
Santa Claus	dæ tɔ	CVCV	d/s, t/kl			n,z	

TABLE 4.2 *(continued)*
Abbreviated Speech Sample for a Preschool Child

Gloss	Transcription	Canonical Form	Substitutions I	Substitutions F	Omissions I	Omissions F	Distortions
Christmas tree	dɪmə dɪ	CVCVCV	d/kr,d/tr			s,s	
sleep	di	CV	d/sl			p	
carrot	tɛwə	CVCV	t/k,w/r			t	
duck	dʌ	CV				k	
yellow	wɛo	CVV	w/j		l		
bathtub	bætʌ	CVCV				θ,b	
bath	bæ	CV				θ	
jump rope	dʌwo	CVCV	d/dʒ,w/r			mp,p	

Summary

Word Structures	Substitutions I	Substitutions F	Omissions I	Omissions F	Distortions
V	p/f	ə/l	ð	p	
CV	d/θ	ə/r	l	b	
CVV	d/ð	ə/ɚ	r	m	
CVCV	d/s	ʌ˞/ɝ	tʃ	f	
CVCVCV	d/z		g	v	
VVCV	w/l			θ	
	t/tʃ			t	
	d/dʒ			d	
	d/ʃ			n	
	w/r			s	
	w/j			z	
	t/k			l	
	d/g			tʃ	
	p/pl			k	
	d/tr			ŋ	
	d/dr			mp	
	d/st				
	t/kl				
	d/kr				
	d/tr				

Phonemic Repertoire
1. Always used correctly: w,h
2. Used correctly in some context: p, b, m, w, t, d, n, h
3. Appearing; not used correctly: none
4. Not represented in sample words: ʒ

Processes
1. Final consonant deletion—all phonemes
2. Stopping
3. Liquid simplification
4. Vocalization
5. Cluster reduction
6. Fronting

TABLE 4.3

The International Phonetic Alphabet (Symbols ɝ and ɚ included)

	Bi-labial	Labio-dental	Dental and Alveolar	Retroflex	Palato-alveolar	Alveolo-palatal	Palatal	Velar	Uvular	Pharyngal	Glottal
Plosive	p b		t d	ʈ ɖ			c ɟ	k g	q ɢ		ʔ
Nasal	m	ɱ	n	ɳ			ɲ	ŋ	N		
Lateral Fricative			ɬ ɮ								
Lateral Non-fricative			l	ɭ			ʎ				
Rolled			r						ʀ		
Flapped			ɾ	ɽ					ʀ		
Fricative	ɸ β	f v	θ ð s z	ʂ ʐ	ʃ ʒ	ɕ ʑ	ç j	x ɣ	χ ʁ	ħ ʕ	h ɦ
Frictionless Continuants and Semi-vowels	w ɥ	ʋ	ɹ				j (ɥ)	(w)	ʁ		

CONSONANTS

VOWELS

			Front Central Back
Close	(y ʉ u)		i y ɨ ʉ ɯ u ɪ ʏ ʊ
Half-close	(ø o)		e ø ɤ o
Half-open	(œ ɔ)		ɛ œ ɜ ʌ ɔ æ
Open	(ɒ)		a ɐ ɑ ɒ

(Secondary articulations are shown by symbols in brackets.)

Other Sounds.—Palatalized consonants: ƫ, ɖ, etc. Velarized or pharyngalized consonants: ɫ, d̴, z̴, etc. Ejective consonants (plosives with simultaneous glottal stop): p', t', etc. Implosive voiced consonants: ɓ, ɗ, etc. ř fricative trill. σ, ǫ (labialized θ, ð, or s, z). ʅ, ʓ (labialized ʃ, ʒ). ɺ, ɕ, ʘ (clicks, Zulu c, ǂ, x). ɺ (a sound between r and l). ʍ (voiceless w). ɪ, ʏ, ʊ (lowered varieties of i, y, u). ɜ (a variety of ə). ɐ (a vowel between ø and o).

Affricates are normally represented by groups of two consonants (ts, tʃ, dʒ, etc.), but, when necessary, ligatures are used (ʦ, tʃ, ʤ, etc.), or the marks ‿ or ͡ (t͡s or t͡ʃ, etc.). c, ɟ may occasionally be used in place of tʃ, dʒ. Aspirated plosives: ph, th, etc.

Length, Stress, Pitch.—ː (full length). · (half length). ' (stress, placed at beginning of the stressed syllable). ͵ (secondary stress). ˉ (high level pitch). ˗ (low level); ' (high rising); ͵ (low rising); ˋ (high falling); ͵ (low falling); ˆ (rise-fall); ˇ (fall-rise). See *Écriture phonétique internationale*, p. 9.

Modifiers.— ~ nasality. ͺ breath (l̥ = breathed l). ˬ voice (s̬ = z). ' slight aspiration following p, t, etc. ˔ specially close vowel (e̝ = a very close e). ˕ specially open vowel (e̞ = a rather open e). ̫ labialization (ŋ̫ = labialized n). ̪ dental articulation (t̪ = dental t). ̑ palatalization (z̑ = ʑ). ˔ tongue slightly raised. ˕ tongue slightly lowered. ̹ lips more rounded. ̜ lips more spread. Central vowels ï (= ɨ), ü (= ʉ), ë (= ə̈), ö (= ɵ), ë (= ə˔), ö (= ɔ̈); ˌ (e.g. n̩) syllabic consonant. ̯ consonantal vowel. ʆ variety of ʃ resembling s, etc.

Source. C. M. Wise, APPLIED PHONETICS, © 1957, p. 31. Reprinted by permission of Prentice-Hall, Inc., Englewood Cliffs, N.J.

Analyzing the Sample

Distinctive Feature Approaches. Grunwell (1982) lists five criteria that the analysis of a speech sample should satisfy. It should (a) describe the patterns used by the speaker, (b) identify the ways in which these patterns differ from those used by normal speakers, (c) determine the implications of these disordered patterns for effective communication, (d) provide the necessary information for developing treatment goals and guidelines, and (e) provide a basis for assessing changes during treatment (p. 198).

Distinctive feature theory, which initially gave impetus to the development of multiphonemic therapy approaches, is one attempt to meet these criteria. As explained in chapter 2, distinctive feature theory groups sounds into classes according to the common features which define them. For example, according to the system used by Singh and Polen (1972), the following phonemes share the features +continuant, −sonorant, −nasal: /f, v, θ, ð, s, z, ʃ, ʒ/. If for all of the above phonemes the child substitutes sounds that change one of the features, it might be assumed that he has difficulty with the group of sounds that are characterized by that feature. Rather than treating his problem as if he had eight separate errors, it might be more economical to try to establish the missing feature. The child might then learn to produce all eight phonemes.

If the child made the substitutions noted in Table 4.2, there would be evidence that the feature +continuant did not appear in conjunction with −sonorant, −nasal sounds; e.g., the child substitutes p/f, d/θ, d/ð, d/s, d/z, d/ʃ. Based on this observation, it seems reasonable that teaching the child to produce continuancy might result in correction of all eight phonemes. Table 4.4 illustrates this information.

Speech-language pathologists may find the use of distinctive features unwieldy for analyzing children's articulation. One criticism is that the features proposed by Chomsky and Halle (1968) or Jakobson, Fant, and Halle (1963) were designed as a theoretical model to describe the language, not the language user (Parker, 1976; Walsh, 1974). Chomsky (1968) has maintained that the generative-transformational grammar model is not a production model. Therefore, the features may not be meaningful in describing a child's errors.

The features used in Table 4.5 (Singh & Polen, 1972) represent one of many feature systems proposed by linguists and speech scientists. It is abbreviated compared to Chomsky and Halle's (1968) or Jakobson, Fant, and Halle's (1963) feature systems, but it is practical in that it is closely related to speech production and speech perception.

The features used in this system are defined by Costello (1975, p. 66) as follows:

- *front/back:* articulated in front of or against the alveolar ridge versus behind the aveolar ridge
- *nonlabial/labial:* articulated without the lips as the place of articulation versus with the lips
- *nonsonorant/sonorant:* articulated with a restricted airflow versus with an unrestricted airflow and spontaneous voicing
- *nonnasal/nasal:* presence of oral versus nasal resonance

TABLE 4.4
Distinctive Feature Analysis of a Preschool Child's Substitutions for Fricatives

Substitutions	Similar Features in Target and Substituted Sounds	Different Features in Target and Substituted Sounds	
		Target	Substituted
p/f	−voice −nasal −sibilant +front −sonorant +labial	+continuant	−continuant
d/θ	−nasal −sibilant +front −sonorant −labial	+continuant −voice	−continuant +voice
d/ð	+voice −nasal −sibilant +front −sonorant −labial	+continuant	−continuant
d/s	−nasal +front −sonorant −labial	+continuant +sibilant −voice	−continuant −sibilant +voice
d/z	+voice −nasal +front −sonorant −labial	+continuant +sibilant	−continuant −sibilant
d/ʃ	−nasal −sonorant −labial	+continuant +sibilant −front −voice	−continuant −sibilant +front +voice

Maintained features shared by all target phonemes
−nasal
−sonorant
Error feature for all target phonemes
+continuant

- *stop/continuant:* articulated by abrupt termination of airflow versus continuous airflow
- *nonsibilant/sibilant:* frictionless airflow versus presence of high-frequency friction
- *voiceless/voiced:* absence versus presence of voicing

TABLE 4.5
Distinctive Features System

0 1	Front Back	Nonlabial Labial	Nonsonorant Sonorant	Nonnasal Nasal	Stop Continuant	Nonsibilant Sibilant	Voiceless Voiced
p	0	1	(0)	(0)	0	(0)	0
b	0	1	0	0	0	(0)	1
t	0	0	(0)	(0)	0	(0)	0
d	0	0	0	0	0	(0)	1
k	1	(0)	(0)	(0)	0	(0)	0
g	1	(0)	0	0	0	(0)	1
f	0	1	(0)	(0)	1	0	0
v	0	1	0	0	1	0	1
θ	0	0	(0)	(0)	1	0	0
ð	0	0	0	0	1	0	1
s	0	0	(0)	(0)	1	1	0
z	0	0	0	0	1	1	1
ʃ	1	(0)	(0)	(0)	1	1	0
tʃ	1	(0)	(0)	(0)	0	1	0
dʒ	1	(0)	0	0	0	1	1
j	1	(0)	1	0	(1)	(0)	(1)
r	1	(0)	1	0	(1)	(0)	(1)
l	0	0	1	0	(1)	(0)	(1)
w	1	1	1	0	(1)	(0)	(1)
m	0	1	1	1	(1)	(0)	(1)
n	0	(0)	1	1	(1)	(0)	(1)
h	1	(0)	(0)	(0)	1	0	(0)

Source: "Use of a Distinctive Feature Model in Speech Pathology" by S. Singh and S. Polen, 1972, *Acta Symbolica, III*, p. 22. Copyright 1972 by *Acta Symbolica*. Reprinted by permission.

Costello (1975) used this system for distinctive feature analysis in preparation for remediation. She advocated sampling the child's articulation by administering the following measures: (a) Fisher-Logemann Test of Articulation Competence (Fisher & Logemann, 1971), (b) Goldman-Fristoe Test of Articulation Sounds in Words Subtest, Stimulability Subtest, and Sounds in Sentences Subtest (Goldman & Fristoe, 1969), (c) a spontaneous speech sample, (d) the McDonald Deep Test of Articulation (McDonald, 1964), and (e) the Sound Production Tasks (Elbert, Shelton, & Arndt, 1967). After plotting the resulting data, the most common substitution for each error phoneme is determined and used as the basis for distinctive feature analysis. Table 4.6 shows this analysis re-using part of the data in Table 4.2. Those features that account for the largest number of errors can easily be examined by noting the circles on the matrix. Again, failure to use continuancy is the primary error shown.

Although the traditional phonetic description terms do not provide a neat binary model, they can be used to analyze generalizations in much the same way as distinctive features, and they may more adequately describe the process of articulation. Singh and Frank (1979) used such a model to analyze the substitutions in children's speech. Table 4.7 shows the consonants of English described in traditional terms. Analysis of the substitutions of the child de-

TABLE 4.6
Distinctive Feature Analysis of Substitutions Using Singh and Polen's (1972) Model as Described by Costello (1975)

ERROR	0 Front 1 Back	Nonlabial Labial	Nonsonorant Sonorant	Nonnasal Nasal	Stop Continuant	Nonsibilant Sibilant	Voiceless Voiced
p/f	0–0	1–1	0–0	0–0	⟨0–1⟩	0–0	0–0
d/θ	0–0	0–0	0–0	0–0	⟨0–1⟩	0–0	⟨1–0⟩
d/ð	0–0	0–0	0–0	0–0	⟨0–1⟩	0–0	1–1
d/s	0–0	0–0	0–0	0–0	⟨0–1⟩	⟨0–1⟩	⟨1–0⟩
d/z	0–0	0–0	0–0	0–0	⟨0–1⟩	⟨0–1⟩	1–1
d/ʃ	0–1	0–0	0–0	0–0	⟨0–1⟩	⟨0–1⟩	⟨1–0⟩

Source: "Articulation Instruction Based on Distinctive Features Therapy" by J. Costello, 1975, *Language, Speech and Hearing Services in Schools*, 6, p. 68. Copyright 1975 by the American Speech-Language-Hearing Association. Adapted by permission.

scribed above can be charted as in Table 4.8. Examination of this table shows that many substitutions occur in the fricative row and change the manner of production to the stop category. Place of articulation is maintained as nearly as possible. As with the distinctive feature analysis described above, we find that the child is making one type of error which accounts for all fricative misarticulations.

Phonological Process Analysis.   Another method for describing immature patterns in the speech of normal children developing language and of individuals with multiple articulation errors is the phonological process analysis. Phonological processes simplify groups of sounds and eliminate sound contrasts. Young children exhibit processes on the way to developing adult articulation. The processes most frequently used by normal children have been described by Ingram (1976) and are discussed in chapter 2. Shriberg and Kwiatkowski (1980) refer to those processes that commonly occur during the period of

TABLE 4.7
Traditional Description of Consonants

Manner of Articulation	Place of Articulation						
	Bilabial	Labiodental	Dental	Alveolar	Palatal	Velar	Glottal
Stop	p b			t d		k g	
Fricative		f v	θ ð	s z	ʃ ʒ		h
Affricate					tʃ dʒ		
Glide	w				j		
Liquid				l	r		
Nasal	m			n		ŋ	

TABLE 4.8
Correct Sounds and Substitutions Described by Place and Manner of Articulation

Manner of Articulation	Place of Articulation						
	Bilabial	Labiodental	Dental	Alveolar	Palatal	Velar	Glottal
Stop	p b			t d		t/k d/g	
Fricative		p/f	d/θ d/ð	d/s d/z	d/ʃ		h
Affricate					t/tʃ d/dʒ		
Glide	w						
Liquid				w/l	w/r		
Nasal	m			n			

normal language acquisition and occur across many languages as *natural processes*. These also tend to be most common in the speech of individuals with articulatory disorders. A number of authors (Ingram, 1981; Hodson, 1980; Lund & Duchan, 1983; Shriberg & Kwiatkowski, 1980; Weiner, 1979) have proposed methods for analyzing phonological processes and have outlined the processes to be examined. Compton and Hutton (1978) have devised a test which results not in phonological processes, but in generative rules as described in chapter 2. Each of these methods will be described briefly.

Procedures for the Analysis of Children's Language.   Ingram (1976) listed the following processes as common in the developing speech of normal children:

- Syllable Structure Processes
  Final consonant deletion
  Unstressed syllable deletion
  Reduplication
  Cluster reduction
- Assimilatory Processes
- Substitution Processes
  Stopping
  Fronting
  Gliding of liquids
  Frication
  Vocalization
  Deletion

Ingram's (1981) analysis examines a number of aspects of the individual's rule system. The phonological process analysis is one of these. The following are the components of Ingram's analysis:

1.   The *phonetic analysis* determines the total number of sounds that the child uses and the frequency of use of phonemes in the initial,

medial, and final position of words. Ingram provides a formula for determining a criterion of frequency in order to say that a given phoneme is included in the child's repertoire. The formula is based on the number of different words in the sample and the number of different phonemes the child uses in producing these words. For example, in a given sample, it might be necessary for the child to produce a phoneme four times in order to consider it as having been acquired. Also analyzed in this component are the child's syllable structures and word structures. The child's two most frequent syllable structures are noted, and the percentages of monosyllables and closed syllables (syllables with final consonants) are obtained. A large phonetic repertoire and a variety of syllable and word structures should mean greater intelligibility.

2. The *homonymy analysis* examines forms that sound alike but have different meanings. A percentage of homonymous forms is obtained, which plays a large part in determining the degree of intelligibility. The extent of homonymy is largely determined by the number of different phonemes in the child's repertoire. If a very limited number of phonemes are used, then many words sound the same. For example, if the child used only the consonants /b, p, m/, he might have the following productions:

ball	/bɔ/	pie	/pa /	me	/mi/
gone	/bɔ/	tie	/pa /	knee	/mi/
dog	/bɔ/	kite	/pa /		

This is an example of a high percentage of homonymy.

3. The *substitution analysis* identifies the types of substitutions for adult forms and their frequency of occurrence.
4. The *phonological process analysis* calculates the percentage of use of 27 different phonological processes. The analysis also allows for the inclusion of other less common processes.

Ingram states that his method is designed to be applicable for both clinical and research purposes. His procedure is meant to meet five goals: (a) It is complete, (b) it is flexible regarding sample type and size, (c) it is adaptable for different children (the entire analysis does not have to be completed for each child), (d) it is cumulative in that the analysis provides new information at each step, and (e) it is normative for comparing results.

Ingram's workbook includes eight recording forms to aid in making the analysis. The major strength of the format is its completeness. However, the practicing clinician may criticize the amount of paperwork required.

Phonological Analysis: A Multifaceted Approach.   Like Ingram, Lund and Duchan (1978, 1983) advocate the analysis of a variety of aspects of the child's phonological system. They call their procedure a *multifaceted approach* because they propose to discover more than just phonological processes. The analyses that they suggest include (a) feature analysis of substitutions, (b) analysis of context-sensitive patterns, (c) syllable structure analysis, (d) analysis of idiosyncratic structures, and (e) analysis of possible phonological strategies.

Lund and Duchan advocate narrow phonetic transcription to identify feature changes in those errors usually described as distortions. They analyze feature changes according to manner, place, and voicing, and then describe patterns in terms that other authors call phonological processes: stopping, frication, nasalization, affrication, gliding, and vocalization for manner errors; fronting, backing, alveolarizing, labializing, and velarizing for place errors; and voicing and devoicing for voicing errors.

Under context-sensitive patterns, they examine assimilation, coalescense (the collapsing of two syllables into one, e.g., *spaghetti*–[skɛti]), and transposition of sounds (e.g., *asked*–[ækst]).

Possible problems with the syllable structure of words include weak-syllable deletion (*pajamas*–[dʒaməs]), reduplication of syllables (*baby*–[bibi]), addition of syllables (*book*–[bʊki]), and restricted syllable structure, including cluster reduction (*drum*–[dʌm]) and final consonant omission (*cat*–[kæ]).

Finally, Lund and Duchan consider it important to look for patterns that are not common among children with normally developing or delayed speech and therefore not listed above. In addition, some children may use strategies that are the result of the application of a number of rules. For example, cluster reduction, final consonant omission and weak-syllable deletion may result in the child producing only CV structures for words. Other possible strategies include avoidance or selection of certain words based on their phonological structure.

The authors advocate completing the analysis in the following order:

1. Transcribe a formal articulation test using narrow transcription.
2. Obtain a narrow transcription of a sample of spontaneous speech.
3. Examine the effects of context on misarticulations.
4. Identify syllable structure patterns.
5. Examine unusual whole-word configurations to identify idiosyncratic patterns.
6. Examine all of the above information in order to discover the existence and strength of patterns.
7. Make an inventory of the sounds that the child produces, whether or not they match the target.
8. Complete a substitution analysis.

Lund and Duchen provide sample charts for steps 6 and 7.

Like the procedures to be described at the end of this chapter, this analysis offers the possibility of obtaining thorough information regarding the child's phonological system without the need to purchase specific testing and charting materials. Some will see this as an advantage for cost and flexibility; others may prefer the structure that specific materials provide.

Natural Process Analysis.   Shriberg and Kwiatkowski (1980) use only the following eight natural processes in their analysis: (a) final consonant deletion,

(b) velar fronting, (c) stopping, (d) palatal fronting, (e) liquid simplification, (f) cluster reduction, (g) assimilation, and (h) unstressed-syllable deletion. They base their choice of these natural processes on three factors:

1. The process must have phonological reality based on the fact that (a) it changes a more complex articulatory structure to a less complex one, and (b) it occurs across languages.
2. It must frequently occur in children with delayed speech.
3. It must be able to be scored reliably by clinicians.

This last criterion caused Shriberg and Kwiatkowski to omit one process that is well established in the phonological literature: voicing–devoicing. Further, distortions and omissions are considered to be phonetic errors and are not included in the Natural Process Analysis. The final difference between this method and most process analyses is that only one process is allowed to account for a given sound change. Rule ordering is not included. This means that if the child substituted t/ʃ, only stopping would be coded. Palatal fronting would not be noted for this substitution.

Shriberg and Kwiatkowski advocate obtaining a sample of approximately 200 to 225 words and using the first 90 different words for analysis. The analysis is to be completed in specific order, scanning the sample for each of the eight processes in the order listed. This procedure is based on the assumption that this order best demonstrates the most likely processes to occur. For example, if a child produces the word *dog* as /dɔd/, the substitution of d/g would automatically be counted as velar fronting rather than progressive assimilation because all instances of velar fronting are to be coded before assimilation is assessed for remaining uncoded forms. The authors recommend that following the process analysis, the clinician re-examine the data for phonetic errors (distortions and omissions) and for uncoded deletions and substitutions. The clinician should also determine the variables associated with inconsistent process use.

The Shriberg-Kwiatkowski analysis is more streamlined and less time-consuming than the Ingram analysis. However, one criticism is that some useful data may be lost due to the analysis of only 90 different words and to the prescribed order for conducting the analysis.

The Assessment of Phonological Processes.   Hodson's Assessment of Phonological Processes (1980) uses 55 single-word responses to toys. All English consonants are tested in the prevocalic and postvocalic positions, and 31 consonant clusters are assessed. Following transcription of the sample words, the data are transferred to a phonological process assessment sheet where applicable processes are checked off across the row. Hodson uses the following classification of processes:

Process	*Example*	
Basic Phonological Processes		
Syllable Reduction	/teto/	for *potato*
Cluster Reduction	/pun/	for *spoon*

Process		*Example*
Obstruent Singleton Omission	/u/	for *shoe*
	/bʌ/	for *bus*
Stridency Deletion	/i/	for *see*
	/ti/	for *see*
Velar Deviations	/dʌn/	for *gun*
Miscellaneous Phonological Processes		
Prevocalic Voicing	/do/	for *toe*
Postvocalic Voicing	/bæd/	for *bat*
Glottal Replacement	/kæʔ/	for *cat*
Backing	/kʌg/	for *tub*
Stopping	/dʌm/	for *thumb*
Affrication	/tsi/	for *see*
Deaffrication	/ʃiz/	for *cheese*
Palatalization	/ʃu/	for *sue*
Depalatalization	/su/	for *shoe*
Coalescense	/fok/	for *smoke*
Epenthesis	/təres/	for *trace*
Metathesis	/æks/	for *ask*
Sonorant Deviations		
Liquids		
Omission	/aɪt/	for *light*
	/aɪt/	for *right*
Gliding	/waɪt/	for *light*
	/waɪt/	for *right*
Vowelization	/wiə/	for *wheel*
	/beə/	for *bear*
Nasals	/bĩ/	for *bean*
Glides	/eɪt/	for *wait*
Vowels	/it/	for *it*
Assimilation		
Nasal	/nʌ̃n/	for *sun*
Velar	/gɔg/	for *dog*
Labial	/fwɛtɚ/	for *sweater*
Alveolar	/tɝtɪ/	for *turkey*
Articulatory Shifts		
Substitution of /f,v,s,z/		
for /θ,ð/	/fʌm/	for *thumb*
Frontal Lisp	/θʌn/	for *sun*
Dentalization of /t,d,n,l/	/ðu/	for *do*
Lateralization	/s̪up/	for *soup*

The number of occurrences and percentage of occurrence for each of the above processes are recorded on a summary sheet. A list of phonemes produced by the child is also included on this sheet.

Hodson also provides a screening instrument, which includes 20 words. The phonemes in these words are examined for the basic processes and for liquid deviations. The screening test is designed for screening large numbers of children or for administration prior to determining the need for the full assessment.

The number of processes to be examined in the complete analysis may be somewhat unwieldy, and the therapeutic value of dividing them into such small categories is questionable. However, the analysis procedure is simple and clear enough that the large number of processes can be checked in a reasonable amount of time. Only single-word stimuli are used for the analysis. Hodson justifies this decision on the basis of the difficulty of understanding spontaneous speech produced by children with severe articulation disorders. This is an important consideration in working with highly unintelligible children. Hodson's analysis, as well as the next two to be described, may be particularly useful for assessing children with low intelligibility. The use of toys and allowing the child to select and name them in the order that he chooses are advantages for use with young children. This strategy is also likely to elicit some connected speech.

The Phonological Process Analysis.   Weiner's procedure (1979) includes a protocol for obtaining the sample to be analyzed as well as a system for analysis. Action pictures are used to elicit phonemes in single words and in sentences through delayed imitation. For example, the response "back" is elicited by saying:

> Here is Uncle Fred's back. An elephant is standing on Uncle Fred's _____ [back].
>
> What is the elephant doing? [Standing on Uncle Fred's back.]

Forms are provided for identifying 16 processes in the sample obtained from the pictures. The processes are grouped under the general headings of (a) syllable structure processes, which simplify the structure of syllables, (b) harmony processes, which are based on assimilation, and (b) feature contrast processes, which account for substitutions that are not related to neighboring sounds. The syllable structure processes are deletion of final consonants, cluster reduction, weak-syllable deletion, glottal replacement. The harmony processes are labial assimilation, alveolar assimilation, velar assimilation, prevocalic voicing, final consonant devoicing, manner harmony, and syllabic harmony (reduplication). Feature contrast processes include stopping, affrication, fronting, gliding of fricatives, gliding of liquids, vocalizations, denasalization, and neutralization.

The data are summarized by profiling the child's phonetic inventory, determining the proportion of occurrence of the 16 processes in the test words and in non-test words, and deciding whether or not the process operates in the child's speech. Weiner sets the criterion for inclusion in the phonetic inventory at four or more examples of the phoneme, but gives no clear-cut criteria for determining the presence of a process.

One advantage of Weiner's model is that it includes a strategy for eliciting the sample. However, despite the fact that it is time-consuming to administer, this strategy may not produce a sample that is fully representative of the child's speech due to the fact that the speech is imitated. A second advantage is that the process analysis is simple and straightforward. Excessive paperwork is avoided. This analysis is also available as a computer program.

Bankson and Bernthal (1982b) examined the phonological processes that were identified through the delayed word imitation task and the delayed sentence imitation task on this test, and found that the two procedures did not differ significantly. They concluded that the clinician may obtain the same results by using only one of the two procedures. They suggest that completing both provides a more in-depth sample, but supplementing one of the two with another method of elicitation would provide a more varied sample.

Compton-Hutton Phonological Assessment.   Compton and Hutton (1978) devised a 50-item picture-naming test for phonological assessment. It is not a process analysis, but a phonological or generative rule analysis. Forms are provided for recording responses to the test words, examining error patterns, and identifying phonological rules. For the error pattern analysis, phonemes are grouped according to word position and manner classes: stops, nasals, frictions (fricatives), affricates, liquids, glides, vocalics, final clusters, and initial blends. After marking the errors for each of these classes of sounds, the clinician circles phonological rules which apply for each class. The rules are expressed in the form:

$$\begin{bmatrix} b \\ d \\ g \end{bmatrix} \rightarrow \begin{bmatrix} p \\ t \\ k \end{bmatrix}$$

The Compton and Hutton model does not discuss the phonological analysis in terms of processes. Although the information obtained is basically the same, the process analyses discussed above may provide greater generalization in some cases. For example, the rules

$$\begin{bmatrix} k \\ g \end{bmatrix} \rightarrow \begin{bmatrix} t \\ d \end{bmatrix} \qquad \begin{bmatrix} \int \\ 3 \end{bmatrix} \rightarrow \begin{bmatrix} s \\ z \end{bmatrix} \qquad \begin{bmatrix} l \\ r \end{bmatrix} \rightarrow w$$

indicate a general pattern of fronting, but because these rules are examined under three separate manner classes, that generalization might be lost. On the other hand, generative rules may be more accurate because they can describe specific contexts in which a sound change occurs. For example, a generative rule may specificy that /t/ is substituted for /k/ only when it precedes a front vowel.

The testing format for this analysis can be criticized because it includes only single-word productions. However, the authors do note the value of transcribing and analyzing any spontaneous speech or non-test words that may occur during testing in order to observe any inconsistencies between single-word and connected-speech productions.

Benjamin and Greenwood (1983) compared the results obtained from two of the assessment procedures described above, The Assessment of Phonological Processes (Hodson, 1980) and Procedures for the Phonological Analysis of Children's Language (Ingram, 1981) and a third, the Phonological Process

Protocol (Khan & Lewis, 1982). They used these procedures to measure the percentage of occurrence of five processes in 18 children. The processes were final consonant deletion, cluster reduction, stopping, fronting and gliding. They found good agreement among the three procedures despite the fact that different samples were used for each. Gliding was the least consistent across analyses. The authors suggest that reliability need not be a major factor in choosing a test to evaluate the major processes, so that the clinician may consider issues such as time needed for completion, number of processes to be evaluated, type of sample available or obtainable, and intelligibility and interest level of the child.

A Procedure for Completing Phonological Analysis. It is not necessary to use a published procedure for analysis. The following method for doing a phonological process analysis incorporates elements from the systems already discussed. The data in Table 4.2 are used to illustrate this analysis.

1. Transcribe the sample phonetically as a list of words as described earlier (Table 4.2). The beginning clinician may then find it useful to group the words according to their initial and final consonants. However, this step may seem wasteful to the experienced clinician, who may prefer to scan the original transcript for phonemes, word structures, and substitutions.

2. Analyze the syllable structures. A list of the different word structures found in the sample should be made. Prior to tabulation, the beginning clinician may want to list the word structure beside each word as in Table 4.2. With experience comes the ability to list the different patterns while scanning the sample. The word structures for this example are V (5), CV (9), CVV (5), CVCV (7), VVCV (1), and CVCVCV (1). From the analysis, two things become obvious: (a) There is a limited repertoire of word structures, and (b) syllable-final consonants are omitted. One other detail should be examined. There is a relatively large number of CVV word structures in the sample considering the rarity of this form in English. This should alert the clinician to examine the origin of the CVV structures. It can be seen that they come from two sources: (a) two omissions of intersyllable consonants, and (b) three vocalizations (substitution of a vowel for a consonant) of final consonants. The second issue will appear later in the analysis.

3. Analyze substitutions and omissions. They can be recorded on the transcription sheet. Omissions should be recorded as syllable-initiating or syllable-terminating. An attempt should be made to code errors as substitutions rather than distortions whenever possible because substitution data provide greater opportunity for examining consistencies. For example, a narrow phonetic transcription might reveal the following substitutions: ʃ/s, ʒ/z, ç/ʃ, j/ʒ, c/t, ɟ/d (see Table 4.3). Inspection of these substitutions reveals that all of the phonemes are produced further back in the mouth than normal. If a broad transcription had been used, most of these phonemes would have been coded as

distorted. Marking them as such gives no information about the pattern of error.

Once all substitutions and omissions have been recorded, a summary list can be made. In this case, substitutions are: p/f, d/θ, d/ð, d/s, d/z, w/l, t/tʃ, d/dʒ, d/ʃ, w/r, w/j, t/k, d/g, p/pl, d/tr, d/dr, d/st, t/kl, d/kr, ə/l, ə/r, ə/ɚ, ʌᵊ/ɝ. All final consonants in the sample are deleted. Semi-vowels become vowels.

4. Following the listing of substitutions, omissions, and distortions, examine the data for phonemes in the child's repertoire. The distortion column is ignored for this analysis. The following lists of sounds should be made: (a) phonemes always used correctly, (b) phonemes used correctly anywhere in the sample (note word position), (c) phonemes appearing in the sample as substitutions, but never used correctly, and (d) phonemes that were not represented in the sample words.

5. Examine the substitution and omission columns for phonological processes. The distortion column continues to be ignored at this point. The following order of analysis is suggested: (a) Scan the omission column for final consonant deletion, number of times it does and does not occur, and phonemes for which it applies, and (b) scan the substitutions for stopping, fronting of palatals and/or velars, gliding or liquid simplification, cluster reduction, assimilation, voicing or devoicing, and other processes. Notation should be made of which phonemes are affected.

Examination of the number and kinds of processes will enable the clinician to predict the degree of homonymy in the child's speech and the level of speech intelligibility (already known from listening). A greater number of processes will produce more homonymy and therefore less intelligibility. However, the specific types of processes also contribute differentially to intelligibility. For example, the child who exhibits deletion processes and stopping will have more homonymous forms than children who exhibit other processes. The clinician who desires a more precise measure of homonymy can use the procedure outlined by Ingram (1981).

The relative importance of determining the phonemic repertoire and analyzing the phonological processes may vary from child to child. The phonemic repertoire determination may include the most important information for a child with a very severe articulation problem. For children who exhibit articulation characteristic of the first 50 words described by Ingram (1976), the process analysis would reveal many processes, but the more meaningful information might be that the child uses only four consonants. For example, examine the sample below:

ball	bɔ	*zipper*	dɪbə
cat	dæ	*pretty*	bɪdɪ
candy	dænɪ	*drum*	dʌ
light	aɪ	*broke*	bo

down	dɑʊ	*go*	do
no	no	*put*	bʊ
there	dɛ˟	*that*	dæ
tummy	dʌmɪ	*cheese*	di
Mama	mɑmɑ	*Daddy*	dædɪ
rabbit	æbɪ	*sit*	dɪ
show	do	*shoe*	du

Assuming this to represent the child's complete repertoire, his consonant inventory includes /b/, /d/, /m/, and /n/.

Process analysis would reveal the following processes operating in his speech: stopping, velar fronting, palatal fronting, final consonant deletion, cluster reduction, voicing, and deletion of initial liquids. This analysis tells us that the child uses most major processes and needs work on eliminating all of them. It may fail to account for the absence of liquids because initial consonant omission is not a commonly discussed process.

Although the information can be expressed either way, it may be equally useful in this case to describe the features of the phonemes that the child uses rather than the changes made. The full repertoire includes only the following classes of sounds:

Manner	Place
stop	bilabial
nasal	alveolar
voiced	

Only voiced bilabial and alveolar stops and nasals are used, and only in syllable-initiating positions. The feature analysis indicates that the child needs help in developing fricatives, glides and liquids, palatals, velars, and unvoiced sounds.

Neither analysis may represent the information as clearly as simply saying that the child uses only four consonants (/b, m, d, n/), in only the syllable-initiating position. Obviously, this repertoire needs expansion in many directions. The real decision is the ordering of features to be learned or processes to be eliminated. The phonemic repertoire data have given the clearest picture of the child's current status. The process or feature analysis will help to direct the therapeutic procedures.

6. Analyze the child's phoneme preferences. Weiner (1981) suggests that some children may demonstrate a preference for the use of certain phonemes not necessarily consistent with the child's phonological processes. Such preferences may look like processes at first glance, but closer analysis shows that the preference is more widespread than the process would predict. For example, Weiner mentions a child who substituted /θ/ for all initial fricatives, affricates, liquids, and glides. Weiner points out that initially this child's sample might be interpreted as exhibiting a fronting process, but the substitution

of /θ/ for /f/ and /w/ does not reflect fronting. In addition /g/ is produced correctly. Based on the children he observed, Weiner gives four characteristics of sound preferences: (a) One or a few phonemes were substituted for a manner class, (b) sound preference was more common in the initial position, (c) sound preference was more likely to affect non-labial and voiceless sounds, and (d) fricatives were more often affected than other manner classes. This does not mean that a given substitution must meet all of these characteristics to reveal a sound preference. When a particular sound is especially prevalent as a substitution and it does not fit with the child's phonological patterns, sound preference is a possibility.

For children with severe articulation disorders, what may initially look like exceptions to a phonological process may be better explained by sound preference. It is important to examine the possibility of sound preference because different therapeutic techniques are indicated for remediation of processes and sound preferences (Weiner, 1981).

Using the Assessment Results

The value of any assessment procedure lies in its usefulness in planning remediation and making predictions about success. One problem in using diagnostic results to plan therapy is the difficulty of determining exactly where an observed breakdown actually occurs in the phonological-articulatory system. Winitz makes this point in chapter 9, and provides the following example. Consider the difficulty that exists in trying to establish whether a child's difficulty has resulted from a breakdown in the phonological system or whether it is a motor planning or production problem. Often a phonological rule can be used to describe the consistency of an articulation error, but it does not necessarily follow that the primary cause of difficulty lies in a defective phonological system. For example, a rule which states that a target sound is omitted in consonant blends may define a generalization that exists because a breakdown has occurred at any of a number of points in the sound production process. A radiologic or spectrographic examination may reveal unusual articulatory relationships that suggest errors in timing or overall coordination of the component sounds of blends. In this particular case, the phonological rule describes the consistency of the patterned error on blends; it does not adequately explain it, and furthermore, this interpretation might mislead one to believe that the primary reason for the error is at the underlying phonological level and not elsewhere. For this reason, it is important to examine all aspects of the phonological-articulatory system and to be open to all possible explanations for a given problem.

Making predictions is the second important outcome of assessment. In early sections of this chapter, research regarding the predictive value of tests of stimulability and discrimination was discussed. A third factor in making predictions involves the severity of the articulation problem itself. Van Riper and Erickson (1969) used this as a basis for the Predictive Screening Test of Articulation, which was designed to predict which first-grade children would correct their articulation errors by third grade without clinical intervention. This prediction was based on the number of errors on the screening test.

In addition to the number of errors the child exhibits, the types of errors may also be related to the severity of the problem. Renfrew (1966) discusses the great difficulty encountered in therapy with clients who use consonants correctly in initial position of words but omit medial and nearly all final consonants. She refers to these omissions as a persistent "open-syllable" pattern and describes intelligent children who become aware of their disability to the extent of adding a consonant, which is usually incorrect, after giving a one-word response. This added consonant is produced as a separate syllable, and Renfrew reports that such children seem to find it impossible to make the transition from vowel to consonant in the same syllable.

Panagos (1974) explained the open-syllable problem identified by Renfrew as but one symptom of a more generalized language disorder in which children with delayed language development systematically reduce syllable complexity. He relates the problem to deeper levels of cognitive and linguistic development and discusses it in terms of simplified rule systems by which the child operates. A number of studies have suggested this relationship between language and articulation disorders (Leonard, Miller, & Brown, 1980; Matheny & Panagos, 1978; Menyuk & Looney, 1972; Schwartz, Leonard, Folger, & Wilcox, 1980; Shriner, Holloway, & Daniloff, 1969; Whitacre, Luper, & Pollio, 1970). In general, it has been found that children with articulation errors score more poorly on formal tests of syntax (Marquardt & Saxman, 1972; Saxman & Miller, 1973; Smit & Bernthal, 1983). There is also a relationship between phonological errors and other syntactic measures, such as morphological omissions (Menyuk, 1964; Smit & Bernthal, 1983; Paul & Shriberg, 1982) and sentence structure complexity (Menyuk, 1964; Paul & Shriberg, 1982). It has been shown that linguistic complexity may promote articulation errors (Dunn & Barron, 1982; Panagos, Quine, & Klich, 1979) and that phonological complexity and syntactic complexity may interact in producing errors in both domains (Paul & Shriberg, 1982).

Campbell and Shriberg (1982) also found an interaction between phonological errors and pragmatics. The children in their study demonstrated more phonological processes on unstressed words than on unstressed and on those stressed words that were topics rather than those that were comments. The comment is the new information in the sentence, and may be considered to be more necessary to communicate clearly. Likewise, stressed words usually carry important information.

This suggested relationship between phonological errors and other linguistic deficits indicates need for evaluating the language of children with articulation problems. Description of language evaluation procedures is not within the realm of this text, but it is important to note here that the clinician should be aware of the potential language problems of articulation-disordered children and be prepared for such assessment.

Shriberg (1982) and Shriberg and Kwiatkowski (1982a, 1982b) have attempted to develop procedures for assessing severity of articulatory involvement and deriving a classification system. They examined the contributions of four factors in determining severity: (a) percentage of consonants correct, (b) severity ratings of judges, (c) percentage of intelligible words, and (d) supraseg-mental ratings (loudness, quality, phrasing, stress, rate, pitch). They found that percentage of consonants correct was the major predictor of the judges' sever-ity ratings, but they were also influenced by age and suprasegmentals. The authors suggested the following procedures for classifying clients as mild, moderate or severe:

1. Tape a continuous speech sample. Repeat the client's utterances for subsequent analysis.
2. Calculate percentage of consonants correct from the tape.
3. Score the six suprasegmentals on a 3-point rating scale.
4. Use percentage of consonants correct as the major weighting factor, but also account for age and suprasegmentals.

SUMMARY

Thorough and accurate assessment is a necessary prerequisite for any remediation program, but assessment is not an activity that is complete before therapy begins. Continual evaluation and reevaluation is important throughout the remediation process in order to determine the appropriateness of ongoing procedures, to suggest needed changes, and to make decisions regarding termination.

This chapter has presented a variety of procedures to be used for assessment. Any evaluation of articulation includes obtaining an adequate sam-ple of speech, which generally includes both single-word productions and spontaneous conversation. Traditional methods have usually analyzed substitu-tions, omissions, and distortions in single-word samples. Tests that evaluate sounds in a variety of phonetic contexts are also available.

Linguistic approaches to analyzing articulation are based on examination of the child's rule system. Distinctive-feature analysis and phonological-process analysis are two methods of describing the child's rules and determining how they differ from the standard system.

In addition to the articulation test or phonological analysis, a thorough evaluation should include any or all of the following, depending on the child's symptoms and needs: oral-facial examination, stimulability testing, and perhaps auditory discrimination testing. Other aspects of any communication assessment such as case history, hearing evaluation, language assessment, etc., have not been discussed here.

Each clinician must select those evaluation strategies that are appropriate for a particular situation. The best assessment protocol is one that is based on the kind of careful attention to detail that goes into developing formal tests, but is designed by the clinician to fit the needs of the client and the therapeutic program.

Appendix 4.1

ASSESSMENT INSTRUMENTS AVAILABLE COMMERCIALLY

Articulation Tests

Arizona Articulation Proficiency Scale (AAPS), Janet Barker Fudala. Los Angeles: Western Psychological Services, 1963, 1970, 1974. Cost: $27.80 per set of cards, 25 record booklets, 25 survey test forms and manual. Time: approximately 20 minutes, administration.

Articulation Testing and Treatment: A Sensory-Motor Approach, Eugene T. McDonald. Pittsburgh, PA: Stanwix House, 1964. Cost: $18.00; individual record sheet, screening (50 sheets per pad), $.75; teacher report form, screening (50 sheets per pad), $1.25.

Austin Spanish Articulation Test (ASAT), Elizabeth Carrow. Allen, TX: Teaching Resources Corporation, 1974. Cost: $19.00; examiner's manual and test stimuli, 130 pages; test booklet, 4 pages. Time: 25 minutes.

C-PAC: Clinical Probes of Articulation Consistency, Wayne Secord. Columbus: Charles Merrill Publishing Co., 1981. Cost $45.00; examiner's manual only, $14.95. Time: 3–5 minutes per probe.

A Deep Test of Articulation, Picture Form, Eugene T. McDonald. Pittsburgh, PA: Stanwix House, 1964. Cost: $18.00; individual record sheet, screening (50 sheets per pad), $.75; teacher report form, screening (50 sheets per pad), $1.25.

A Deep Test of Articulation, Sentence Form, Eugene T. McDonald. Pittsburgh, PA: Stanwix House, 1964. Cost: $13.50; individual record sheet, screening (50 sheets per pad), $.75; teacher report form, screening (50 sheets per pad), $1.25.

Clinical Probes of Articulation Consistency (C-PAC), Storytelling Manual, Wayne Secord & Roxie M. Ball. Columbus: Charles E. Merrill Publishing Co., 1981. Cost: $14.95. Time: 3 minutes per story.

The Denver Articulation Screening Examination (DASE), Amelia F. Drumwright. Denver: Ladoca Project and Publishing Foundation, Inc., 1971. Cost: $6.50, Denver Articulation Manual Workbook; picture cards (per set), $1.25; test forms (per 25), $1.75; 1-hour training and proficiency film, $400.00; 1-hour training and proficiency video cassette, $150.00; rental of training and proficiency film (per week), $50.00; rental of training and proficiency video cassette (per week), $40.00. Time: Picture form, 20–45 minutes; sentence form, 8–10 minutes, administration; 10–20 minutes, scoring.

Goldman-Fristoe Test of Articulation (GFTA), Ronald Goldman and Macalyne Fristoe. Circle Pines, MN: American Guidance Service, Inc., 1969, 1972. Cost: $37.50; examiner's manual, 27 pages; 50 responses forms, 2 pages. Time: 45 minutes, administration and scoring.

Integrated Articulation Test, Orvis C. Irwin. Published in Orvis C. Irwin, *Communication variables of cerebral palsied and mentally retarded children.* Springfield, IL.: Charles C. Thomas, 1972. Two equivalent forms, Part Tests A through E and Alternate Part Tests A through E. Cost: $29.75. Manual and test forms are not available except as a part of the book.

Photo Articulation Test (PAT), Kathleen Pendergast, Stanley E. Dickey, John W. Selmar, and Anton L. Soder. Danville, IL: Interstate Printers and Publishers, Inc., 1969. Short and long forms available. Cost: $14.75. Manual, 19 pages; score sheet, 1 page. Time: 5 minutes or less, administration and scoring.

Predictive Screening Test of Articulation (PSTA) (3rd ed.), Charles Van Riper and Robert L. Erickson. Kalamazoo, MI: Western Michigan University, Continuing Education Office, 1973. Cost: $1.50. Manual, 18 pages; score sheet, 5 pages. Time: 7–8 minutes, administration and scoring.

Screening Speech Articulation Test (SSAT), Merlin J. Mecham, J. Lorin Jex, and J. Dean Jones. Salt Lake City, UT: Communication Research Associates, Inc., 1970. Cost: manual, 30 pages, $4.50; score sheets, $2.50 for pad of 25; test booklet, 30 pages. Estimated time for administration and scoring: Picture portion: 5 to 8 minutes; consonants in sentences: 3 to 5 minutes; vowels in sentences: 2 minutes; blends in words: 1 minute.

Screening Deep Test of Articulation, Eugene T. McDonald. Pittsburgh, PA: Stanwix House, 1968. Cost: $18.00; individual record sheet, screening (50 sheet pers pad), $.75; teacher report form, screening (50 sheets per pad), $1.25.

The Templin-Darley Tests of Articulation (2nd ed.), Mildred C. Templin and Frederic L. Darley. Iowa City: University of Iowa Bureau of Educational Research and Service, (sound edition), 1969. Cost: $6.00, manual, 38 pages, Appendix A (test words), Appendix B (test sentences); reusable overlays for scoring, $1.00 set of nine; test response forms, 4 pages, $.10 each; specimen set, $6.00 postpaid. Time: Variable; no time limit.

Test of Minimal Articulation Competence (T-MAC), Wayne Secord. Columbus: Charles E. Merrill Publishing Co., 1981. Cost: $25.95.

Descriptions and evaluation of these tests may be found in Newman (1979).

Phonological Assessment Procedures

The Assessment of Phonological Processes, Barbara W. Hodson. Danville, IL: The Interstate Publishers and Printers, Inc., 1980. Cost: $24.95. Extra recording forms (pad of 48), $2.50; extra phonological analysis summaries (pad of 48), $7.50; extra screening forms (pad of 96), $3.75.

Compton-Hutton Phonological Assessment, Arthur J. Compton and Stanley Hutton. San Francisco: Carousel House, 1978. Cost: $35.00. Additional forms (set of 25), $4.25.

Natural Process Analysis, Lawrence Shriberg and Janet Kwiatkowski. New York: John Wiley and Sons, 1980. Cost: $29.95.

Phonological Analysis: a Multifaceted Approach, described in Nancy J. Lund and Judith F. Duchan, *Assessing children's language in naturalistic contexts.* Englewood Cliffs, N.J.: Prentice-Hall Inc., 1983. Cost: $19.95.

Phonological Process Analysis, Frederick Weiner. University Park Press, 1979. Cost: $19.95.

Procedures for the Phonological Analysis of Children's Language, David Ingram. University Park Press, 1981. Cost: $15.95. Scoring forms, $9.95.

Computer Programs for Phonological Assessment

Blache Phonemic Inventory with Sound Substitution Analysis, Stephen Blache. San Diego: College-Hill Press. Cost: $65.00.

Lingquest 2, Phonology Analysis, copyright 1982, Michael W. Palin and Dennis R. Mordecia, distributed exclusively by Charles E. Merrill Publishing Co., Columbus, Ohio. Cost: $495.00.

Minimal Contrast Therapy, Frederick Weiner. State College, PA: Parrot Software. Cost: $49.95.

Phonological Analysis by Computer Programs, Frederick Weiner. State College, PA: Parrot Software. Cost: $49.95.

Programs to Examine Phonetic and Phonological Evaluation Records, Lawrence D. Shriberg. San Diego: College-Hill Press. Cost: $295–$695 depending on options.

REFERENCES

Aungst, L. F., & Frick, J. V. (1964). Auditory discrimination ability and consistency of articulation of /r/. *Journal of Speech and Hearing Disorders, 29*(1), 76–85.

Bankson, N. W., & Bernthal, J. E. (1982a). Articulation assessment. In N. J. Lass, J. L. Northern, D. E. Yoder, & L. V. Reynolds (Eds.), *Speech, language and hearing* (Vol II). Philadelphia: W. B. Saunders, 1982.

Bankson, N. W., & Bernthal, J. E. (1982b). A comparison of phonological processes identified through word and sentence imitation tasks of the PPA. *Language, Speech and Hearing Services in Schools, 13,* 96–99.

Bankson, N. W., & Bernthal, J. E. (1983). In the defense of the traditional articulation test battery. In J. L. Locke (Ed.), *Assessing and treating phonological disorders: Current approaches. Seminars in speech and language, 4.* New York: Thieme-Stratton, Inc.

Benjamin, B. J., & Greenwood, J. L. (1983). A comparison of three phonological assessment procedures. *Journal of Childhood Communication Disorders, 7,* 19–27.

Bernstein, D. K. (1978, November). *More of the same about different.* Paper presented at the American Speech Language Hearing Association Annual Convention, San Francisco.

Bernthal, J. E., & Bankson, N. W. (1981). *Articulation disorders.* Englewood Cliffs, NJ: Prentice-Hall, Inc.

Campbell, T., & Shriberg, L. (1982). Associations among pragmatic functions, linguistic stress, and natural phonological processes in speech-delayed children. *Journal of Speech and Hearing Research, 25,* 547–553.

Carter, E. T., & Buck, M. W. (1958). Prognostic testing for functional articulation disorders among children in the first grade. *Journal of Speech and Hearing Disorders, 23,* 124–133.

Chomsky, N. (1968). *Language and mind.* New York: Harcourt, Brace & World.

Chomsky, N., & Halle, M. (1968). *The sound pattern of English.* New York: Harper and Row, Publishers.

Compton, A. J., & Hutton, J. S. (1978). *Compton-Hutton phonological assessment.* San Francisco: Carousel House.

Costello, J. (1975). Articulation instruction based on distinctive features theory. *Language, Speech and Hearing Services in Schools, 6,* 61–71.

Curtis. J. F. (1956). Disorders of articulation. In W. J. Johnson, S. Brown, J. Curtis, C. Edney, & J. Keaster (Eds.), *Speech handicapped school children* (Rev. ed., pp. 92–153). New York: Harper & Row.

Curtis, J. F., & Hardy, J. C. (1959). A phonetic study of misarticulation of /r/. *Journal of Speech and Hearing Research, 2,* 244–257.

Diedrich, W. M. (1983). Stimulability and articulation disorders. *Seminars in Speech and Language, 4*(4), 297–311.

Dubois, E. M., & Bernthal, J. E. (1978). A comparison of three methods of obtaining articulatory responses. *Journal of Speech and Hearing Disorders, 43,* 295–305.

Dunn, C., & Barron, C. (1982). A treatment program for disordered phonology: Phonetic and linguistic considerations. *Language, Speech, and Hearing Services in Schools, 13,* 100–109.

Dworkin, J. (1978). Differential diagnosis of motor speech disorders: The clinical examination of the speech mechanism. *Journal of the National Student Speech and Hearing Association, 8,* 37–62.

Dworkin, J., & Culatta, R. (1980). *D-COME: Dworkin Culatta oral mechanism examination.* Nicholasville, Kentucky: Edgewood Press.

Elbert, M., & McReynolds, L. (1978). An experimental analysis of misarticulating children's generalization. *Journal of Speech and Hearing Research, 21*(1), 136–150.

Elbert, M., Shelton, R., & Arndt, W. (1967). A task for evaluation of articulation change: 1. Development of methodology. *Journal of Speech and Hearing Research, 10,* 281–288.

Faircloth, M. A., and Faircloth, S. R. (1970). An analysis of the articulatory behavior of a speech-defective child in connnected speech. *Journal of Speech and Hearing Disorders, 35,* 51–61.

Farquhar, M. S. (1961). Prognostic value of imitative and auditory discrimination tests. *Journal of Speech and Hearing Disorders, 26,* 342–347.

Fisher, H., & Logemann, J. (1971). *The Fisher-Logemann test of articulation competence.* Boston: Houghton Mifflin.

Gallagher, T. M., & Shriner, T. H. (1975a). Articulatory inconsistencies in the speech of normal children. *Journal of Speech and Hearing Research, 18,* 168–175.

Gallagher, T. M., & Shriner, T. H. (1975b). Contextual variables related to inconsistent /s/ and /z/ production in the spontaneous speech of children. *Journal of Speech and Hearing Research, 18,* 623–633.

Goldman, R., & Fristoe, M. (1969). Test of articulation. Circle Pines, MN: American Guidance Service.

Goldman, R., Fristoe, M., & Woodcock, R. (1970). *The Goldman-Fristoe-Woodcock test of auditory discrimination.* Circle Pines, MN: American Guidance Service.

Grunwell, P. (1982). *Clinical phonology.* Rockville, MD: Aspen Systems Corporation.

Ham, R. E. (1958). Relationship between misspelling and misarticulation. *Journal of Speech and Hearing Disorders, 23,* 294–297.

Hodson, B. W. (1980). The assessment of phonological processes. Danville, IL.: The Interstate Printers and Publishers, Inc.

Hoffman, P. R., Schuckers, G. H., & Ratusnik, D. L. (1977). Contextual-coarticulatory inconsistency of /r/ misarticulation. *Journal of Speech and Hearing Research*, *20*, 631–643.

Hoffman, P. R., Stager, S., & Daniloff, R. G. (1983). Perception and production of misarticulated /r/. *Journal of Speech and Hearing Disorders*, *48*, 210–215.

Ingram, D. (1976). *Phonological disability in children.* New York: Elsevier.

Ingram, D. (1981). *Procedures for the phonological analysis of children's language.* Baltimore: University Park Press.

Jakobson, R., Fant, C. G. M., & Halle, M. (1963). *Preliminaries to speech analysis.* Cambridge: M. I. T. Press.

Johnson, J. P., Winney, B. L., & Pederson, O. T. (1980). Single word versus connected speech articulation testing. *Language, Speech, and Hearing Services in the Schools*, *11*(3), 175–179.

Jordan, E. P. (1960). Articulation test measures and listener ratings of articulation defectiveness. *Journal of Speech and Hearing Research*, *3*(4), 303–319.

Khan, L., & Lewis, N. (1982). *Phonological process protocol.* Field Test Edition.

Kisatsky, T. J. (1967). The prognostic value of Carter-Buck tests in measuring articulation skills of selected kindergarten children. *Exceptional Children*, *34*(2), 81–85.

Kresheck, J. D., & Socolofsky, G. (1972). Imitative and spontaneous articulatory assessment of four-year-old children. *Journal of Speech and Hearing Research*, *15*, 729–733.

Leonard, L., Miller, J., & Brown, H. (1980). Consonant and syllable harmony in the speech of language disordered children. *Journal of Speech and Hearing Disorders*, *45*, 336–345.

Locke, J. L. (1980a). The inference of speech perception in the phonologically disordered child. Part I: A rationale, some criteria, the conventional tests. *Journal of Speech and Hearing Disorders*, *45*, 431–444.

Locke, J. L. (1980b). The inference of speech perception in the phonologically disordered child. Part II: Some clinically novel procedures, their use, some findings. *Journal of Speech and Hearing Disorders*, *45*, 445–468.

Lund, N. J., & Duchan, J. F. (1978). Phonological analysis: A multifaceted approach. *British Journal of Disorders of Communication*, *13*, 119–126.

Lund, N. J., & Duchan, J. F. (1983). *Assessing children's language in naturalistic contexts.* Englewood Cliffs, N. J.: Prentice-Hall, Inc.

Madison, C. L. (1979). Articulatory stimulability reviewed. *Language, Speech, and Hearing Services in Schools*, *10*(3), 185–190.

Marquardt, T., & Saxman, J. (1972). Language comprehension and auditory discrimination in articulation deficient kindergarten children. *Journal of Speech and Hearing Research*, *15*, 382–389.

Mason, R., & Simon, C. (1977). An orofacial examination checklist. *Language, Speech and Hearing Services in Schools*, *8*, 155–163.

Matheny, N., & Panagos, J. M. (1978). Comparing the effects of articulation and syntax programs on syntax and articulation improvements. *Language, Speech and Hearing Services in Schools*, *9*, 57–61.

McDonald, E. T. (1964). *A deep test of articulation–picture form.* Pittsburgh: Stanwix House, Inc.

Menyuk, P. (1964). Comparison of grammar of children with functionally deviant and normal speech. *Journal of Speech and Hearing Research*, *7*, 109–121.

Menyuk, P., & Looney, P. (1972). Relationships among components of the grammar in language disorder. *Journal of Speech and Hearing Research*, *15*, 395–406.

Milisen, R. (1954). A rationale for articulation disorders. In R. Milisen & Associates (Eds.), The disorder of articulation: A systematic and clinical and experimental approach. *Journal of Speech and Hearing Disorders*, Monograph Supplement 4, 5–18.

Monnin, L. M., & Huntington, D. A. (1974). Relationship of articulatory defects to speech-sound identification. *Journal of Speech and Hearing Research, 17*, 352–366.

Moore, W. H., Burke, J., & Adams, C. (1976). The effects of stimulability on the articulation of /s/ relative to cluster and word frequency of occurrence. *Journal of Speech and Hearing Research, 19*(3), 458–466.

Newman, P. W. (1979). Appraisal of articulation. In F. L. Darley (Ed.), *Evaluation of appraisal techniques in speech and language pathology* (pp. 89–119). Reading, MA: Addison-Wesley.

Olmsted, D. L. (1971). *Out of the mouth of babes: Earliest stages in language learning.* The Hague: Mouton.

Panagos, J. M. (1974). Persistence of the open syllable reinterpreted as a system of language disorder. *Journal of Speech and Hearing Disorders, 39*, 23–31.

Panagos, J. M., Quine, M. E., & Klich, R. J. (1979). Syntactic and phonological influences on children's articulation. *Journal of Speech and Hearing Research, 22*, 841–848.

Parker, F. (1976). Distinctive features in speech pathology: Phonology or phonemics? *Journal of Speech and Hearing Disorders, 41*, 23–29.

Paul, R., & Shriberg, L. (1982). Associations between phonology and syntax in speech delayed children. *Journal of Speech and Hearing Research, 25*, 536–547.

Paynter, E. T., & Bumpas, T. C. (1977). Imitative and spontaneous articulatory assessment of three-year-old children. *Journal of Speech and Hearing Disorders, 42*(1), 119–125.

Powers, M. J. (1957). Functional disorders of articulation: Symptomatology and etiology. In L. E. Travis (Ed.), *Handbook of speech pathology.* New York: Appleton-Century-Crofts, Inc.

Renfrew, C. E. (1966). Persistence of the open syllable in defective articulation. *Journal of Speech and Hearing Disorders, 31*, 370–373.

Sander, E. K. (1972). When are speech sounds learned? *Journal of Speech and Hearing Disorders, 37*(1), 55–63.

Saxman, J., & Miller, J. (1973). Short term memory and language skills in articulation deficient children. *Journal of Speech and Hearing Research, 16*, 721–730.

Schwartz, R., Leonard, L., Folger, M., & Wilcox, M. (1980). Early phonological behavior in normal-speaking and language-disordered children: Evidence for a synergistic view of linguistic disorders. *Journal of Speech and Hearing Disorders, 45*, 357–377.

Secord, W. (1981a). *C-PAC: Clinical probes of articulation consistency.* Columbus: Charles E. Merrill.

Secord, W. (1981b). *T-MAC: Test of minimal articulation competence.* Columbus: Charles E. Merrill.

Shelton, R. L. (1978). Speech sound discrimination in the correction of disordered articulation. *Allied health and behavioral sciences, 1*, 176–194.

Shriberg, L. D. (1982). Diagnostic assessment of developmental phonological disorders. In M. A. Crary (Ed.), *Phonological intervention: Concepts and procedures.* San Diego: College-Hill Press, Inc.

Shriberg, L. D., & Kwiatkowski, J. (1980). *Natural process analysis.* New York: John Wiley and Sons.

Shriberg, L. D., & Kwiatkowski, J. (1982a). Phonological disorders I: A diagnostic classification system. *Journal of Speech and Hearing Disorders, 47*, 226–241.

Shriberg, L. D., & Kwiatkowski, J. (1982b). Phonological disorders III: A procedure for assessing severity of involvement. *Journal of Speech and Hearing Disorders, 47*, 422–456.

Shriner, T. H., Holloway, M. D., & Daniloff, R. G. (1969). The relationship between articulatory deficits and syntax in speech defective children. *Journal of Speech and Hearing Research, 12*, 319–325.

Siegel, G. M., Winitz, H., & Conkey, H. (1963). The influence of testing instruments on articulatory responses of children. *Journal of Speech and Hearing Disorders, 28,* 67–76.

Singh, S., & Frank, D. C. (1979). A distinctive feature analysis of the consonantal substitution pattern. In H. H. Walsh (Ed.), *Phonology and speech remediation: A book of readings.* Houston: College Hill Press.

Singh, S., & Polen, S. (1972). Use of a distinctive feature model in speech pathology. *Acta Symbolica, 3,* 17–25.

Smit, A., & Bernthal, J. (1983). Performance of articulation-disordered children on language and perception measures. *Journal of Speech and Hearing Research, 26,* 124–136.

Smit, A. B., & Bernthal, J. E. (1983). Voicing contrasts and their phonological implications in the speech of articulation-disordered children. *Journal of Speech and Hearing Research, 26*(4), 486–499.

Smith, M. W., & Ainsworth, S. (1967). The effects of three types of stimulation on articulatory responses of speech defective children. *Journal of Speech and Hearing Research, 10,* 333–338.

Snow, K., & Milisen, R. (1954). The influence of oral versus pictorial presentation upon articulation testing results. *Journal of Speech and Hearing Disorders,* Monograph Supplement 4, 29–36.

Sommers, R. K., Leiss, R. H., Delp, M. A., Gerber, D. F., Smith, R. M., Revucky, M. V., Ellis, D., & Haley, V. A. (1967). Factors related to the effectiveness of articulation therapy for kindergarten, first, and second grade children. *Journal of Speech and Hearing Research, 10*(3), 428–437.

Spriestersbach, D. C., & Curtis, J. F. (1951). Misarticulation and discrimination of speech sounds. *Quarterly Journal of Speech, 37,* 483–491.

St. Louis, K., & Ruscello, D. (1981). *The oral speech mechanism screening examination.* Baltimore: University Park Press.

Templin, M. C. (1947). Spontaneous versus imitated verbalization in testing articulation in preschool children. *Journal of Speech and Hearing Disorders, 12,* 293–300.

Templin, M. C. (1957). Templin speech sound discrimination test. In M. C. Moore (Ed.), *Certain language skills in children.* Minneapolis: University of Minnesota Press.

Travis, L. E. (1931). *Speech pathology.* New York: D. Appleton-Century Company, Inc.

Travis, L. E., & Rasmus, B. (1931). The speech-sound discrimination ability of cases with functional disorders of articulation. *Quarterly Journal of Speech, 17,* 217–226.

Turton, L. J. (1980). Developmental bases of articulation assessment. In W. D. Wolfe & D. J. Goulding (Eds.), *Articulation and learning* (2nd ed.) Springfield, IL: Charles C. Thomas Publisher.

Van Riper, C., (1947). *Speech correction principles and methods* (2nd ed.). New York: Prentice-Hall, Inc.

Van Riper, C. (1972). *Speech correction principles and methods* (5th ed.) Englewood Cliffs, NJ: Prentice-Hall.

Van Riper, C., & Erickson, R. (1969). A predictive screening test of articulation. *Journal of Speech and Hearing Disorders, 34,* 214–219.

Van Riper, C., & Irwin, J. (1958). *Voice and articulation.* Englewood Cliffs, NJ: Prentice-Hall.

Walsh, H. (1974). On certain practical inadequacies of distinctive feature systems. *Journal of Speech and Hearing Disorders, 39,* 32–43.

Weiner, F. F. (1979). *Phonological process analysis.* Baltimore: University Park Press.

Weiner, F. (1981). Systematic sound preference as a characteristic of phonological disability. *Journal of Speech and Hearing Research, 46,* 281–285.

Weiner, P. S. (1967). Auditory discrimination and articulation. *Journal of Speech and Hearing Disorders, 32,* 19–28.

Weismer, G., Dinnsen, D., & Elbert, M. (1981). A study of the voicing distinction associated with omitted, word-final stops. *Journal of Speech and Hearing Disorders, 46*(3), 320–327.

Wepman, J. (1973). *Auditory discrimination test* (rev. ed.). Palm Springs: Language Research Association, Inc.

Whitacre, J. D., Luper, H. L., & Pollio, H. R. (1970). General language deficits in children with articulation problems. *Language and Speech, 13*, 231–239.

Winitz, H. (1975). *From syllable to conversation.* Baltimore: University Park Press.

Wise, C. (1957). *Applied phonetics.* Englewood Cliffs, NJ: Prentice-Hall.

Woolf, G., & Pilberg, R. (1971). A comparison of three tests of auditory discrimination and their relationship to performance on a deep test of articulation. *Journal of Communication Disorders, 3*, 239–249.

Zehel, Z., Shelton, R. L., Arndt, W. B., Wright, V., & Elbert, M. (1972). Item context and /s/ phone articulation test results. *Journal of Speech and Hearing Research, 15*, 852–860.

PART II

General Considerations in Articulation Treatment

As noted in the introduction, the treatment of articulation disorders has a considerable history. During that history a number of different types of approaches have been used, each of them bringing some new contribution to what we know about helping children talk better. This section presents an overview of remediation methods for articulation disorders. The discussion deals with underlying principles, general procedures, and research directed toward identifying effective methods and verifying the value of specific procedures. In this section, four general approaches to therapy will be described: the traditional approach (chapter 5), the behavioral approach (chapter 6), linguistic approaches (chapter 7), and communication-centered therapy (chapter 8). These approaches are not discrete; each of them shares some aspects with the others. It may be that the best approach is one that combines elements of all of them.

This section also considers two areas of special concern. One is the role of auditory factors in articulation learning (chapter 9), and the other is the need for special methods in working with individuals whose articulation problems are caused by organic pathologies (chapter 10).

5 The Traditional Approach to Articulation Treatment

During the first 4 decades of this century, early "speech correctionists" laid the foundations for what we now know as the *traditional approach to articulation therapy.* Pioneers such as Mosher (1929), Scripture and Jackson (1927), Borden and Busse (1929), Ward (1923), Peppard (1925), and Travis (1931) were among the first to set forth their ideas about how to treat clients with articulation problems. They were followed by such experts as West, Kennedy, and Carr (1937), Nemoy and Davis (1937), and Stinchfield and Young (1938).

As this chapter shows, these clinicians emphasized the proper positioning of the articulators, that is, correct phonetic placement and a variety of drill activities for the different speech sounds. They also stressed and taught their clients the importance of good listening skills.

In 1939, Charles Van Riper published the now classic work *Speech Correction: Principles and Methods.* In this book, Van Riper was the first to set forth the *stimulus approach,* a general set of guidelines to be used in articulation therapy, rather than a series of exercises and drills. As he stated, "[although] most texts in speech correction give a host of drill material for the various speech sounds, this text will ignore such drill and will concentrate upon techniques and policies" (Van Riper, 1939, p. 208). His text was the first to describe an organized scheme for articulation treatment.

This chapter was written by **Wayne A. Secord**.

Traditional articulation therapy today is no doubt more closely tied to Van Riper and his stimulus approach than to anyone else, even though the practice of articulation therapy has evolved throughout the years since Van Riper first wrote about it. Since 1939, Van Riper's text has been revised six times (1947, 1954, 1963, 1972, 1978, and most recently in 1984 with Lon Emerick). Clearly, his approach has stood the test of time. It has changed in certain ways over the years because other therapy methods have influenced Van Riper's thinking as well as clinicians' use of his approach. On the other hand, at least some aspects of the traditional approach are incorporated in most if not all other approaches to articulation treatment. One of them, the *discrimination approach*, emerged from the writings of Van Riper.

Van Riper's approach will be discussed in depth later in this chapter. First, other traditional treatment methodologies will be surveyed. Some of these methods were predecessors of Van Riper's approach and served to influence its development. Others were developed afterwards and could be considered spin-offs. For example, one approach focuses primarily on discrimination, while another emphasizes stimulation. Both of these are stressed heavily by Van Riper. Some of these later methods, as well as behavioral and linguistic approaches (discussed in chapters 6 and 7), have had an impact on Van Riper's writings and on clinical practices derived from them.

AN OVERVIEW OF TRADITIONAL METHODS

Phonetic Placement

The *phonetic placement approach*, aspects of which are still being used by speech pathologists today, was first described by Scripture and Jackson (1927). This approach stresses the correct positioning of the articulators and the correct use of the breath stream. It does not rely on listening skills or discrimination training. Assuming that each speech sound is always produced in only one way, the clinician teaches the client how to place the lips, tongue, and jaw and how to breathe for each misarticulated sound. Tongue blades, the clinician's fingers, mirrors, other devices, and diagrams may be used. The approach relies heavily upon drill to stabilize the production of each learned sound. Because the approach requires the client to form each target sound consciously, it may be difficult to transfer the skills learned to conversational speech. The phonetic placement approach can be used with individuals or with groups. According to Van Riper (1978), it maybe particularly useful with people with hearing impairments.

The Moto-Kinesthetic Approach

The *moto-kinesthetic approach* of Edna Young and Sara Stinchfield-Hawk (Stinchfield & Young, 1938), is related to the phonetic placement approach. However, each sound is taught as part of a specified stimulus syllable, word, phrase, or sentence. The client lies down, to encourage relaxation, while the clinician manipulates the client's articulators to stimulate correct production of the target sound. At the same time, the clinician says the sound while the client watches. Thus the client simultaneously receives tactile, kinesthetic, auditory, and visual feedback. Because of the one-to-one nature of the therapy techniques, the kinesthetic approach can only be used on an individual basis. Today this approach is largely used with clients with neurogenic impairments, including cerebral palsy. Aspects of the moto-kinesthetic approach, particularly the stimulations used to elicit new sounds, are often used in traditional therapy, as will be seen later in this chapter.

The Stimulus Approach

The *stimulus approach*, first advocated by Charles Van Riper in 1939, focuses on the single misarticulated target sound. The approach begins with intensive ear training and proceeds to production of the sound in isolation, in syllables, in words, in phrases, in sentences, and in conversation. It includes work to stabilize the correct production of the sound and transfer its use to settings outside of therapy. This method, as it is practiced today, will be discussed in depth later in this chapter.

The Group Method

The *group method* proposed by Ollie Backus and Jane Beasley (1951) emphasizes the client as a whole person with many behaviors, of which speech is only one. Backus and Beasley treated groups of clients with a variety of speech disorders rather than one type of disorder (such as articulation problems). The focus is on using speech in a meaningful context, to communicate with the clinician and other members of the group. In addition to improvement in speech skills, goals include personal adjustment and social-skills growth. The group activities involve conversational practice of the target sound and feedback on misarticulations. The approach is, in part, based on the idea of learning as a process that moves from the whole to the parts and back to the whole. The group communication situation provides the whole, or the starting point, while individual work on speech sounds is the part. An important aspect is the warm, accepting atmosphere of the group and the group's dynamics.

Integral Stimulation

The *integral stimulation approach* advocated by Robert Milisen (1954), like the moto-kinesthetic approach, involves use of as many sources of feedback as possible, particularly auditory and visual feedback. In contrast to the traditional approach of Van Riper, however, it begins with production rather than auditory discrimination. Stress is put on successful production of the first target sounds, which are therefore very carefully chosen for stimulability and frequency in speech (to provide motivation for learning).

Servotheory Approach

Edward Mysak (1959) described the *servotheory approach* to articulation treatment, stressing the need for the client to discriminate the error sound and the correct target. Mysak emphasized *error-sound sensitivity* and *error-sound measuring processes* and the related processes of *correct-sound seeking and approximating* and *correct-sound tracking*. In the first stage of therapy, the client learns to discriminate quickly and accurately correct and incorrect articulations in a variety of linguistic contexts. In the second stage, the client produces the sound in different words until correct production is more and more consistent. Next, the clinician provides direct instruction, until the sound is mastered.

Sensory-Motor Approach

According to Eugene McDonald (1964a), because the syllable is the functional unit of speech production, it is the unit upon which articulation therapy should be based. In all stages of *sensory-motor therapy*, the clinician produces the stimulus syllable(s) and the client imitates. McDonald's approach begins with identification of those contexts in which a target sound can be correctly produced. One drawback of the approach is that it depends on the existence of at least one context in which the sound is correctly produced. If the client consistently misarticulates the sound, there are no procedures recommended for eliciting it.

In the first phase of therapy, the client produces syllables and then describes the position and movement of the articulators involved. In this way, the client becomes aware of the "feel" of correct production of the sound. Activities begin with bisyllables such as /bibi/ with equal stress; eventually the clinician adds different stress patterns, different vowels, different consonants, and trisyllables. The progression is from simple to complex. In the second phase of therapy, the clinician uses the context(s) in which a client can correctly produce a sound. Again, the clinician models the stimulus context and the client imitates. At each point the client may be given the chance to practice and to describe how the sound feels. Eventually the word or syllable combination is used in sentences, which do not have to make sense. In the third phase of therapy, the number of phonetic contexts in which the client uses the word is increased. Again, stress, vowels, and consonants are varied. During the course of therapy, the client may be tested for additional facilitating contexts.

Discrimination Approach

According to Harris Winitz (1969, 1975; Winitz & Bellerose, 1962, 1963), the key to articulation treatment of children is speech sound discrimination. After identifying the contexts in which a client misarticulates a target sound, the clinician teaches the child to discriminate the error sound. When the child can discriminate between the error and the target sounds in sentences, speech production begins. The clinician uses common toys or other objects whose names contain the error and target sounds and gets the child to play with them. The child must use the correct name to obtain the toy. Thus correct articulation is naturally rewarded. In more difficult cases, progressively more difficult sound contrasts might be used. Winitz begins training with the error sound rather than the target sound, and continues to focus on the error sound except when teaching the child to discriminate between his or her own error and the target. For a more complete discussion of the importance of discrimination training in articulation therapy, see chapter 9 of this text.

Nonsense Approach

The goal of the *nonsense approach* developed by Adele Gerber (1973) is to facilitate carry-over of learned target sounds from deliberate use (as in the therapy setting) to spontaneous conversational speech. Thus Gerber does not present techniques for acquiring sounds, except for /r/. Once the client (usually a school-aged child or adolescent) has mastered deliberate production of the target sound, the clinician systematically trains the child to use the target in nonsense materials. The materials start with simple CV, VCV, and VC syllables and proceed gradually to entire conversations in nonsense words and then use of nonsense words in meaningful contexts. At each level, the nonsense material is produced with conversational juncture, speed, stress, and so forth. Once the nonsense words can be produced spontaneously in meaningful sentences, real target words from the child's vocabulary are introduced. Eventually those words are used in sentences and conversational speech. The child is also taught techniques for monitoring his or her own speech. All procedures emphasize conversational speed and prosody.

THE TRADITIONAL APPROACH

This section presents an in-depth look at the traditional approach as it is practiced by speech pathologists today. Before beginning therapy, the clinician performs all necessary assessments, both for diagnosis and intervention planning (see chapter 4 on assessment). A tentative treatment plan and tentative therapy targets are selected, though changes are often made during the course of therapy.

Most clinicians who use the traditional approach direct therapy toward one sound, or at most two sounds, at a time. For example, if /s/ is the target, it is likely that the client also misarticulates its cognate, /z/, at least occasionally. Thus both /s/ and /z/ may be chosen as initial therapy targets. Some clinicians do use a "bombardment" approach; that is, they direct treatment toward many error sounds simultaneously. This, however, is the exception rather than the rule. Typically, clinicians have treated only a small number of sounds at once.

Several factors are involved in deciding which sounds to treat first. Perhaps the most important consideration is the chronological age of the client; the target sound should be developmentally appropriate for the child. A second important factor is the frequency of the sound in English phonology. Sounds that occur frequently make good therapy targets because their remediation may result in noticeable improvements in the intelligibility of the client's speech. Another consideration is stimulability; that is, the clinician looks for sounds that the client can produce correctly by imitating the clinician's exaggerated model. Stimulable sounds usually respond more favorably to treatment than other sounds. Another factor is the extent to which the client produces errors. Sounds that the client can sometimes produce correctly are good targets for therapy because the correct productions provide a point of departure for treatment. Finally, the clinician might consider sounds that the client produces with relatively minor errors. If the client produces the sound with only a very mild distortion of the target, for instance, only a slight "fine tuning" may be needed.

In choosing the initial therapy targets, the clinician takes all these factors, and perhaps others, into consideration. He or she weighs all the possibilities and may trade one advantage for another. For example, a clinician may choose to treat a more severe, unstimulable error over a less severe, stimulable sound because the target sound occurs frequently in English and is also the first sound in the client's name ("Wudy" for "Rudy"). Although it sounds complicated, speech pathologists go through this process frequently. With experience, the decision-making process becomes easier.

Once assessment is complete and the initial therapy targets have been chosen, it is time to begin the actual course of therapy. As mentioned previously, early practitioners stressed procedures for placement of the articulators and use of the breath stream. Therapy was implemented through a series of drills and exercises. Before Van Riper, texts on articulation treatment were filled with diagrams and lists of tongue and speech exercises, as well as exercises for listening for certain acoustic properties of sounds and discriminating between error sounds and the target.

In 1939, Van Riper outlined the first general guidelines, seven steps to use in treating articulation disorders.

> (1) The speech defective[1] must be convinced that he has errors which he must eradicate. (2) The causes of the disorder, if still existent, must be eliminated. If those causes are no longer present, their influence must be counteracted. (3) Through intensive ear training, the old word configurations are broken down so that the correct sound and the error may be isolated, recognized, identified, and discriminated. (4) Through various methods, the speech defective must be taught to produce the correct sound in isolation and at will. (5) The new and correct sound must be strengthened. (6) The new sound must be incorporated within familiar words, and the transition to normal speech must be accomplished. (7) The use of the sound must be made habitual, and the error must be eliminated. (p. 209)

While the traditional approach has evolved through the years, Van Riper's contributions of emphasis on ear training and on stabilizing the new sound and transferring its use to conversational speech are still crucial to the approach. In the seven editions of his book (as well as a text written with John Irwin in 1958), he has assembled a cohesive approach to articulation treatment.

That approach, as practiced today, has four major stages: (a) sensory-perceptual training (ear training), (b) production training (establishment), (c) stabilization, and (d) transfer and carry-over. An important fifth stage is *maintenance*. These stages are summarized in Table 5.1. In the words of Van Riper and Emerick,

> The hallmark of traditional articulation therapy lies in its sequencing of activities for (1) sensory-perceptual training, which concentrates on identifying the standard sound and discriminating it from its error through scanning and comparing; (2) varying and correcting the various productions of the sound until it is produced correctly; (3) strengthening and stabilizing the correct production; and finally, (4) transferring the new speech skill to everyday communication situations.

---

[1]The term *speech defective* is dated and no longer used.

TABLE 5.1
Course of Therapy

1. Sensory-perceptual training (Ear training)
   Identification
   Isolation
   Stimulation
   Discrimination
2. Production training
   Sound establishment/Sound acquisition
3. Production training—Sound stabilization
   Isolation
   Nonsense syllables
   Words
   Phrases
   Sentences
   Conversation
4. Transfer and carry-over
5. Maintenance

This process is usually carried out first for the standard sound in isolation, then in the syllable, then in a word, and finally in sentences. (p. 193)

Thus, this approach has four operational levels—the sound in isolation, the syllable, the word, and the sentence. It can be depicted as a staircase (Figure 5.1), a program of clear-cut levels through which a client must pass on the way to correct production of an error sound. It is useful because it gives both the clinician and the client a clear direction; they know at any time what has been accomplished and what is still to be done. It is not necessary to enter the "Van Riper staircase" at the bottom. If, for instance, a client can say an error sound correctly in isolation and in syllables but not at the word level and beyond, therapy might well begin by training in words.

Sensory-Perceptual Training (Ear Training)

The goal of this stage of therapy is to define a standard for the target sound. The client is not required to actually produce the sound. Rather, the emphasis is on developing an auditory model that will serve as an internal standard against which comparisons can be made. This helps the client become aware that he or she is indeed making errors. When therapy moves to production training, the client will use this image as a basis to vary productions and evaluate them.

Ear training is composed of four phases. They are:

1. Identification
2. Isolation
3. Stimulation
4. Discrimination

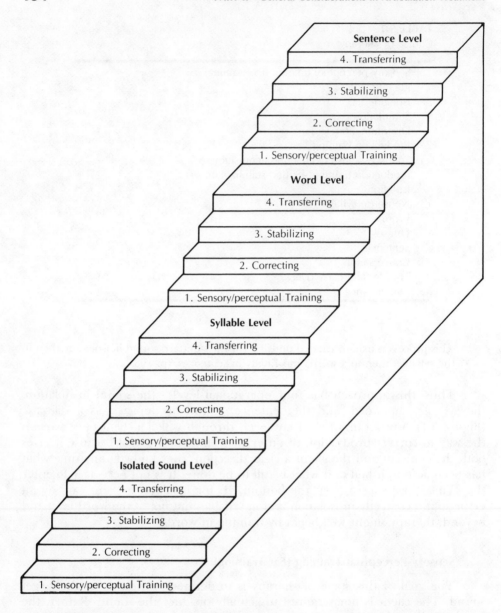

FIGURE 5.1
Design of articulation therapy. (*Source:* Charles Van Riper, Lon Emerick, SPEECH CORRECTION: An Introduction to Speech Pathology and Audiology, 7th Edition, ©1984, p. 194. Reprinted by permission of Prentice-Hall, Inc., Englewood Cliffs, New Jersey.)

Identification.   The goal of this phase of sensory-perceptual training is to teach the client the auditory, visual, and tactile-kinesthetic properties of the target sound. The client learns to identify the target sound in isolation against a background of several possibilities composed of similar and dissimilar properties. Once the client identifies the sound, the clinician describes its inherent acoustic, visual, and movement features. With a young child, the sound /t/ becomes the "ticking sound," the /s/ becomes the "snake sound," and the /k/ becomes the "coughing sound." With older children and adults, much more sophisticated acoustic and anatomical descriptions may be more appropriate and useful. The clinician describes and demonstrates the sight, sound, and feel of the sound. When this phase of ear training is complete, the client should be able to recognize the sound in isolation and perceive, if not describe, a number of its important characteristics.

Isolation. In this phase of ear training, the client is expected to use the new recognition skills to isolate the target sound when it is produced against a backdrop of other speech sounds. That is, he or she must be able to locate the target when the clinician produces a word, phrase, or sentence using it. The clinician might, for example, give a child two cards, one with a happy (smiling) face and one with a sad (frowning) face. The clinician would say, "When I say a word, I want you to show me the happy face if it has your sound in it. If it doesn't, show me the sad face." The clinician then utters words one at a time, and the child responds by displaying the appropriate card after each stimulus word. The clinician can increase the difficulty of the task by presenting a series of words or even a sentence and asking the child to signal each word that contains the target sound. The child can next be asked to identify the position of the target in the stimulus word—initial (beginning), medial (middle), or final (end). This task is quite common in ear training. Again, the focus of this phase is on the location of the target sound in various phonetic contexts.

Stimulation. In this third phase of ear training, the clinician presents the target sound in a variety of ways. The sound may be presented at different intensities (loudnesses), perhaps with the use of a tape recorder. In a group therapy setting, other clients may be asked to produce the target sound. The client is, in effect, bombarded with instances of the target. In addition to varying loudness, the clinician may present samples quickly or slowly, of long or short duration. The client may be asked to listen to sentences or even paragraphs containing several uses of the sound. Even tongue twisters can be used. In each case, the client is asked to identify the target sound as it occurs. The goal of this phase is to elevate the client's sensitivity to the phonetic properties of the sound and further develop a complete, internalized auditory model of the target.

Discrimination. Discrimination, the final phase of ear training, may be the most important because it is the basis for developing the client's learning, detecting, and correcting skills. Therapy is still focused on listening, rather than producing sounds. The task at this point is to make external comparisons; that is, the client listens to the productions of the clinician and compares them to the internal auditory image of the sound that he or she has developed. This is known as an *interauditory* comparison (where the client compares someone else's production with the image), as opposed to an *intra-auditory* comparison (in which the client would compare his own production with the image). This discrimination is the last interauditory skill learned before training shifts to enhancing the client's skill in listening to his or her own speech.

It is important to note that the ability to make external comparisons does not necessarily mean that the client can make accurate internal (intra-auditory) comparisons (Aungst & Frick, 1964). Thus the efficacy of sound discrimination training is a matter of some controversy today (see, for example, Dickson, 1962; Sonderman, 1971; Williams & McReynolds, 1975). The ability to produce a target sound at least inconsistently, that is, to have some internal production model, may be important (Lapko & Bankson, 1975).

While Van Riper presents ear training as a stage that precedes production training, some clinicians feel that sensory-perceptual training and early establishment of production of new sounds should go hand in hand. They feel that the more a client knows about his or her own production, the better will be the auditory image for the target sound.

Van Riper and Emerick (1984) describe two tasks in discrimination training, error detection and error correction. In error detection the client is to uncover errors produced on purpose by the clinician. He may be required, for instance, to stop the clinician whenever the target sound is produced incorrectly. The clinician usually produces a series of target sounds with an intentional mistake, probably of the type most often made by the client. The "mistake" can occur within the context of a series of words, a passage, or even a tongue twister, to make it more difficult if appropriate. These tasks could be called "ear twisters"; they are useful in developing discrimination skills.[2]

Error correction is an extension of error discrimination. At this point the client is asked to explain why the sound was in error and perhaps what needs to be done to correct it. For example, for /s/ the client might say, "You forgot to close your teeth" or "You stuck your tongue out; you have to keep it in your mouth." The clinician might reply, "Okay, how's this?" and then produce the target in the way the client described.

This last phase is often the bridge to the client's first analyses of his or her own productions, the first time the client really begins to take a critical look at how he or she is making errors. The client now has available at least some rudiments of the perceptual equipment needed to begin making internal comparisons, has learned about many aspects of the sound to be learned, and is thus more apt to make good judgments about his or her own productions and to make better judgments more quickly.

In the last phase of ear training, the focus shifts to intra-auditory discrimination. Van Riper and Emerick (1984) contend that this process involves learning how to recall, perceive, and predict errors. As experienced clinicians know, there is a natural time sequence involved in error recognition. At first, most clients will recognize their errors only some time after they have occurred. Clearly, to be able to make the important self-corrections necessary for more automatic accurate production, one needs to be able to detect one's own errors immediately as they occur. What's more, it is necessary to be able to predict the sounds and sound combinations that are likely to lead to errors.

----

[2]Consider carefully the appropriateness of tasks such as these for very young children. This task, in particular, requires a child to be able to use language to comment on the correctness or appropriateness of the language itself (metalinguistic awareness). Although this ability is observed in normally developing children as early as age 4, it is important to consider carefully the age and linguistic abilities of each client.

Thus this last phase of ear training, though often not heavily emphasized, is crucial to the ongoing process of automatic self-monitoring of speech. These skills will also be needed throughout the remainder of therapy, but at this point the emphasis on discrimination is primary rather than secondary.

Teaching intra-auditory discrimination is not easy. Moment-to-moment appraisals of one's own speech are often difficult to learn. Some clinicians use signals to help their clients immediately recognize their errors. Any signal—a light, a tone, slapping the table—that alerts the client that he or she has made an error can be used. Clinicians also use shadowing techniques, such as simultaneous talking with the client. Here the clinician may either speak more loudly at exactly the moment the client makes the error or stop talking altogether. Amplification techniques, especially those where the client can hear his or her own voice but more loudly, are also effective (Van Riper, 1963).

One final aspect of discrimination training is learning how to predict sounds and sound combinations where errors are likely to occur. The clinician may provide activities, such as circling letters in an oral reading passage where an error might occur or speaking more loudly on likely targets in sample words or sentences. In each case, the client must identify the places where errors are most likely to occur. Again, almost any activity that provides practice in predicting errors will help the client develop self-discrimination and correction skills. (For several exercises for all phases of ear training, see Van Riper, 1963.)

Conclusion.   Ear training consists of four phases: identification, isolation, stimulation, and discrimination. While it is the first phase of articulation therapy, it does not end when therapy moves to production training. In reality, training in listening and self-correction often continues throughout the course of therapy. As a new, more difficult production level is undertaken, the problem of intra-auditory discrimination may arise again. The ultimate goal of ear training is to provide the client with the skills necessary to correct his or her own errors throughout the process of therapy. This ability is essential if the client is to learn automatic, correct, and fluent speech.

One final caution: The effectiveness of sound discrimination training is a matter of some dispute today. It is undoubtedly an outgrowth of concern that clinicians and researchers have with regard to the overall efficacy of auditory discrimination testing. For more information on this dispute, refer to the section on assessment of auditory discrimination in chapter 4.

Production Training (Sound Establishment)

The second major stage of treatment usually begins after the client has learned to identify the acoustic features of the new sound to be learned; that is, when the client can recognize the characteristics of the new sound and make some correct judgments about whether a given production is correct or incorrect. (Again, some clinicians who use traditional methods begin with eliciting at least some instances of the sound before training sound awareness.) The focus of production training is to evoke and establish a new sound pattern that will replace the client's error pattern.

It is not necessarily easy to evoke the correct sound. Van Riper and Emerick (1984), as in previous editions of Van Riper's work, stress the notions of *varying* and *correcting* the attempts at the sound. The client must learn to change the way he or she produces the sound. As Van Riper and Emerick say,

> Long-practiced habits are very resistant to change. . . . Variation must precede approximation. By this we mean something similar to what happens when a person learns to shoot an arrow at a target. When he shoots and misses, he must first know that his second shot will have some chance of hitting a different part of the target, preferably a spot closer to the bull's-eye. But he must vary and he must try to correct. This same procedure occurs in articulation therapy. (p. 199)

Thus, no matter what approach the clinician uses to elicit the new sound, the client will most probably have to vary and correct productions of that sound before he or she can produce the sound consistently and accurately.

Secord (1981a) has described in depth several commonly used approaches to eliciting new sounds. They include (a) auditory stimulation/imitation, (b) use of context, (c) phonetic placement, (d) the moto-kinesthetic method, and (e) sound approximation.

Auditory Stimulation/Imitation.   The first method used to elicit new sounds is auditory stimulation (Bernthal & Bankson, 1981; Irwin, 1965; Milisen, 1954; Powers, 1971; Van Riper, 1978; Weiss, Lillywhite, & Gordon, 1980). The clinician provides one or several examples of the target sound and requires the client to repeat it. This widely used technique is probably the best known method (if not the easiest to implement) of eliciting new sounds.

Auditory stimulation can be handled in several different ways. If the sound can be produced in isolation, the clinician might present two or three instances of the correct sound. If the sound can only be produced in a syllable, the clinician would present the target syllable two or three ways. (Some authorities feel that only certain sounds, such as continuants /s, z, f, v, θ/, to name a few, can be produced in isolation, and that others, such as stops and affricates, must be produced in syllables. Others feel that no sound can actually be produced in isolation.) The client then attempts to produce the sound correctly. The clinician may ask the client to say the sound loudly and softly, to prolong it, or produce short bursts of the sound. Next the client might be asked to describe how the sound feels. He or she will definitely be asked to vary productions on the road to producing the correct form.

Auditory stimulation is often combined with other methods for establishing new sounds. For example, the clinician might use phonetic placement (described later) to help the client produce the sound the first few times and then revert to auditory stimulation for practice. It is common clinical practice to use a combination of methods to elicit new sounds.

Again, the clinician must stress varying and correcting. At this point in therapy, the client is trying to learn accurate and deliberate production. Many attempts will fall short of this goal, so the client may need to be encouraged to continue trying. These varying and correcting responses improve the client's internalized model of the correct production. Just as early ear-training responses are unsure and unstable, early production responses will vary. That is, the establishment of an internalized model of the correct sound, be it auditory or motor, requires a great deal of trial-and-error learning.

Use of Context.   Often a client will be able to produce a target sound in some contexts but not in others because of the coarticulatory effects of adjacent sounds. That is, adjacent sounds make it easier for the client to produce a sound in some contexts. Those contexts are called *facilitating contexts* (McDonald, 1964a). They are specific phonetic environments—syllables or words, singularly or in combination—where a sound that is usually produced incorrectly is produced correctly. The clinician may use those contexts in therapy. Two methods of identifying facilitating contexts are deep testing (McDonald, 1964b) and using probes of articulation consistency (Secord, 1981b) (see chapter 4 for a discussion of these two methods).

The facilitating contexts will often be familiar words or word combinations. Correct production in these contexts is used as a point of departure for establishing the sound. For instance, assume that Josh, who lisps, can say /s/ correctly in the word *outside*. A clinician might break *outside* into its components *out* and *side* and use the second part (*side*) as a place to begin training for /s/. Because Josh can already say the sound correctly, the clinician needs to expand on this correct use. (McDonald, 1964a, has described the sensory-motor approach, a complete approach to treatment based on early use of facilitating phonetic contexts.)

Using contexts in words, such as in *outside* for Josh, is important because these words, which Van Riper calls *key words*, become a standard for production. Josh will learn to compare his other attempts to produce the /s/ sound with the /s/ in *outside* and will develop other words from this base. As another example, assume that Sara could correctly say *hats*. The clinician might have her hold the ending sound so long that she, in effect, begins to produce the /s/ by itself (in isolation). Thus, the key word can be, and often is, a starting block for producing the target in isolation.

If the client can produce the sound correctly in several contexts, production training might begin at the word level. However, this would only be the case if the client has relatively accurate and consistent production at the important isolation and syllable levels.

These facilitating context words can also be used as key words in the paired stimuli method of articulation therapy. This specific, behavioral approach is discussed in detail in chapter 12.

Some clients will not present any facilitating contexts and will not be able to produce the target sound in response to auditory stimulation. In that case, the clinician will need to teach the client directly how to say the target sound. The remaining techniques to be discussed are suited to that purpose.

Phonetic Placement.   As we have seen, for years speech clinicians have been using diagrams, instruments, and exercises to show their clients where and how to position their speech organs to pronounce specific sounds correctly. Scripture and Jackson (1927) are probably most responsible for what is today known as the *phonetic placement method*. Clinicians still frequently use this method to help teach clients how to place the articulators correctly, to modify the breath stream, and to voice sounds appropriately. It is designed to give the client as many clues as possible to use in producing a difficult sound. The clinician may use a variety of diagrams, applicators, or instruments to explain the correct production. One very commonly used tool is a mirror, either large or hand-held, to enable the client to see his or her own production of the sound. Weiss and his colleagues (1980, p. 168) have summarized several of the many techniques and devices used in the phonetic placement method.

1. Manipulate or hold the articulators in place with tongue blades and sticks
2. Use [the clinician's] finger to manipulate the client's articulators
3. Describe and instruct verbally
4. Use a breath indicator for mouth and nose
5. Show the client graphic records such as a spectrogram
6. Let the client feel his breath stream with his hand or see its effects on a tissue
7. Have the client observe the clinician and self in a mirror while producing the target sound
8. Have the client feel his own laryngeal vibration
9. Have the client look at diagrams, photographs, or drawings of the articulators while producing target sounds
10. Show the client palatograms of articulators while producing target sounds

The variety of techniques available in the phonetic placement method is limited only by the clinician's imagination.

As mentioned, this method is often used in combination with other methods discussed in this section. For example, a clinician might extract a target sound from a key word and present it several times via auditory stimulation. As the client responds, the clinician could give moment-to-moment phonetic placement instructions to help the client vary and correct the response. For an exhaustive list of phonetic placement techniques, see Secord (1981a). Here are some examples for eliciting /s/. Techniques marked with an *M* are especially effective if a mirror is used; those followed by an asterisk are especially good for lateral /s/.

M Demonstrate the feature characteristics of /s/:
Tongue tip-blade nearly touching the alveolar ridge
Slow release of air over the tongue toward the cutting edges of upper central incisors
Vocal cords silent

M 1. Demonstrate this procedure in a mirror step by step first and then allow the client to demonstrate the same. Tell the client to:
   a. Raise the back of the tongue so he can feel his upper back teeth.
   b. Place the tip of the tongue behind his upper front teeth and then pull it away from them just a bit.
   c. Close his teeth so that they are barely touching. The clinician should then hold the tip of his finger in front of the center of the client's mouth and say: "Blow air slowly over your tongue toward my finger."

M 2. For /s/ with the tongue tip down:*
   a. Back of the tongue to upper back teeth.
   b. Tongue tip placed behind lower central incisors. (You may need a tongue depressor for this.)

      c. Close the teeth.

      d. Initiate /s/.

  3. To develop a central air flow, a variety of techniques are available:*

      a. Draw a small target and hold it in front of mouth. Tell the client to make a bull's-eye with the /s/.

      b. Hold your fingertip about three inches from the client's nose. Ask him to force the /s/ outward and upward toward your finger, or have the client use his own finger.

      c. Have the client close his teeth and direct the air flow for /s/ through a straw.

      d. Use a tongue depressor and trace a line through the center of his tongue to give the client the idea of a trough before attempting /s/.

      e. Have the client brush the lower gums with his tongue while attempting to say /s/.

      f. Tell the client to pucker his lips and then fully retract them. Push the tongue forward and say /s/.

      g. Place the client's finger at the very center of the teeth and have him attempt /s/.

M 4. Use a tongue depressor to explain precise points of contact in the mouth. Then place the tongue depressor just behind the teeth. Ask the client to hold it there with his tongue tip. The small opening created when you remove the tongue depressor is almost the distance necessary for air to pass in order to secure /s/.

  5. Instruct the client to close the teeth and rapidly bring the back of the tongue up against the lower teeth while attempting /s/.

  6. Tell the client to groove the tongue and then attempt /s/.

  7. Tell the client to brush the upper gums with his tongue tip while he attempts /s/.

  8. Instruct him to close his teeth and bring his lips together tightly. Then slowly open the lips to allow the /s/ to escape. (Secord, 1981a, pp. 21–22)

The Moto-Kinesthetic Method. Developed by Edna Young and Sara Stinchfield-Hawk in the late 1930s, the moto-kinesthetic method is similar to phonetic placement. In fact, according to Sommers (1983), it is perhaps the ultimate extension of the general phonetic placement concept. It differs from other phonetic placement techniques, however, in its stress on patterns of movement in articulation and on increasing awareness of kinesthetic movements to guide articulation.

    In this method, the clinician uses his or her own hands to manipulate the client's articulators. In this way the clinician forces the client to notice where the movement begins, how much tension or pressure is needed, the overall shape and direction of the movement, and the timing of the movements. The clinician thus helps the client use the tactile and kinesthetic senses to feel the way the sound is produced. The clinician may also provide visual and auditory stimulation to improve the client's sensory image of the correct production. Here is an example of the correct moto-kinesthetic stimulation for /s/, based on Young and Hawk (1955): Place the thumb and forefinger of your left hand at the corners of the upper lip. Place the thumb and forefinger of your right hand on the corners of the lower lip. If the occlusion is normal, push the lower jaw into the position of a normal bite; then pull the lower jaw down to create an ever so slight opening between the teeth. Ask the client to blow air through the teeth.

More detail on the moto-kinesthetic method can be found in Young and Hawk's 1955 book. A brief summary of each moto-kinesthetic stimulation for all consonants, vowels, and diphthongs can be found in Secord (1981a).

Today the moto-kinesthetic method is primarily used as an adjunct to phonetic placement. In fact, many of the stimulations are no doubt perceived as phonetic placement techniques. The moto-kinesthetic method is used for the most part to evoke correct speech sounds for the first time.

Sound Approximation. *Sound approximation* refers to two similar approaches, progressive approximation and modification of other sounds (Van Riper, 1978). Both involve the behavioral learning principle known as *shaping*. In progressive approximation, the clinician evokes a series of sounds or sound segments that gradually approximate the target response, until the actual target sound is produced. Van Riper described progressive approximation as follows:

> The clinician joins the client and makes the same error the client makes. She then shows the client a series of transitional sounds, each of which comes a little closer to the standard sound until finally the standard sound is produced. Each little modification the client makes that comes a bit closer to the goal is rewarded. Those variations that move away from the target sound are ignored. (1978, p. 188)

Thus the clinician begins with the client's error and gradually modifies it, using his or her own finely tuned discrimination skills to guide the client's productions. Many clinicians know and use this method—for instance, with a client who has a distorted /ɝ/ that resembles the /ʊ/ in *put*. The client initially produces the error /ʊ/ in isolation and is then guided by the clinician's instructions to produce sounds that come closer and closer to the target /ɝ/.

The second type of sound approximation method is modification of other sounds. Here the clinician uses another sound or sounds already in the client's repertoire as a point of departure for the target sound. The clinician instructs the client to produce a known sound and then to adjust the articulators in certain ways while continuing to produce the known sound. Each articulatory adjustment is a movement that comes closer to the position necessary for the target sound. This method is often used with nonspeech sounds such as coughing to elicit a /k/ or growling to elicit /ɝ/. Once the client produces a sound that is close to the target, the clinician can use a variety of other techniques, such as auditory stimulation and further phonetic placement instruction, to bring the production precisely on target. Here are several clinical examples for /s/.

1. Instruct the client to bring his teeth together and "slurp" inhaled air, then exhale this air as /s/.
2. Shape /s/ from /θ/. Instruct the client to prolong /θ/ as in *think*. Tell him or her to gradually bring the tongue into the mouth over the

back of the top teeth and along the alveolar ridge to the vicinity for /s/ while saying /θ/.

    a.   Same procedure but use a tongue depressor to guide the movement.

    b.   Tell the client to do the same but use the tongue tip to "point" to the back of the teeth and the gum ridge.

    c.   Tell the client to say a list of initial-position /θ/ words slowly, pushing the tongue inward and upward to the alveolar ridge as the /θ/ sound is uttered.

3. Shape /s/ from /t/. Instruct the client to make rapid productions of /t/ and prolong the last one into /s/.

4. Shape /s/ from [tʰ]. Tell the client to say /t/ with a great amount of plosion. This considerably aspirated [tʰ] will result in the German affricate /ts/. Ask the client to prolong the second sound in /ts/, resulting in tssssss. Then the /t/ is dropped.

5. Shape /s/ from /i/. Instruct the client to say /i/, then gradually close the teeth and say /s/.

6. Shape /s/ from /ʃ/. Tell the client to say /ʃ/, smile and push the tongue a little forward.

7. Shape /s/ from /z/. Tell the client to whisper a /z/ or hold his hand on his throat while producing /z/, then turn off the voicing.

8. Shape /s/ from /n/. Tell the client to place the tongue at the position for /n/ and then to release the tongue a little bit and force air over the tongue.

9. Shape /s/ from /l/. Tell the client to put the tongue up for /l/, close the teeth and remove the tongue a little bit, and then blow air over the tongue.

10. Shape /s/ from /h/. Instruct the client to close the teeth first, then prolong /h/ while gradually raising the tongue tip.

11. Shape /s/ from /f/. Instruct the client to lift the tongue tip slowly while prolonging /f/ and gradually bringing the front teeth together.

Conclusion. This section has described five ways to establish correct production of an error sound. Most of these eliciting methods have been used for years. For a complete discussion of eliciting techniques, see Nemoy and Davis (1954), Secord (1981a), and Bosley (1981).

Production Training (Stabilization)

When a client has learned to make the target sound accurately though deliberately, the next task is to stabilize that correct response at the simplest level of production—isolation. As shown in Figure 5.1, isolation is the first in a series of stabilization levels that are each assumed to be of increasing complexity and difficulty. The client must master the target sound at each of these levels. The task is *stabilization*, that is, developing the ability to say the target sound relatively easily and quickly.

Not all clinicians begin at the isolation level. Some insist that the syllable level is the appropriate entry point. They point out that evidence suggests that the syllable is the basic element of speech and that, while not all phonemes can be produced in isolation, all can be produced in syllables. Still other clinicians begin stabilization training at the word level because words are more meaningful. After all, phonemes are units used to signal changes in meaning. Advocates of beginning with isolated sounds or syllables, however, believe that there is often too much interference between the client's habitual error sound and the new sound if it is used in a meaningful context (a word). They feel that this interference is reduced by early stabilization work in isolation and/or syllables.

No matter what stabilization level is chosen as the beginning point, as the client enters each level, ability to produce the sound is weak and generally unstable. As the client leaves the level, however, production should be consistently accurate and fluent. Stabilization at one level is considered a prerequisite for entry to the next level, and increases the client's chances for success at that next level.

Isolation.   Beginning with isolation, then, the goal is to develop a stronger, more consistently correct response. This response will serve as a foundation for later, more complicated phonetic alterations. Often the clinician will use a mirror in isolation work. The mirror further extends the visual cues learned in the establishment stage.

The following list presents some common tasks used in isolation training:

1.   practicing prolonging the target
2.   varying the number of productions emitted at any one time
3.   varying the intensity with which the sound is produced
4.   whispering the new sound
5.   starting and stopping production in response to the clinician's signal
6.   simultaneously talking and writing the new sound (This technique has been highly recommended by Van Riper, 1963).
7.   responding to large and small letters that represent the target by using loud or soft sounds depending on the size of the letter cues
8.   playing "speech games" where the child responds by producing his target sound a certain number of times when it is his turn
9.   playing with a deck of cards with different numbers used to indicate to the child the number of times to produce the sound
10.   switching from one sound to another and then back to the target so that the target is said immediately after the client has repositioned the articulators (This technique is used later in training.)

Throughout treatment at this level, the client is instructed to concentrate on how the sound "feels"; that is, on such characteristics as where the tongue is during production, where the airstream is going, what the productions look like in the mirror, and what happens when an error is produced.

Many clients, even young children, become quite adept at analyzing their own productions. They may come to know as much about their error responses as they do about what they need to do to say the sound correctly. Again, the clinician may continue using ear training during stabilization work in isolation. The client who continues to practice varying and correcting isolated productions and to develop auditory self-monitoring skills is likely to progress nicely in this stage.

Toward the end of the isolation phase, most clinicians begin to give tasks that facilitate movement from simple isolated productions to production in syllables. The client whose productions are stable at one level will typically have little trouble moving to the next level, but the smart clinician will prepare the client for this step. For example, the client may occasionally be able to produce a few simple syllables without much trouble. Before the clinician moves on to the syllable level, the training sessions should incorporate a few of the simple syllables to help smooth the transition. One very useful principle here is the behavioral "itsy bitsy" principle—"think small." The steps from one level to the next should be small enough to ensure success for the client.

Nonsense Syllable Level.   During this phase, the goal is to develop more consistently correct productions in a variety of nonsense-syllable contexts. At this point, training in nonsense syllables offers certain advantages over practice in meaningful words. First, the clinician can use nonsense syllables for any target sound to practice the sound in a wide variety of phonetic contexts. For example, for /s/, contexts could include:

/si/	(CV)	prevocalic
/is/	(VC)	postvocalic
/isi/	(VCV)	intervocalic
/sib/	(CVC)	initial
/bis/	(CVC)	final

Any of the stressed vowels could then be substituted for /i/, creating more nonsense syllables to be used in practice. By producing a wide variety of nonsense syllables, the client practices the target sound in all different syllable positions. This practice helps prepare for connected speech, which requires accuracy in sequentially initiating and terminating syllables, as well as in producing the sound between syllables.

The clinician might also use the target sound in nonsense clusters, such as /ipsi/ and /ispi/. This practice helps ready the client to produce complex cluster words. The clinician can develop nonsense clusters that foreshadow real words. If the client is going to have to master the cluster /ts/, as in the word *outside,* for instance, the clinician might provide practice in the nonsense clusters /itsi/, /ætsi/, and /etsi/. This practice builds a stable base of motor readiness for learning cluster contexts (see Winitz, 1975; Secord, 1981b).

A second advantage of using nonsense syllables is reducing the interference of the client's habitual error sound. Just as correct phonemes signal changes in meaning, so can error phonemes signal changes in meaning for the client. Consider a rapid drill activity for Cindy, a 7-year-old who substitutes /θ/ for /s/.

> *Clinician:* Say /saɪ/ five times.
> *Cindy:*   saɪ
>   saɪ

saɪ
saɪ
saɪ
Clinician: Good! Now say /si/.
Cindy: si
si
si
si
si
Clinician: Great! What do you do with your eyes?
Cindy: /θi/ [thee]

It is easier for Cindy to produce the /s/ as a nonsense syllable because there is very little competition from her articulatory programming for /θ/. However, she still uses /θ/ as the meaningful insertion to signify what you do with your eyes; you "thee." Thus, using nonsense syllables allows Cindy to learn to produce /s/ more easily.

To summarize, most clinicians who use traditional methods use nonsense syllables to provide practice in a variety of phonetic contexts and syllabic positions and to reduce interference from the old error. With Cindy, the clinician might use a nonsense-syllable diagram such as the one shown in Figure 5.2. Cindy would be told to say /s/ and combine it with the vowels in the diagram. Thus she might produce:

sa   /se/
se   /si/
si   /saɪ/
so   /so/
soo   /su/

She can also combine the vowels and a following /s/:

as   /es/
es   /is/
is   /aɪs/
os   /os/
oos   /us/

Intervocalic combinations can be created with /s/ between two instances of each vowel or two different vowels.

asa   /ese/
ese   /isi/
oso   /oso/
ase   /esi/
esa   /ise/

The clinician can simply sequentially point to the sounds Cindy is to produce.

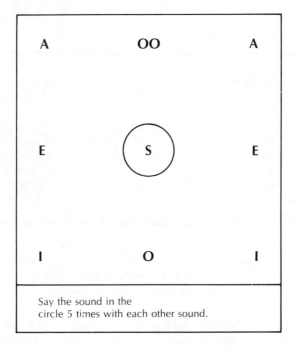

FIGURE 5.2
Nonsense syllable diagram used with a second grade student.

The focus of training might next shift to nonsense words. For example, a clinician might first present an activity where familiar objects are given funny or silly nonsense names that contain the child's target sound. Then the clinician might have the child play a "fill-in" or cloze game where the clinician describes the object and the child tells its nonsense name. The purpose here is to get the child accustomed to using the target sound as part of a nonsense word that has a referent, the object described.

Next, Cindy might use the nonsense words in simple phrases or sentences to increase the length of utterance that she can say containing her target sound. From there the focus of training might shift to nonsense words used in a conversational or even storytelling frame. A clinician might conduct a session using silly names created for characters in a child's story or for puppets. For example, the clinician might say,

"Tell me about /sæbo/ and /sæbi/, the two pirates who searched for buried treasure," or

"This is /sibɑ/, a little lost puppy. Tell me how /sibɑ/ got home."

Thus the child continues to use nonsense words, but the activity resembles tasks that will later be accomplished with real words.

Some clinicians carry nonsense training quite far. They may have the client tell a story using a wide variety of nonsense words or use nonsense words in conversational responses. The only difference between these activities and

TABLE 5.2
Substages of Word-Level Stabilization Training

Substage	Syllables	Examples for /s/
1. Initial prevocalic words	1	sun, sign, say
2. Final postvocalic words	1	glass, miss, pass
3. Medial intervocalic words	2	kissing, lassie, racer
4. Initial blends/clusters	1	star, spoon, skate
5. Final blends/clusters	1	lost, lips, rocks
6. Medial blends/clusters	2	whisper, outside, ice-skate
7. All word positions	1–2	[any of above]
8. All word positions	any	signaling, eraser, therapist
9. All word positions; multiple targets	any	necessary, successful

those used later for sentence and conversation stabilization training is the set of target words. Again, using nonsense words helps make the transition to the word level easier and increases the chances of success.

Words.   When the client is able to produce the target sound in nonsense syllables relatively easily and quickly, therapy moves to stabilization training in words. Table 5.2 outlines a series of substages commonly used in this phase, though some clinicians use even smaller steps. The treatment plan moves from simple, one-syllable words to complex, multisyllable examples. While this scheme may be varied in practice, it is typical of the progression most frequently used. The goal is to teach the client to produce the target sound in the almost endless variety of phonetic contexts in which it can occur in words. He or she must be able to say the sound when it abuts a number of other consonants and vowels, as well as in the simplest CV, VC, or CVC words.

Clearly, the task is a challenging one. The client needs to learn not only simple words like *so, say,* and *us,* but also complex words such as *successful* or even *necessary.* It is equally challenging for the clinician, who must assure that the client can *fluently* produce these numerous contexts in order eventually to stabilize all those complex productions in even longer and more complex connected speech utterances.

Again, some clinicians will skip early stablization training in isolation and/or syllables and begin with words. They may attempt to elicit correct productions first in simple VC or CV one-syllable words or may begin with words or word contexts produced correctly during the initial assessments. Those words may be used as a beginning point for treatment, the first training words from which other, similar words are developed. As mentioned before, these clinicians may feel that words are a more useful, natural beginning point because they are everyday communication tools.

Once an initial corps of correctly produced words is established, the clinician may return to the scheme shown in Table 5.2. Ear-training procedures may be used before or concurrently with further work on production. The clinician may also continue to stress self-monitoring throughout the remaining course of treatment.

The clinician's first task in word stabilization training is to choose the corps of target words. Some clinicians prefer to use a small group of highly familiar, meaningful words, adding a few words at a time as the client masters the first ones. Others begin with a few words and then add a great many more when the client can consistently produce the first targets accurately. The first practice group often will consist of names of familiar people, objects, or pets, or familiar slang words. Because the client will use these frequently occurring words relatively often, the new, correct production can be reinforced by parents, friends, and other people. These words will also be of greater interest to the client and no doubt will be more meaningful than a group of randomly chosen words.

Throughout this stage, ear-training activities should be used at least occasionally so that the client continues to develop the ability to monitor his or her own productions of the target words and correct errors where necessary. With both adults and children who cannot monitor their own productions well, it is best to use a very small group of words at the outset, perhaps 10 to 15 words at each substage (prevocalic, postvocalic, and intervocalic). The client should practice only those words and the clinician should reinforce only those words when produced correctly, ignoring errors in all words other than the 30 to 45 targets. This procedure helps clients to remember the specific words they can say and are responsible to monitor. It also lets parents and other family members be more aware of the specific words to reinforce or remind the client to correct. When a small group of words is used, it is easier to develop "speech awareness" in the client. Frequently the correct production of this small target group will easily generalize to other words; the client's ability to self-monitor also often improves.

One commercially available program (discussed in chapter 6) using this approach of a very small group of initial training words is the S-PACK (Mowrer, Baker, & Schutz, 1968). This behavioral instructional program uses only about 30 words, which have been programmed for use up to and including conversational tasks. Mowrer has demonstrated considerable improvement using only this small group of training words.

Some clients simply do not have any beginning words in which they can produce their targets correctly, even though they can produce them correctly in nonsense syllables. They find the competition from the error response too great. In this case, the clinician must again "think small," using techniques that gradually step over the gap from nonsense syllables to teach the client how to produce the target sound in words. Van Riper and Emerick (1984) list three types of techniques used for this purpose:

1. reconfiguration,
2. simultaneous talking and writing, and
3. signaling,

to which we can add:

4. creating simple words from complex contexts.

The idea behind *reconfiguration* is to teach the client "that words are made up of sound sequences and that these sound sequences can be modified without losing the unity of the word" (Van Riper & Emerick, 1984, p. 208). Again, with Cindy (who lisps, substituting /θ/ for /s/ at the beginning of words), the clinician might use a sentence involving initial /s/: *Cindy has a dog named Sir.* First, Cindy is told to substitute another sound, perhaps /p/, for one of her nonerror sounds: *Cindy has a pog named Sir.* Next, she uses her new, target sound for other sounds, but not in the error words: *Cindy has a ssssog named Sir.* She then substitutes /p/ for the initial /s/ in the sentence: *Pindy has a dog named Pir.* The next step is to speak the sentence but omit all instances of initial /s/: _indy has a dog named _ir. Finally, Cindy is instructed to use her new sound in the blank spaces: *SSSS[C]indy has a dog named SSSSir.*

In *simultaneous talking and writing,* the clinician again chooses words using the target sound. The client says and writes the sound, first by itself, then in one-syllable words, then in the first syllable of multisyllable words, then in whole words. Next the client may alternate the letter and the whole word, and finally may write only the letter as he or she pronounces the whole word.

Signaling techniques use "preparatory sets" to allow the client to combine the target sound with the rest of the word. The client might draw out the target sound until the clinician gives a prearranged signal; then a vowel or the rest of a word is added. For instance, Cindy may sit with her eyes closed saying *sssss.* When the clinician rings a bell, Cindy immediately and automatically says *ir.* Van Riper and Emerick (1984, p. 208) recommend requiring the child to say the word twice, *sssss* [bell] *irsir.*

If Cindy says the target correctly but then produces the error before the rest of the word (*sthir*), the clinician may ask her to begin by forming her mouth for the vowel that begins the rest of the word (*ir*). This simple task of preforming the mouth often solves the problem, as may the use of pairs of words in which the first ends with the vowel of the second. (For more on these three techniques, see Van Riper & Emerick, 1984, pp. 208–209.)

Creating simple words from complex contexts is another form of using context. The clinician uses the results of deep testing (McDonald, 1964b) or a test of articulation consistency (e.g., Secord, 1981b) to identify those contexts in which the target can be produced correctly. To use the example of the child who can correctly say *outside,* the clinician may be able to break that word in half, retaining the second syllable, *side.* Using this word as a key word, as in the paired stimuli method (see chapter 12), the clinician can pair *side* with other words such as *out, sign, sight,* and *sigh.* Once the client can use his sound in a few words, development of other words becomes much easier.

Activities used in word-level stabilization training have several goals. One important goal is eliciting a large number of responses to give the client practice in production and evaluation. A second purpose is to provide a wide variety of exercises to keep the therapy sessions from becoming meaningless drill (though, unfortunately, considerable drill work is often needed). Some emphasis is usually placed on self-correction skills, with continued reminders and special practice on judging correct and incorrect productions. Clinicians usually reward self-correction skills at this point because treatment will soon move to much longer and phonetically more complex utterances. It is then much more difficult to give immediate reinforcement for correct responses.

The therapy tasks may include speech games, making things, drill work, speech dittoes, and so forth. For examples of some commonly used activities, see the list of activities in Appendix B.

To summarize, there are three main purposes of stabilization training at the word level:

1. to provide numerous opportunities for practice in a variety of increasingly more complex word contexts
2. to stabilize correct sound productions at each substage (initial, final, medial, etc.)
3. to develop further the ability to self-monitor correct and incorrect sound productions

As in other levels, the ultimate goal of training is consistent, correct production of the target sound with ease and speed.

Phrases.   At this point some clinicians choose to work on stabilization training using the target sound in short (two- to four-word) phrases. This practice is in keeping with the "think small" philosophy. It may help ensure that the jump from words to sentences is not so great that the client encounters difficulty. Again, it is important for the client to be successful (to some degree) at each stage. Thus, many clinicians insert one or more sessions of phrase work between work on words and sentences, while others consider phrases to be a level equal in stature (and possibly in time devoted) to words and sentences. Usually, however, the client who has mastered stabilization at the word level is ready to proceed to sentence practice, and most clinicians will begin the sentence level with short sentences in any case.

Sentences.   Once the client is able to produce the target sound consistently in words, the likelihood of breakdown at the sentence level is reduced. In a few cases, stabilization training may begin at the sentence level. This is likely only when the client cannot produce the target sound at any simpler level but can produce it in certain contexts in running speech. For example, Don may be able to produce /r/ correctly only when it occurs after the word *are,* as in *The boys are running.* In that case, the clinician might build on that base.

Just as practice at the word level is carefully sequenced to ensure success, practice at the sentence level is also structured by level of difficulty and complexity. Table 5.3 outlines a simple scheme for structuring sentence practice. Following such a scheme will enable the client to make steady progress in producing sentences and to become more skilled at monitoring his or her own productions as the utterances become more complex. In other words, the difficulty of the exercises must be carefully sequenced to develop both production and perception skills.

In addition to controlling the level of complexity of the practice sentences, the clinician should control the phonetic environment. Early sentence practice might use simple one-syllable words and then move to examples of more complex clusters.

TABLE 5.3
Substages of Sentence-Level Stabilization Training

Sentence Description	Instances of Target Sound
1. Simple short sentence	1
2. Sentences of various lengths	1
3. Simple short sentence	2 or more
4. Sentences of various lengths	2 or more

Some clients may have difficulty making the transition to sentences. In that case the clinician may choose to have the client practice only a limited number of words that he or she knows well in the various word positions (initial, medial, and final). Van Riper (1978) listed several techniques the clinician can use to help establish production in sentences: slow-motion speech, echo speech or shadowing, unison speaking, the corrective set, and role playing.

In *slow-motion speech*, the clinician and the client say the target sentence together, but very slowly. This oral drill may be preceded by performing simple motor tasks, such as walking, in slow motion. For the speech exercise, the clinician may sit behind and slightly above the client so that the client can hear the difficult words clearly.

Shadowing is one form of echo speech. In this activity, the client repeats the clinician's speech as quickly and automatically as possible, one word at a time. Interestingly, children can learn to do this more easily than adults can. A second form of *echo speech* has the client repeat a series of words, a phrase, or a sentence, after the clinician has given a signal. The signal should include a gesture or prompt which the client also repeats.

Unison speech employs sentences or phrases that have already been identified. Often using hand tapping or other signals of rhythm, the clinician and client speak in unison. Again the client follows the clinician's physical movements and the prosody of the clinician's speech. Each phrase or sentence is spoken several times.

An activity that most children enjoy is correcting the clinician. The *corrective set* uses this practice. The clinician will do or say something obviously wrong and ask the child to correct it. When the child is beginning to enjoy correcting the clinician's mistakes, the clinician produces some utterances that contain the child's common error. Often the child will be able to say the sentence accurately in order to correct the clinician.

Some children are able to speak correctly when they are acting or *role playing*, though they cannot produce their target sounds in sentences when they are "being themselves." Thus dramatics, theater, and story-telling may all be vehicles for getting a child to become involved in another role and therefore to speak correctly.

When the client can fluently produce the target sound in sentences and can skillfully monitor his or her own speech, it is time to tackle even longer connected speech utterances. It is time for conversation.

Conversation.   Most clinicians today do at least some work on stabilizing production in conversation in the therapy setting before moving on to settings outside the treatment room. This conversational therapy usually moves from very structured tasks, where the responses are planned or known, to unstructured tasks, as in everyday speech.

In structured tasks, the clinician controls the task so that only specific words using the target sounds are practiced. One such task is telling silly stories. The clinician might create a deck of cards picturing objects whose names contain /s/ in different positions. The child turns five cards face up and then must tell a story using all five of the objects. He or she is responsible for saying the target sound correctly in all of the object names but not in any other words. If the client makes errors in other words, the clinician pays little, if any, attention to those mistakes.

Another structured activity involves using a simple map where all of the locations and street names contain the client's target sound. Figure 5.3 shows a map highlighting the sound /s/. The clinician asks the client questions that require the sound in the answer.

> *Clinician:*   Now you're on Ca*s*s Street at the Bu*s* Station. How do you get to the ca*s*tle?
>
> *Child:*   You go up *S*easide Drive and turn left on Ra*ce* Street till you get to the Big *S*ea. The ca*s*tle is on top of *S*ailboat Point looking out on the Big *S*ea.

Here again the clinician has structured the task so that the client uses the target in known contexts within a "conversation." The client is aware of when

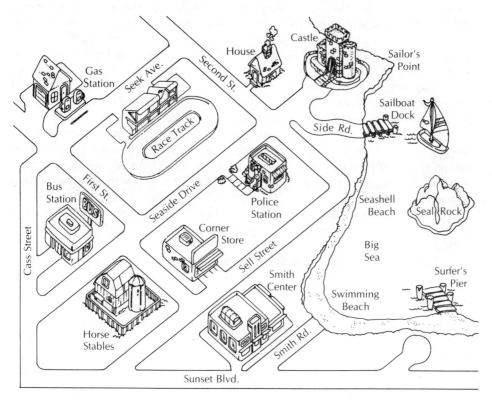

FIGURE 5.3
Map incorporating /s/ for structured conversation training.

the sound will be used, which helps with both production and self-monitoring.

There are myriad structured tasks like these and the ones described in Appendix B. The point is to structure the task so that the specific response opportunities are known to both clinician and client.

Once the client can perform the structured tasks without trouble, it is time to attempt use of the target sound in conversation, where no constraints are placed on the client. That is, the client's responses will consist of connected speech on any topic. The client is now asked to monitor his or her own speech and to correctly produce all occurrences of the target sound.

For some clients, however, the jump from structured conversational tasks to unstructured ones may be too large. In keeping then with our "think small" philosophy, it might be appropriate to provide some intermediate steps which consist of a combination of structured and unstructured activities. This will help to sequence the difficulty level gradually. If the client's productions at the unstructured conversational level are consistently poorer than at the level before, then some of this bridging work should be provided.

Typical unstructured therapy tasks include answering open-ended questions. "Tell me the things you would do if you won a million dollars in the state lottery." "What movies have you seen lately? Tell me about them." "What did your family discuss at dinner last night?"

If the client can read fairly well, reading can be used for conversational training (both unstructured and structured). It elicits continuous, flowing speech, and the extent of structure can easily be controlled. For example, the clinician could choose a reading passage and have the client go through it and circle all instances of the target. Then the client reads the passage out loud. This task is highly structured because all instances are known ahead of time. Later the client can perform the unstructured task of reading the passage out loud without looking it over first. Finally, the client can tell the clinician what the passage was about—a completely unstructured task.

The clinician can also prepare preset reading passages incorporating several instances of the client's sound. Those instances can be marked in boldface, in a different color, or with a capital letter. Again, this task is very structured. The same passages can later be given to the client with the signals removed.

When the client has acquired the ability to converse in unstructured conversation easily and rapidly, most of the treatment within the therapy setting is finished.

The focus of therapy now shifts to enlarging the therapy setting.

Transfer and Carry-over

Consider the child who has just carried on a completely unstructured conversation in therapy and made no errors. As he leaves the room at the end of the session, he turns to the clinician and says, "Thee you Friday, Mr. Thecord"—100% correct in conversation during therapy, 100% *incorrect* at the door! Unfortunately, this is not an uncommon experience. It almost seems as if an aura of correct speech surrounds the client during therapy and disappears at the door.

The clinician's challenge, then, is to enlarge the therapy situation to include all important settings in the client's life; to expand the learning environment so that the client recognizes cues to correct speech outside the therapy room. This process is called *transferring* the newly learned skills. The term *transfer*, first used in the traditional approach in the late 1960s and early 1970s, was borrowed from the behavioral approach. It refers to the extension of learned behaviors from the original setting to other settings. (Chapter 6 has a more complete discussion of transfer. See also Mowrer, 1982.)

Carry-over refers to the ability to use the new sound in conversation. It is not unusual to hear a clinician complain that "the sound just doesn't carry over" or "there is little carry-over." What the clinician means is that the client performs well in therapy but cannot remember to say the sound correctly at home or with friends. The cues that help control the almost automatic correct production in therapy either do not exist outside the therapy setting or are not strong enough to help maintain the learned skill in other situations.

Many clinicians use the terms *transfer* and *carry-over* interchangeably. However, some use *carry-over* to refer to only the conversation stage of therapy. To still others, *carry-over* signifies retention of the skill after therapy work on the sound is complete.

Again drawing on Van Riper and Emerick (1984, pp. 213–216), there are several techniques the therapist can use to develop the client's transfer and carry-over skills. One simple activity is giving *speech assignments*. The clinician designs very specific assignments for the client to carry out at home, in school, in the office. The assignments should be individually designed for the client's ability levels and environments. The clinician should also ask for a report on how the client fared during the next therapy session. This simple tactic often provides the motivation necessary for the client to succeed.

A second useful practice is to have the client or someone else, perhaps a classmate, *check* the client's speech and record errors.[3] The client could simply mark an index card every time an error is produced during dinner conversation. Another possibility is to assign a simple *penalty* for each error. However, "painful and highly emotional penalties should not be used" (p. 214). Instead, the penalties could be game-like. One variation is to give rewards (points, stars on a card) for correct production and take those rewards away (one at a time) for errors. (Behaviorists call this *response cost*; see chapter 6).

The clinician can also, with the help of the client's family, set up *nucleus situations* in which correct speech is required. Everyone makes speech errors. Requiring the client to have perfect speech at all times can have the effect of making him or her nervous and too self-conscious, possibly causing the errors to increase. Therefore, certain situations can be chosen to be targets for correct speech. The reading group for a second grader or all coffee breaks for an adult might be good choices. When the client makes a mistake in the nucleus situation, it should be penalized "good-naturedly but emphatically" (p. 214). Most clients will be able to transfer correct speech to this limited number of situations, and the correct speech often generalizes to other situations.

---

[3]A word of caution is given here concerning the use of peers as speech monitors. This can sometimes be a socially touchy situation and should therefore be handled carefully.

Yet another approach is *negative practice,* requiring the client occasionally to say the word incorrectly. Research shows that the occasional deliberate production of a habitual response a person is trying to eradicate helps make him or her more conscious of the habit and helps make it more vivid. It also has the same effect as providing a penalty for the error, even though no penalty is given. This approach should not be taken until the client can consistently produce the correct sound when asked.

It is very important to *use the new sound in various types of speaking.* The client must be able to use the new sound in sending messages, in interacting socially, in thinking, in expressing emotions. The clinician may need to set up a nucleus situation for each of these types of expression to ensure the client's facility in each of them.

Finally, the client must learn to use the proprioceptive sense to monitor his or her own speech. That is, it is not enough to be able to hear whether a production is correct; the client must also be able to feel it. Exercises to increase proprioceptive awareness of the correct positions and movements of speech include speaking with ear plugs, speaking while wearing earphones that supply a masking noise, whispering, and speaking in pantomime. In schools, contrived tasks, such as talking with teachers, meeting with the janitor to give a specific message, or talking in reading groups while self-monitoring, can be used. Some clinicians use parents or other paraprofessional speech aides to work with students outside the clinical setting. In addition, there are some commercially available programs that can be used in transfer work.

Maintenance.   A last part of therapy that is often neglected is *maintenance* (another concept drawn from behaviorists). *Maintenance* refers to retention of the newly learned skill after the course of therapy is complete. Some clinicians do not dismiss their clients after all transfer work has been completed. Instead, they see the client on a decreasing basis, perhaps once a week for a month, and then once a month for few months, then once every 3 months, every 6 months, and so on, for periodic checks. Some clinicians who practice in schools make periodic checks in the child's classroom for some months and then check back once a year. These checks serve as a clinical reminder to the client to continue to use the new skills.

SUMMARY

This chapter has presented an in-depth look at the traditional approach to articulation therapy. One hallmark of this approach is its flexibility. As we have seen, over the years it has been influenced by a variety of other approaches— the sensory-motor approach, the moto-kinesthetic approach, the behavioral approach, and others. Clinicians who advocate these and other approaches often use many aspects of the traditional approach with their individual clients. And in practice today, they continue to pick and choose from the best techniques available to tailor a therapy plan.

To summarize, the path of traditional therapy involves the stages of ear training, over which there is considerable dispute today, sound establishment, stabilization, transfer, carry-over, and maintenance. These processes are implemented through a wide variety of specific techniques, which may involve listening, imitating, physical modeling, and lots of drill and practice. Training almost always focuses on one sound at a time. When one sound is corrected, another, if necessary, is treated and so forth until all error sounds have been corrected. As you will see later, more contemporary approaches often treat several sounds at one time. Even though the stages of traditional therapy are clearly structured, the practice of therapy itself is often highly creative. Combining techniques and activities and responding to the individual needs of each client provides a highly stimulating and satisfying challenge.

REFERENCES

Aungst, L., & Frick, J. (1964). Auditory discrimination ability and consistency of articulation of /r/. *Journal of Speech and Hearing Disorders, 28*, 76–85.

Backus, O., & Beasley, J. (1951). *Speech therapy with children.* Boston: Houghton Mifflin.

Bernthal, J., & Bankson, N. (1981). *Articulation disorders.* Englewood Cliffs, NJ: Prentice-Hall.

Borden, R., & Busse, A. (1929). *Speech correction.* New York: F.S. Crofts.

Bosley, E. (1981). *Techniques for articulatory disorders.* Springfield, IL: Charles C. Thomas.

Dickson, S. (1962). Difference between children who spontaneously outgrow and children who retain functional articulation disorders. *Journal of Speech and Hearing Research, 5*, 263–271.

Gerber, A. (1973). *Goal: Carryover.* Philadelphia: Temple University Press.

Irwin, R. (1965). *Speech and hearing therapy.* Pittsburgh: Stanwix House.

Lapko, L., & Bankson, N. (1975). Relationship between auditory discrimination, articulation stimulability and consistency of misarticulation. *Perceptual and Motor Skills, 40*, 171–177.

McDonald, E. (1964a). *Articulation testing and treatment: A sensory-motor approach.* Pittsburgh: Stanwix House.

McDonald, E. (1964b). *A deep test of articulation.* Pittsburgh: Stanwix House.

Milisen, R. (1954). The disorder of articulation: A systematic clinical and experimental approach. *Journal of Speech and Hearing Disorders*, Monograph Supplement 4.

Mosher, J. (1929). *The production of correct speech sounds.* Boston: The Expression Co.

Mowrer, D. (1982). *Methods of modifying speech behaviors.* Columbus, OH: Charles E. Merrill.

Mowrer, D., Baker, R., & Schutz, R. (1968). *S-programmed articulation control kit.* Tempe, AZ: Educational Psychological Research Associates.

Mysak, E.D. (1959). A servomodel for speech therapy. *Journal of Speech and Hearing Disorders, 24*, 144–149.

Nemoy, E., & Davis, S. (1937). *The correction of defective consonant sounds.* Boston: The Expression Co.

Nemoy, E., & Davis, S. (1954). *The correction of defective consonant sounds* (Rev. ed.). Boston: The Expression Co.

Peppard, H. (1925). *The correction of speech defects.* New York: Macmillan Co.

Powers, M. (1971). Clinical and educational procedures in functional disorders of articulation. In L. Travis (Ed.), *Handbook of speech pathology and audiology.* Englewood Cliffs, NJ: Prentice-Hall.

Scripture, M., & Jackson, E. (1927). *A manual of exercises for the correction of speech disorders.* Philadelphia: F.A. Davis Co.

Secord, W. (1981a). *Eliciting sounds: Techniques for clinicians.* Columbus, OH: Charles E. Merrill.

Secord, W. (1981b). *C-PAC: Clinical probes of articulation consistency.* Columbus, OH: Charles E. Merrill.

Sommers, R. (1983). *Articulation disorders,* Englewood Cliffs: NJ: Prentice-Hall.

Sonderman, J. (1971, November). *An experimental study of clinical relationships between auditory discrimination and articulation skills.* Paper presented at the convention of the American Speech and Hearing Association, San Francisco.

Stinchfield, S., & Young, E. (1938). *Children with delayed or defective speech: Motor-kinesthetic factors in their training.* Stanford, CA: Stanford University Press.

Travis, L. (1931). *Speech pathology.* New York: D. Appleton-Century Co.

Van Riper, C. (1939). *Speech correction: Principles and methods.* Englewood Cliffs, NJ: Prentice-Hall.

Van Riper, C. (1947). *Speech correction: Principles and methods* (2nd ed.). Englewood Cliffs, NJ: Prentice-Hall.

Van Riper, C. (1954). *Speech correction: Principles and methods* (3rd ed.). Englewood Cliffs, NJ: Prentice-Hall.

Van Riper, C. (1963). *Speech correction: Principles and methods* (4th ed.). Englewood Cliffs, NJ: Prentice-Hall.

Van Riper, C. (1972). *Speech correction: Principles and methods* (5th ed.). Englewood Cliffs, NJ: Prentice-Hall.

Van Riper, C. (1978). *Speech correction: Principles and methods* (6th ed.). Englewood Cliffs, NJ: Prentice-Hall.

Van Riper, C., & Emerick, L. (1984). *Speech correction: An introduction to speech pathology and audiology.* Englewood Cliffs, NJ: Prentice-Hall.

Van Riper, C., & Irwin, J. (1958). *Voice and articulation.* Englewood Cliffs, NJ: Prentice-Hall.

Ward, I. (1923). *Defects of speech.* New York: E.P. Dutton.

Weiss, C., Lillywhite, H., & Gordon, M. (1980). *Clinical management of articulation disorders.* St. Louis: C.V. Mosby.

West, R., Kennedy, L., & Carr, A. (1937). *The rehabilitation of speech.* New York: Harpers.

Williams, G., & McReynolds, L. (1975). The relationship between discrimination and articulation training in children with misarticulations. *Journal of Speech and Hearing Research, 18,* 401–412.

Winitz, H. (1969). *Articulatory acquisition and behavior.* Englewood Cliffs, NJ: Prentice-Hall.

Winitz, H. (1975). *From syllable to conversation.* Baltimore: University Park Press.

Winitz, H., & Bellerose, B. (1962). Sound discrimination as a function of pretraining conditions. *Journal of Speech and Hearing Research, 5,* 340–348.

Winitz, H., & Bellerose, B. (1963). Effects of pretraining on sound discrimination learning. *Journal of Speech and Hearing Research, 6,* 171–180.

Young, E., & Hawk, S. (1955). *Moto-kinesthetic speech training.* Stanford, CA: Stanford University Press.

6

The Behavioral Approach to the Treatment of Articulation Disorders

One of the most important things speech-language pathologists do is help others change some aspect of their communicative behavior. Treatment programs should be evaluated primarily in terms of the efficiency and permanency of behavioral change. Of course, clinicians perform many other important duties, such as making referrals to other professionals, administering diagnostic tests, and so forth, but the largest task is to help people change specific behaviors.

This chapter focuses on procedures found to be highly successful in controlling and modifying behavior. The procedures described are the result of research conducted by such noted learning theorists as J. Watson, E. L. Thorndike, C. Hull, and, more recently, B. F. Skinner. The primary intent of these psychologists was to discover laws of learning that hold true for all living organisms, chiefly, laws that govern human learning. Their research procedures were modeled after those used by scientists in the fields of physics, biology, chemistry, and medicine. In all these fields, once lawful relationships are determined, predictions can be made about future events.

What the learning theorists were seeking was a formula that would explain how humans learn. They wanted an explanation analogous to Graham's (1951) mathematical equation,

Donald E. Mowrer, Ph.D., is a professor of speech pathology in the Department of Speech and Hearing Disorders, Arizona State University, Tempe, Arizona.

$$y = f(x) \text{ under } c,$$

where *y* is an event like the bursting of a rubber balloon, = means "is," *f* means "a function of" or "directly related to," (*x*) is a specified amount of air pressure sufficient to rupture the balloon, and *c* stands for the conditions, such as strength of the rubber and atmospheric pressure. What the law says in this case is that if you continue to blow up a balloon, you will reach the point when the balloon can no longer resist the air pressure and it will rupture. The amount of air pressure needed to rupture the balloon can be specified in advance when the physical properties of the balloon are known. Laws of this type are common in physics. They allow us to predict the occurrence of many events in our daily lives. For example, a specified amount of pressure applied to the brakes of your car will bring the car to a halt in a specified number of feet, water becomes gaseous when it is heated to 212° at sea level, and a ball will attain a specified speed when rolling down a 12-inch plane inclined at an angle of 45°. Under prescribed conditions, these events always occur as predicted.

Assuming lawful relationships observed in the natural sciences also occur in human learning, Skinner (1956) sought to discover if similar relationships exist in the behavior of animals in certain learning situations. He conducted a series of experiments designed to identify the variables responsible for behavioral change. After he and his colleagues accumulated massive amounts of data from a series of experiments and analyzed these data, their conclusions were published in an impressive text entitled *Cumulative Record* (Skinner, 1959). From these observations, Skinner formulated a number of laws that seemed to govern behavior. One of these laws dealt with the effect consequences have upon rate of behavior. Simply stated, when a desired event (such as food) follows a specific behavior (such as a bar press), that behavior is more likely to occur in the future. Conversely, when a behavior (bar press) is followed by an aversive event (such as shock), that behavior is less likely to occur in the future. This latter condition was described as *punishment*.

What Skinner and others were seeking could be expressed as a modification of the formula Graham used to describe observed relationships in the natural sciences. The functional relationship of stimuli and responses in a learning situation could be expressed as $R = f(S)$ *under c*. The response, *R*, is a function of the stimulus, (*S*), under specified conditions. A pigeon can be trained to peck (response) at a red disk (stimulus) when food (a condition) is presented immediately following each peck at the disk. If shock (a different condition) follows a peck (response) when a green disk (stimulus) is presented, soon the pigeon will not peck at the green disk but will peck repeatedly only when a red disk is presented. By controlling the consequences of the pecking response in each of the two situations, the experimenter can literally control the frequency of pecking behavior on these two stimulus conditions. The pigeon has learned to react differently to the two stimulus conditions, that is, it has learned to discriminate between red and green. Any similar pigeon can be taught this discrimination task. (Of course, the pigeon must be hungry.) If all pigeons learn this discrimination task when the consequences are controlled in this manner, we can make a general statement about pigeon learning. If rats, pigs, goats, cockroaches, and humans also learn this red-green discrimination task under similar conditions, then we can formulate a law of learning for discrimination tasks.

Once the stimulus-response relationships are identified, we can predict and control behavior by manipulating the consequences of the behavior. This was one of Skinner's major findings, and it is the framework upon which the treatment of articulation, as described in this chapter, is founded. Put simply, those who control the consequences of a behavior control the behavior. Thus, we can increase or decrease the number of speech sounds an individual produces simply by controlling the consequences of these sounds. In this way we can bring about prescribed changes in articulation. As stated in the first paragraph of this chapter, causing changes in articulation patterns is our chief goal. The client who comes to us substituting /t/ for /k/, distorting /r/, and lisping should leave our treatment program articulating /k/, /r/, and /s/ correctly in all situations. Knowing how to change behavior is the key to effective articulation treatment programs. In the following sections of this chapter, we will draw heavily from the research findings of the learning theorists in an attempt to apply a scientific rationale to the treatment of articulation errors.

IDENTIFYING THE TARGET BEHAVIOR

Assuming lawful relationships exist between stimuli and responses during the learning process, how can we apply the information derived from the learning theorists to an articulation treatment program? The first step is to define the behavior in its present state, the incorrectly articulated sound. We may observe acoustic elements of the sound, air stream direction, tongue placement, etc. Above all, our observation must be objective, and we must observe a behavior or product of a behavior that can be counted. Subjective descriptions of articulation patterns such as "sloppy speech," "slurred consonants," or "lazy tongue" are not suitable because they are not countable and may mean different things to different people. Terms such as *interdental lisp, /ə/ for /ɚ/ substitution, lateral emission of the airstream,* and *omission of* /s/ are features of behavior that can be measured objectively.

The correct behavior, often called the *target behavior,* also must be specified. It is possible to describe /s/, for example, as a sound having certain acoustic properties, central airstream direction, and a specified tongue position. When these criteria are met, the listener perceives /s/. Clinicians are also interested in the context in which the sound occurs, as well as the speaking situation. When articulation is sampled and described as it occurs in a wide variety of situations that may occur over a period of several days, these data are called the *baseline.* The baseline data provide a description of the present state of the speech behavior. Often clinicians sample a sound in the initial, medial, and final position using only three test words to evoke responses. Such tests would be considered an inadequate baseline. McDonald's (1965) Deep Test of Articulation provides more complete information about how a sound is produced in a variety of phonemic contexts. It is also important to sample the sound as it occurs in conversational speech situations. Much of the information obtained from thorough diagnostic testing can be used to describe the status of the behavior before treatment. A baseline of the behavior is taken so that changes in behavior can be ascertained once the treatment program is initiated.

The first two steps, then, are to describe the client's present behavior and to specify the type of behavior the client should exhibit when the treatment program has been completed. In the next section, two of the most important aspects of the instructional process, antecedent and consequent events, will be considered.

ROLE OF ANTECEDENT EVENTS

Antecedent events are stimuli that evoke a response from the client. They include the use of *cues* and *prompts. Cues* provide hints as to what the response should be, whereas *prompts* specify the exact response. The prompt "Say /k/" specifically identifies the response that is expected. The cue "Say it again" suggests what the response should be. Three types of cues and prompts can be used:

1. Auditory stimuli include spoken instructions and models of sound.
2. Visual stimuli include visual models in which the clinician shows a certain tongue, lip, or teeth positioning by using a hand cue, a picture, written material, diagram, or live demonstration of the position or movement.
3. Kinesthetic stimuli involve manipulation of part of the client's speech mechanism and may include touching the cheeks, holding the jaw open, using a tongue blade to position the tongue, or pressing on the rib cage. Placing peanut butter on the alveolar ridge would be considered a kinesthetic cue.

These stimuli, cues and prompts, determine the nature of the response. They serve to evoke the desired response. Skinner and his associates, however, did not have the advantage of using explicit cues and prompts with animals. You cannot tell a rat to press the bar; neither can you show a pigeon how to peck the desk. In most animal research, a target behavior was chosen on the basis of the animal's ability to perform the task. If it was likely the rat would press a bar when it was placed at a reachable level, then presence of the bar would be the antecedent stimulus designed to evoke the response of pressing the bar. Visual cues were used almost exclusively in animal research; hence, we have limited knowledge about the value and use of other types of cues and prompts with animals.

ROLE OF CONSEQUENT EVENTS

Stimuli presented following a response are classified as consequent events. Skinner and his associates focused on the effects of these events in much of their animal research. The current emphasis on behavior modification techniques in education has drawn heavily from the information gained by meticulous observation of the effects of these events upon animal behavior. The core of behavioral research during the 1950s and '60s centered around variables that affected rate of behaviors, that is, the conditions that increased, decreased, or had no effect upon rate of the behavior.

Increasing Behavior Rate

Skinner identified two procedures that produced an increase in behavior rate; the one to be discussed here is *positive reinforcement*. Positive reinforcement was said to occur when rate of behavior increased from the baseline rate when a particular stimulus, usually one that satisfied a need, was presented immediately following the behavior. In most experiments, food pellets were chosen as the stimulus most likely to serve as a reinforcer. The animal was deprived of food, causing body weight to decrease to a prescribed level.

Body weight served as a definition of a "hungry" animal. When the animal was placed in a cage, it would immediately begin to search for food or escape. Consider a rat placed in a cage containing a lever. It is likely that the rat will depress the lever in its search for food. When this behavior occurs, a mechanism dispenses a food pellet, which the hungry rat consumes. Within a short time, lever-pressing behavior occurs with increasing frequency. The relationship that exists between the frequency of response (lever pressing) and the presentation of the stimulus (food pellet) can be expressed by Graham's formula, $R = f(S)$ *under c*. The rat's behavior is controlled by the consequences of its behavior.

Although food is considered the primary reinforcer, soon just the click of the pellet-dispensing mechanism becomes a reinforcer. The click sound, having been paired with the presentation of the food pellet, takes on the properties of a reinforcer and is called a *secondary reinforcer*. Pavlov (1927) demonstrated how an auditory stimulus (bell) when paired with a primary reinforcer (meat powder) could produce a similar response (salivation) when the two stimuli are presented in rapid succession. Humans quickly learn that money, a secondary reinforcer of little value in itself, can be used to procure food, shelter, and many other primary reinforcers. Words such as *good, fine,* and *right* serve as secondary reinforcers to humans when paired with approval behaviors.

When we analyze the reinforcement paradigm, it is evident that two conditions are necessary for it to be effective. First, a state of need or desire must exist within the organism. This need can be manifested as thirst, hunger, desire for social recognition, or some similar state. Second, the experimenter must be able to control the presentation of a stimulus that satisfies this need. Skinner (1957) called such a stimulus a *positive reinforcer*.

One does not know whether a stimulus is a positive reinforcer until behavior rates are observed. For example, if you have conditioned a rat to depress a lever by following each lever press with a food pellet, lever-pressing behavior will occur at a high rate until the rat is no longer hungry. When the rat becomes satiated with food pellets, lever-pressing behavior terminates. In this case, food no longer serves as a reinforcer.

Sometimes it is difficult to predict what stimulus might serve as an effective reinforcer for some humans. I recall an instance of a teacher who was helping a 12-year-old boy with a reading problem. She used a hand tally counter to keep a record of each word he read correctly. He was told he could exchange points earned on the counter for items of his choice like a flashlight battery, pen, knife, etc. But instead of cashing in his points at the end of each session, he preferred to save them, supposedly for a more expensive item. This went on for several weeks until the tutoring was completed. He had earned several thousand points, enough to buy a radio or a bicycle, which, by the way, his teacher could not afford. When asked what he wanted, he said "the counter."

The principle of positive reinforcement, when applied to human learning, is one of the most effective means of controlling behavior. In spite of this, the concept has received little attention from most authors who describe procedures for treating articulation problems. Texts usually recommend that an occasional friendly pat, smile, or positive verbal statement be used as a reward for the client's efforts, but no explanations are provided regarding type, frequency, or latency of these rewards. Clinicians are encouraged to use game activities to capture the child's interest and maintain attention, but there is little reference to precise management of consequent events of the type Skinner described in his animal research. If human learning is governed by the same principles as animal learning, and if lawful relationships exist between stimulus and response events, then clinicians should pay careful attention to the administration of consequent events.

Choosing Reinforcers

Recall that a reinforcer must satisfy some need or drive state. To ensure that a need exists, children in institutional settings sometimes have been deprived of breakfast and lunch. During the afternoon training sessions, one can be assured that food will serve as an effective reinforcer. But we are usually unable or unwilling to control food intake of our clients in this manner. Assuming the client desires sugar, candy can be selected as a reinforcer. But if the client is allowed to consume the candy immediately, the desire for candy declines and sweet items lose their effectiveness as reinforcers. Other disadvantages of using candy are the potential damage to tooth enamel and the undesirable effects from a nutritional point of view. Food is usually not the best choice for a reinforcer because of the ethics involved in creating a state of deprivation or in providing desired but non-nutritious sweets.

The clinician, then, must find other reinforcers. As mentioned earlier, Pavlov found that if a neutral stimulus (bell) is repeatedly paired with a response-evoking stimulus (meat powder), the neutral stimulus acquires the properties of the response-evoking stimulus, that is, the bell alone evokes salivation. Similarly, certain words in our language often are paired with other direct methods of evoking responses. The word *no* is often paired with a smack on the bottom; *good* may be paired with caressing or comforting responses. It would seem likely that certain words could be used as potential reinforcers with children whose histories reflect association of positive events with these words. If a response increases when immediately followed by words such as *good, right, swell,* and so on, then we conclude that these words are reinforcers. If the behavior does not increase, then they cannot be considered as reinforcers. Often, children labeled as autistic show little response to verbal praise. In this case, social praise first must be paired with primary reinforcers until it acquires secondary reinforcement value.

Even if positive verbal statements serve as reinforcers, they may lose their effectiveness when used continually during an intense training period. The child may become satiated with positive statements. During some stages of an articulation treatment program, the clinician may evoke more than 300 responses in a 15-minute session. Listening to a smiling clinician say *good* or its equivalent 300 times may become very tiring to both child and clinician. Thus, these verbal statements may no longer serve as effective reinforcers to the child.

Use of Tokens

An alternative to the exclusive use of verbal statements as reinforcers is to pair verbal praise with presentation of a token such as a pencil mark, a plastic chip, or some similar marker. Thus, through association, the child learns the value of yet another secondary reinforcer. These tokens acquire a greater value if it is explained they can be exchanged for things of value to the child, such as toys, candy, privileges, activities, and the like. For example, if toys are chosen as redeemable items, then a variety of toys are presented to a child. The child is told that these items can be purchased with tokens earned by responding correctly. Each toy is assigned a value corresponding to a certain number of tokens. A comb may be worth 100 tokens, a bracelet 200 tokens, a car 300 tokens, a ring 150 tokens, and so on. Opportunities to participate in certain activities, such as throwing darts, being first in the cafeteria line, coloring a picture, receiving a colored star, and so on could also be purchased.

The situation is analogous to animal research experiments. The rat, deprived of food, seeks to acquire food. Food is obtained when the rat accidentally depresses a lever. The rat continues to press the lever as long as it is hungry. Similarly, suppose the child has limited access to toys. We assume a state of deprivation for toys exists. The child discovers that by responding correctly, toys can be acquired. The child continues to respond correctly until toys are no longer desired.

Self-Reinforcement

It should now be clear how the principle of positive reinforcement, derived from the study of animal behavior, is applied directly to human learning situations. It would be naive to conclude that learning occurs only when one is reinforced for making certain responses. Obviously, there are many ways learning can occur. Skinner (1953) postulates that simply knowing one has made a correct response is sufficient to modify behavior. Perhaps you have enrolled in a course in which a programmed text was used. Typically the student reads a statement and is asked to answer a question about the statement or fill in a missing word. Immediately after responding, the student compares his/her answer with the correct answer printed in the text. If the two answers match, the student's satisfaction is presumed to be the reinforcer. If the material to be learned is presented in small sequential steps and the student responds correctly throughout the program, the prescribed information is learned in accordance with the original intent of the program writer. In this situation, one literally rewards oneself.

A practical example of how self-reinforcement was observed in a treatment program may help clarify this concept. I administered to 30 children an instructional program designed to correct lisping (Mowrer, 1964). Children were divided into two equal groups. The program consisted of some 300 stimulus items, delivered during three 15-minute sessions. Children in one group were informed whether their responses were correct or incorrect immediately following each response and simultaneously given a redeemable token following each correct response. Those in the other group were given no information about the accuracy of their responses and no tokens were provided. A 30-item criterion test was given before and after the program to evaluate accuracy of /s/ production as taught in the program. Children in the first group obtained significantly higher scores than those in the second group.

However, inspection of individual scores revealed that a few children in the second group who received no information about the adequacy of their responses obtained near-perfect scores on the criterion test! Since feedback was not provided to these children in the form of knowledge of results or tokens, what could account for learning correct /s/ production? Some children may be very perceptive of subtle cues. For example, the fact that they were never told they made a mistake may have led them to assume they were performing the task correctly; their teacher was simply stingy with rewards. The learning histories of some children are such that they do not expect rewards. They simply do what they are told to do. These children are often described as "conscientious children." Thus, if the instructions are sufficient to enable the child to figure out what behaviors are expected, and if the child desires to please the teacher, then positive reinforcement in the form of tokens or verbal praise may not be required in order to change the behavior. If, on the other hand, the instructions alone are insufficient to help the child establish correct /s/ productions, it may be likely the child would not score as well on the criterion test. Thus, antecedent events alone often play an important role in task acquisition.

Clearly, it is difficult to establish a single set of procedures that will be effective with all children. Clinicians should view with considerable caution instructional procedures that demand a standard set of procedures be used for all children regardless of their educational histories or special needs. Although we have learned much from data gathered in research with animals, often it is not possible to apply simple solutions derived from this research directly to situations involving human learning. The child comes to us not as a *tabula rasa* but as a sophisticated learner whose behaviors have been shaped in many different ways. This might help explain the fact that even though a clinician seems to violate many of the principles of operant conditioning, some children learn the prescribed task because they have learned to be very perceptive in picking out salient characteristics of a learning task. On the other hand, some children may not be as perceptive and require far more intensive instruction and feedback.

As an article published in the newsletter of the Harvard Center for Research and Development on Educational Differences (1964) stated, relatively little is known about the complex factors of aptitude, ability, interest, and motivation or about their interactions or effects on learning. It is well known that differences in these areas exist, but education has seldom focused much on them.

Schedules of Reinforcement

The frequency with which a reinforcer is presented contingent upon the correct response seems to influence how well the response is maintained when reinforcement is discontinued. Skinner (1957) investigated the effects of four schedules of reinforcement in his animal research. He discovered that each schedule seemed to affect behavior frequencies differently. In one schedule, frequency of reinforcement depends on a fixed number of responses called *fixed ratio*. For example, one reinforcer may be delivered following two consecutive correct responses (FR-2) or after every six consecutive correct responses (FR-6). In a similar schedule called a *variable ratio*, a reinforcer is provided following an average number of correct responses. For example, the following sequence of correct responses would reflect a VR-3 schedule: 2 correct—R^+ (reinforcer), 4 correct—R^+, 3 correct—R^+, 5 correct—R^+, 2 correct—R^+, 2 correct—R^+. In this sequence, a total of 18 correct responses were made in 6 groups. Eighteen divided by 6 equals 3, the average number of correct responses each group contained.

Examples of fixed and variable ratio schedules of reinforcement are easy to find in our daily lives. The strawberry picker who is paid 25 cents for every three baskets of berries picked works on a fixed ratio schedule (FR-3). The car salesman who averages one sale for every ten people who inquire about cars is on a variable ratio schedule (VR-10). Both schedules result in high response rates in animal behaviors. Some important differences in the persistence of the response have been noted with regard to the frequency of reinforcement (Skinner & Ferster, 1957). If an FR-1 (continuous reinforcement) schedule is used, once reinforcement is terminated, response rate increases briefly, then drops sharply and soon returns to its preconditioned rate. This is called *extinction*. If a reinforcement ratio such as FR or VR of 5 or 10 is selected, then the response is maintained at a high rate for a much longer period. However, if a very large ratio is selected early during the skill-learning period, the response may extinguish before the next reinforcement can be delivered. This is called *ratio strain*.

Another useful observation about schedules of reinforcement pertains to the choice of schedule. It appears that when a new task is being learned, the reinforcer should be delivered frequently, as often as FR-1. As the task is mastered, the ratio can be gradually increased to a variable ratio of perhaps 3, then 6, then 9, and so on. Once the new behavior is firmly established, the reinforcer can be eliminated and the behavior will continue.

The practical application of this information to articulation learning seems obvious, although there is little research data to substantiate the effects of using various reinforcement schedules in treatment programs. Probably, substantial individual differences exist among various children so that it would be difficult to recommend one method of administering schedules over another method.

In spite of the lack of empirical data, most authors who advocate behavior therapy for the treatment of articulation errors recommend using continuous reinforcement when a new skill is taught. Once the new behavior is produced many times without error, a variable ratio schedule is introduced beginning with a VR-2 followed by a VR-4 and later a VR-8 or -10 schedule. Boone and Prescott (1972) recommend a VR-4 once the treatment program is under way. Observations of the amount of verbal praise provided by their student clinicians in numerous treatment sessions indicated a VR-4 schedule was frequently used. We cannot, however, be certain this is the best possible schedule to use with all clients.

Two additional types of schedules were identified by Skinner (1959), but they seldom are used in articulation treatment programs. These schedules are based on time dimensions rather than rate of response. One schedule is fixed, the other is variable. If you provide a reinforcer every 3 minutes, this is called a *fixed interval* (FI-3) schedule. In the other schedule, *variable interval,* a reinforcer is delivered after an average time period, e.g., after 2 minutes, then 4 minutes, then 3 minutes, for average of 3 minutes. Skinner (1959) found that both these schedules generate much lower response rates than the variable ratio schedules. The lowest rate occurred under a variable interval schedule.

There is still much to learn about the effects different reinforcement schedules have on learning articulation skills. We can extract some general principles from animal research and the few studies of human learning, but beyond that, we must rely upon the data we gather from working with individual children.

Decreasing Behavior Rate

Extinction. Skinner was equally interested in stimulus conditions that decreased behavior rate. One technique, *extinction,* has already been mentioned. This principle was discovered by Skinner (1956) quite by accident when his food-dispensing apparatus jammed one night. He arrived in his laboratory early the next morning to discover a steady decrement in the rate of behavior on the cumulative recorder printout. Immediately after the apparatus stopped functioning, there was a burst of responses followed by a gradual decrement in response rate. Finally, response returned to its preconditioned rate. What Skinner discovered from countless repetitions of this experiment was that response rate decreases when reinforcement is removed. One can virtually eliminate a response by withholding reinforcement.

In subsequent studies, it was discovered that some behaviors persist in spite of the fact that reinforcement is eliminated. If the behavior has been practiced thousands of times and a "lean" variable ratio schedule was used, say VR-100, then the behavior continues in spite of the fact that the reinforcer is eliminated. In this case, the behavior is said to be highly resistant to extinction. This is exactly what we want to happen during the articulation treatment program, that is, we want to make the correct speech response highly resistant to extinction. To do this, a "lean" schedule of intermittent reinforcement of the correct response is used, such as VR-20 or -30.

When a motor behavior is practiced thousands of times, changes occur in the neural pathways and the information is stored more or less permanently. Consequently, reinforcement is no longer required to learn the response. Suppose you are reinforced for hitting a tennis ball; you receive good instruction from a tennis coach. With continued practice you become a proficient tennis player. Then you move to Greenland for 10 years where there are no tennis courts. Upon return to your native country, you find you can still play a fair game in spite of the absence of any reinforcement or practice for 10 years. Extinction does not occur in one's *ability* to perform. On the other hand, suppose you didn't move to Greenland; you played tennis daily, but soon you felt no challenge in the game and you were making no progress. Due to lack of interest (lack of reinforcement) you took up another sport. You showed up less and less at the tennis court. Finally, you stopped playing tennis altogether. Extinction of the behavior occurred; you no longer play tennis.

It is uncommon for a person who has learned correct articulation to revert later to the previous pattern, although this might occur in certain individuals who have deep-seated psychological problems. Of course, many children learn to discriminate between correct and incorrect articulation patterns but do not use the correct pattern in all situations. In the speech clinic they are reinforced for using correct articulation, but in the classroom, where they have not been reinforced for correct articulation, the error sound will be used. This is not an example of extinction in the technical sense but a result of discrimination. The response class has not generalized from the speech clinic to other speaking situations.

Time-Out.   A procedure that has been used to reduce the frequency of some behaviors is called *time-out.* In this case, all opportunities for obtaining reinforcers are eliminated; the child may be placed in another room or totally ignored for a certain time. Although this procedure has been used successfully in reducing disruptive behaviors (Patterson & White, 1969), as well as echolalia (Lovaas, 1966), stuttering (Costello, 1975), and similar deviant behaviors, it does not seem to be appropriate in treating misarticulations.

Punishment.   Punishment is a third procedure used to reduce unwanted behaviors. Considerable research is available on this subject. Punishment exists when a stimulus presented immediately following a response results in a decrement in response rate. As in the case of reinforcement, a punisher is defined in terms of its effect upon response rate; it cannot be defined until behavior rate is observed to decrease.

The following example should clarify the concept of punishment. A child in Ms. Smith's classroom had the habit of leaving his seat frequently. Ms. Smith, tired of this behavior, decided to eliminate or at least reduce it by punishing the child for leaving his seat. Each time the child left his seat without permission, Ms. Smith told him to sit down. Her remarks became more emphatic. She threatened to send him to the principal, force him to stay after school, or inform his parents of his misbehavior. In spite of her reprimands and threats, the child was observed to leave his seat even more frequently than before. "I can't understand this," said Ms. Smith to her supervisor. "I keep punishing Terry for leaving his seat, but it doesn't seem to work." If the behavior increased as a consequence of her remarks, then her reprimands acted as a reinforcer, not a punisher. Even though verbal threats would seem to be punishing events, they did not serve as punishers in this case. More likely, the child sought attention from his teacher. He received plenty of it when he left his seat!

Should we punish children for making the incorrect speech response? Here again, we have little empirical data regarding the role of punishment in suppressing misarticulations. I think most speech-language pathologists would agree that punishment in the form of aversive stimuli such as a threat, slap, or reprimand is not appropriate. Informing the child that a response is incorrect may be helpful, especially if this is followed by an instructive comment such as, "No, you forgot to close your teeth," or "No, your tongue stuck out," or "No, you didn't put your tongue high enough." Technically these comments would be classified as punishers if, as a result of using them, the incorrect response decreased.

Response Cost.   Finally, a fourth type of consequent event found to be effective in decreasing behaviors is *response cost*. In this case, a reinforcer is removed following an incorrect response. If you give tokens following correct responses and take them away following incorrect responses, you are using a response cost procedure. Conley (1966) used this procedure with one group of children who misarticulated /s/. He compared their performance on a speech test with that of a similar group of children whose tokens were not removed following incorrect responses. He found that using response cost procedures decreased errors significantly. McReynolds and Huston (1971) found token loss *per se* did not function as an effective punisher, i.e., did not reduce the number of incorrect responses. Until more is known about the effects of this procedure upon reducing certain speech behaviors it is probably wise not to use it when treating articulation disorders.

USE OF ANTECEDENT AND CONSEQUENT EVENTS IN ARTICULATION TRAINING

Generally, antecedent events determine the type of response the child will produce, and consequent events serve to increase or decrease the likelihood a response will occur in the future. Often it is difficult to change articulation patterns using one event exclusively. I remember Bruce Ryan and I attempted to teach correct /ɜ˞/ production to children who distorted /ɜ˞/. The only antecedent information we provided was to request them to produce the sound differently. They were told to produce /ɜ˞/, but after that no instructions were provided regarding how to produce the sound. We thought we could control articulation by differential feedback at the consequent level. When the children made a sound that was close to /ɜ˞/, we would say "good" or "better." If the sound was unlike /ɜ˞/, we depressed a buzzer, and said, "No, make it different." We were unsuccessful in our attempts. Had we provided important antecedent events like, "Curl your tongue up and back," or "Make it sound like this, /ɜ˞/," we would have been able to evoke /ɜ˞/ with little difficulty. Sometimes it may be wise to ignore the incorrect response, especially during the initial treatment sessions. Some children react negatively to criticism. Following 10 consecutive "nos" they may burst into tears and refuse to continue.

Analyzing Effects of Antecedent and Consequent Events

Boone and Prescott (1972) outlined a procedure to help clinicians analyze their use of antecedent and consequent events. They classified antecedent events into two categories: (a) explaining and describing goals or procedures, and (b) modeling the desired behavior or instructing the person how to produce it.

Consequent events were of two types: (a) good evaluations (clinician evaluates client response as correct and indicates verbal or nonverbal approval), and (b) bad evaluations. The last category was a neutral-social category that included the remarks made by the clinician that did not pertain to achieving the goals of the treatment program. Responses of the client were noted. After observing many clinicians, Boone and Prescott concluded that clinicians who were most effective followed rather consistent patterns in their use of antecedent and consequent events. First, the effective clinicians presented a model or instruction, which was followed by the client's response. The client was then informed whether the response was correct or incorrect. This was followed by another model or instruction, and the process was repeated. Poor clinicians provided insufficient cues and inappropriate consequences, and engaged in conversations that were unrelated to goals of the treatment program. Boone and Prescott present one of the few systems available to help clinicians analyze treatment sessions objectively by determining the relative importance to the client's progress of using antecedent and consequent events.

Observing and Recording Behaviors

There is no way of knowing whether one's use of antecedent and consequent events is effective unless accurate records of the client's behavior are kept. A clinician may have an elaborate system of cues designed to evoke correct responses, a well-planned schedule of reinforcement, plus highly desirable reinforcers, but unless behavioral change occurs, the treatment program is ineffective. The effectiveness of procedures is reflected in the client's performance. The chief value of recording responses is to provide guidance in the use of antecedent and/or consequent events.

The obvious way to evaluate behavior is to use a binary system; a response is either right or wrong. There are numerous ways of recording these responses. Many clinicians tabulate correct and incorrect responses using a score sheet similar to the one shown in Figure 6.1. Others use a hand tally counter or simply count up the number of tokens given plus number of wrong responses that have been tallied separately.

Computing Percentage of Correct Responses

After tallying responses, the clinician can determine the percentage of correct responses. For example, if 220 responses are correct and 40 incorrect,

Name: _____

Date: _____

Task: _____

	1	2	3	4	5	6	7	8	9	10	1	2	3	4	5	6	7	8	9	10	1	2	3	4	5	6	7	8	9	10	
																																30
																															60
																															90
																															120
																															150
																															180
																															210
																															240

Time (Min): _____

Key: X Correct
      O Incorrect

Response Summary   _____   _____   _____
                    Correct   Incorrect   Total Responses

FIGURE 6.1
Tally sheet for recording correct and incorrect speech responses.

172

TABLE 6.1
Data from Six Sessions Reflecting Accuracy of Response, Session Length, and Rate Information

Session	Number of Correct Responses	Number of Incorrect Responses	Duration of Session	Percent Correct	Correct Response Rate per Minute	Total Response Rate per Minute
1	58	8	10 min	87%	5.8	6.6
2	30	9	15 min	77%	2	2.6
3	180	10	20 min	95%	9	9.5
4	48	0	8 min	100%	6	6.0
5	20	1	20 min	95%	1	1.05
6	160	72	32 min	69%	5	7.25

the percentage correct would be 85% (220 ÷ 260). Thus, it is possible to determine how accurately the client performed. By converting the number of correct responses into a percentage, we can make comparisons among treatment sessions that differ in time. Look at the data in Table 6.1. Although each session differed in length and number of responses, performance can be compared using correct response percentage figures.

These data can be recorded graphically. Letting the ordinate represent percentage correct in increments of 10% and the abscissa represent session, the percentage correct can be plotted for each session. Through connection of these points, the client's progress or lack of it can be portrayed. Figure 6.2 shows the percentage correct presented in Table 6.1 represented as a line graph.

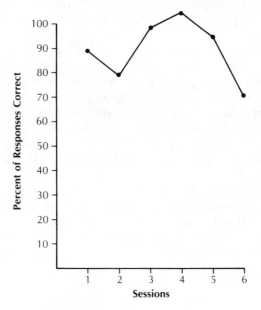

FIGURE 6.2
Percentage of responses produced correctly during each of six sessions, shown as a line graph.

Computing Rate of Response

Although calculating the percentage of correct responses provides us with important information about the accuracy of a client's performance, it ignores rate of behavior. Suppose the number of correct responses produced by clients A and B was 90%. Client A, however, produced 90 correct and 10 incorrect responses during a 5-minute session, whereas client B produced only 9 correct and 1 incorrect response during the same session. By calculating rate of response, we can determine how often the response occurred. In this example, rate of correct response per minute was 18 (90 responses ÷ 5 minutes) for client A, but only 1.8 (9 ÷ 5) for client B.

In order to obtain accuracy information, we also must compute either total response rate per minute (total number of responses divided by number of minutes) or error rate (number of errors divided by number of minutes) and compare one of these rates to the correct rate. Choosing total rate, we find that total rate is 20 (100 ÷ 5) for client A and 2(10 ÷ 5) for client B. We conclude that although response accuracy was the same for both clients, client A produced 10 times as many responses in the same time period as did client B.

Rate information is important to clinicians who attempt to change articulation skills because the articulation of speech sounds involves motor acts (Milisen, 1954). Considerable practice is required to learn motor skills such as typing, playing a musical instrument, mastering sport activities, and so on. Hundreds of movement patterns must be practiced before the skill becomes automatic. Coordination of tongue and jaw movements required for precise articulation also requires considerable practice. The more a client practices a speech response in a variety of contexts, the more likely the response will become automatic. McDonald (1964) emphasized practicing certain speech patterns as an essential part of his sensory-motor approach to the treatment of articulation errors.

Not only the rate of responding but also the overtness of the response is important. In an attempt to evaluate the importance of making overt responses, I asked one group of lisping children to respond overtly to a series of instructional items (Mowrer, 1964). Another group of children who lisped simply listened to the instructions. Following completion of 45 minutes of instruction, most of the children who responded overtly were able to produce /s/ correctly on a criterion task, whereas none of the children who simply listened to the instructions produced /s/ correctly. This demonstrates the importance of making overt responses.

The clinician who insists that the client produce many correct speech responses per unit of time should experience a greater success rate in terms of articulation change than one who evokes but a few responses. Several years ago I reported a study of the number of target responses seven public-school speech clinicians evoked from their clients (Mowrer, 1969a). I was amazed to find the average rate of response per minute was only 2.5. I also noted that some clinicians evoked an average of only .3 responses per minute, whereas others evoked as many as 16 per minute. The average rate of responses evoked using an instructional program to correct lisping (S-PACK) was 7.5 per minute, three times that of the average response rate evoked by traditional treatment methods (Mowrer, Baker, & Schutz, 1968).

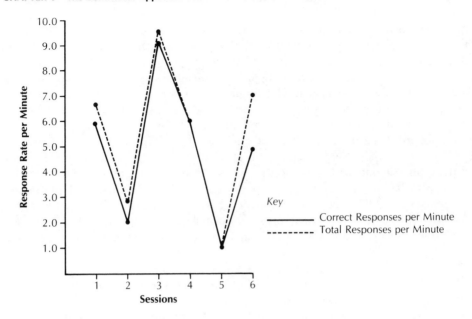

FIGURE 6.3
Response rate per minute plotted for six sessions on an equal-interval graph.

The important point to be made here is that unless we keep accurate records of response data and relate this information to behavioral change, we are unable to determine the effectiveness of specific treatment procedures. The careful observation and recording of events are a fundamental part of every science. If the treatment of communication problems is to become a science (as opposed to an art), then we must keep accurate accounts of our observations of the behavior we are attempting to modify. By analyzing correct and total response rates, we assess the accuracy and frequency of a client's response, two variables that reflect the effectiveness of our treatment procedure (Drash, Caldwell, & Liebowitz, 1970). Using data from Table 6.1, correct and total response rates plotted on the equal interval graph are shown in Figure 6.3.

It is readily apparent that some sessions were better than others with respect to rate of response. If you compare sessions 3 and 5 shown in Figure 6.2, you might conclude that the two sessions were equal because accuracy was about 95% in both instances. But look at these same sessions as shown in Figure 6.3. It can be seen that the activities during session 3 resulted in a high rate of correct response. The client practiced the correct response often, and there were many opportunities for reinforcement to occur. But in session 5, the client produced few responses, and thus there was limited chance for reinforcement to occur. If practice makes perfect, then clearly session 3 was better than session 5.

Notations about Response Class

By making notations about what occurred during the session, we can summarize the nature of the responses. During session 3, the client was required to produce the sound in a variety of phonemic contexts in different words and phrases. In contrast, although most of the responses produced during session 5 were correct, the client received minimal practice saying the sound in a variety of contexts. The client repeatedly asked permission to spin an arrow mounted on a card. The single phrase *May I spin the spinner* was used as the carrier for the desired response, /ɚ/. Obviously, the type of response required in the two sessions differed greatly. Thus, in addition to rate and accuracy information, a third factor emerges as an important event to record: the type of response produced. The child who says the same word 50 times during one session with 90% accuracy has not made the same progress as the child who has used the target sound 50 times in a wide variety of phonemic contexts with 90% accuracy. Also, the child who practices saying the target sound only in the initial position of monosyllabic words has limited practice learning co-articulation skills that will help the response generalize to other words.

If the clinician is interested in changing articulation patterns, he or she must observe and record the accuracy of the client's response, the frequency of the correct and incorrect response, and the context in which the response occurs. If these data are not recorded, the clinician can only guess what is happening as a result of the treatment program. He or she cannot make effective changes in the treatment program because decisions are based only on intuition or feelings about the progress achieved by the client. One could hardly call such a procedure a science.

Behavioral Probes.   Recording all responses may not always be practical. An alternate procedure is to sample the behavior periodically. Such samples are called *probes*. Both Diedrich (1971) and Elbert, Shelton, and Arndt (1967) describe procedures for assessing behavioral change based on an articulation test given at the end of a treatment session. The test items may include the target sound(s) embedded in many contexts or, in the case of the 10-item criterion test used in the S-PACK treatment program (Mowrer, Baker, & Schutz, 1968), only in the phonemic contexts taught during a particular session.

The data from these behavioral probes are graphically recorded. These data provide a representative sample of progress being made during the treatment sessions.

Logarithmic Graphing Techniques.   A more precise procedure for assessing behavioral change was introduced to educators by Lindsley (1964). Rather than dividing the ordinate into equal intervals, he felt increments of behavior should be shown as equal ratios. The audiogram is an example of an equal-ratio-increment graph because sound intensity increases by logarithmic ratios, not by equal intervals. Behavior rates are recorded as points on this graph in the same manner as they are recorded on the equal-interval graph shown in Figure 6.3. The correct response rate from Figure 6.3 is plotted on a logarithmic graph in Figure 6.4.

The logarithmic graphing procedure offers several advantages over other graphing techniques. A greater range of behaviors of widely differing rates can be depicted, and several different behaviors can be recorded. Up to 140

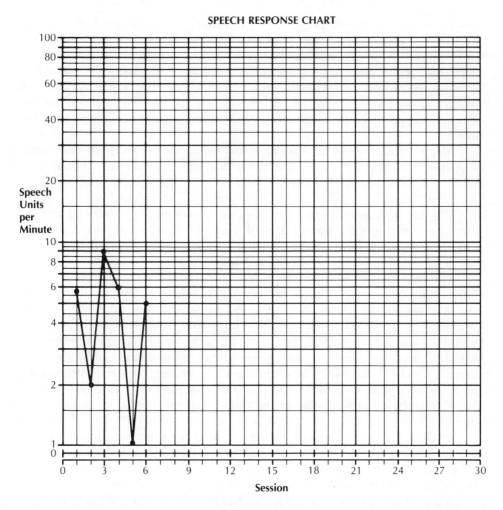

SPEECH RESPONSE CHART

FIGURE 6.4
Correct response rate per minute plotted for six sessions on a logarithmic graph.

calendar days can be included. The equal ratio is more sensitive to behavioral change, and length of session also can be shown. White and Haring (1976) describe in detail how educators can use the logarithmic graphing technique to improve their teaching. Both Diedrich (1971) and Mowrer (1969b) describe how the logarithmic graph can be used when recording various speech behaviors. The reader who is interested in this procedure is encouraged to consult these references.

PREPARING INSTRUCTIONAL OBJECTIVES

Treatment programs based on vague, poorly stated objectives are often ineffective. Much valuable teaching time is lost if the clinician has no clear understanding of what must be accomplished during the brief time the client is seen for treatment. Supervisors of clinical training programs are well aware of the value of requiring student clinicians to write lesson plans. Students are usually asked to specify in detail planned activities for the treatment sessions. Once this careful planning is done, the execution of treatment programs can be more systematic and effective than if one has only a general idea of what should occur during the treatment process. In many states, speech clinicians are required by law to specify behavioral objectives for their teaching programs.

Mager (1962) wrote an easy-to-follow procedure for writing behavioral objectives. He specified three conditions that must be met for a goal to be considered a behavioral objective.

The Do Statement.   First, the clinician must describe objectively exactly what he or she wants the learner to do during the treatment period. It must be possible to count or measure the behavior. If it cannot be counted, there is no way to determine if it has occurred or changed.

For example, if the objective is to make the client *aware* of the correct sound, how could one count the number of times the client was aware? Awareness is a condition that is inferred to be present, but it can't be counted. Instead, it is necessary to choose something countable that indicates that a person is aware. The indicator becomes the *do statement*. Suppose the clinician asks the client to signal by raising his or her hand immediately after the clinician says /s/ in words. If the client signals by raising the hand immediately following each utterance of /s/, then the clinician infers the child is aware of the /s/. Hand raising serves as an indication that the person is aware of the sound.

In the treatment of articulation, the desired behavior most often involves an articulated response. The target behavior is a motor speech response involving the correct production of a sound or sounds in a variety of contexts; therefore, the verb *to say* frequently is used as the do statement.

The following verbs, used as do statements, may be the indicators of some other target or they may be the target behavior themselves:

to say	to produce	to describe
to put	to write	to vocalize
to repeat	to co-articulate	to name
to point	to read aloud	to count

The Conditions Statement.   The second ingredient of a behavioral objective is a brief statement describing the *conditions* present when the behavior is to occur. Obviously, there is no need to specify all the conditions present, such as the color of the room, the construction of the table, or the hair style of the clinician. We need only specify the conditions relevant in evoking the response. If pictures are used to evoke the response, this needs to be stated, as well as whether the target sound will be articulated in the final position of words, in blends, or in various positions of polysyllabic words.

The client may be able to articulate /s/ correctly while the clinician shows a group of pictures that were used in the treatment program, but may be unable to do so when the parent asks him or her to name a group of unfamiliar pictures at home 2 weeks later. The relevant conditions are: the person showing the pictures, the familiarity of the pictures, the place where the pictures are displayed, and the time at which the pictures are shown.

The Accuracy Statement.   A statement about how well the client is expected to perform comprises the third requirement that Mager lists as an important part of a behavioral objective. This part of the statement deals with the accuracy of the client's response, and is usually expressed in terms of a percentage correct or rate of correct response. Often, a time limit is specified as part of the accuracy statement; i.e., a certain number of correct responses are to be produced within a specified number of minutes. Dates may be included if the clinician specifies a time when articulation responses should be correct.

Types of Instructional Objectives

When an objective describes the client's articulation at the time of dismissal, it is called a *terminal objective*. These statements are broad in scope and usually specify an approximate date when the objective should be accomplished. An example of a terminal objective would be: "By May 1, 1984, Sue will correctly articulate /r/ and /l/ at all times as they occur in all positions in words in her spontaneous unmonitored speech." Individual segments of this objective can be identified as follows:

Do Statement: Articulate /r/ and /l/.

Conditions Statement: In all positions in words in spontaneous unmonitored speech.

Accuracy Statement: Correct at all times by May 1, 1984.

Another type of objective, of which there can be many, is called a *sub-objective* or *transitional* objective. These objectives also have been referred to as *short-range goals*. The same three statements must be included in these objectives, that is, the do statement, the conditions statement, and the accuracy statement. These objectives are very specific with respect to the skill to be learned. The following illustrates a sub-objective one might write for a client who is beginning a treatment program for correction of /k/: "Pat will say the /k/ in the final position of 10 words after being shown 10 pictures by the clinician. He will not be told whether his responses are right or wrong. /k/ must be produced correctly in 9 out of 10 words." A summary of the important statements of this sub-objective is as follows:

Do statement: Say /k/.

Conditions Statement: In the final position of words. Ten pictures shown by the clinician. Not informed of results of response.

Accuracy Statement: 90% correctly articulated /k/ sound.

Task Analysis

Before writing behavioral objectives, the clinician must analyze the task to be learned. A series of skills are needed to perform complex tasks. For example, tying a bow in a shoe lace involves numerous precise movements that must be performed in proper sequence. First, the laces must be crossed. Then the overlapping lace is threaded through the lower ∧-shaped opening. The two ends are pulled in opposite directions to form a bow. A loop is formed in the left lace, and so it goes until the bow is completed. A behavioral objective can be written for each step in the series of movements. When teaching a child to tie a bow, a mother proceeds through these steps with her child until each step is learned in proper sequence. One cannot skip steps or try to complete them out of order.

Similarly, if you need to change the front tire of your car, first you must take off the hubcap, loosen the wheel nuts or studs, lift the car with a jack, then remove the wheel nuts or studs. If you do not follow this sequence, that is, if you lift the car first, then try to loosen the wheel nuts, the wheel will simply spin and you will be unable to loosen the nuts. You must follow the correct sequence. The same is true for sequences involved in learning complex mathematical skills. Learning to divide requires prior mastery of skills such as addition and subtraction. One cannot learn multiplication and division until the basic skills are learned.

Most speech clinicians follow a similar procedure of sequencing skills in the remediation of articulation problems. Van Riper (1939) clearly identified the educational taxonomy of learning articulation skills when he specified that the client must be aware of the speech problem first. Then discrimination skills must be taught, followed by production of the target sound in isolation, in nonsense syllables, in words with the target sound in the initial position, final position, and medial position. Phrases that incorporate the target sound are then introduced. Polysyllabic words and blends are introduced, followed by sentence practice and using the sound in spontaneous speaking situations. This taxonomy follows an analytic approach to building a sequence of behaviors. The task, articulating a sound correctly in spontaneous speech, is broken into smaller components that are taught in a specific sequence.

Backus and Beasley (1951) devised a different sequence to teach articulation skills by presenting a complex task, a sentence, first. If the client is unable to produce the sound correctly in this context, a smaller segment of the task is presented, a word. If this proves to be too difficult, the client is encouraged to produce the sound in isolation. This synthetic approach can be broken into a series of tasks in much the same manner as the analytic technique. Similarly, behavioral objectives can be written for each step in the series.

An example of a task analysis of learning to produce /s/ in spontaneous speech is illustrated in the flow chart I devised for a lisp correction program (Mowrer, 1964). This flow chart, shown in Figure 6.5, depicts a sequential series of steps, each presumably more complex or difficult than the previous one. The effect of mastering each task is cumulative in that saying /i/ facilitates saying /is/, which in turn aids production of /s/ in isolation. Once the isolated

Flow Chart for θ/s Correction

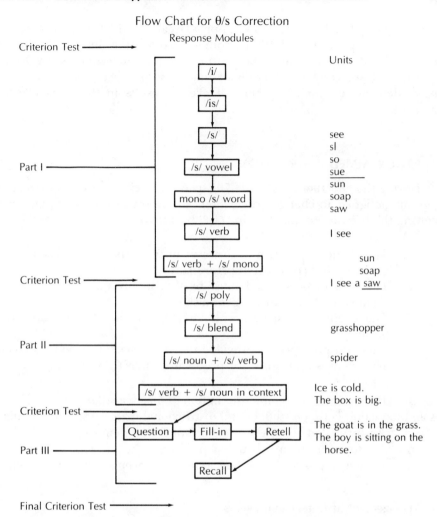

FIGURE 6.5
Flow chart for three-part lisp correction program used in S-PACK. (*Source: Methods of Modifying Speech Behaviors*, 2nd ed. (p. 302) by Donald E. Mowrer, 1982, Columbus: Charles E. Merrill Publishing Company. Copyright © 1982 by Bell & Howell Company. Reprinted by permission.)

sound is produced, a vowel is added, and when this is mastered a final consonant is added, yielding a monosyllabic word. Just as changing a tire requires following a prescribed sequence, the same holds true for learning articulation skills.

Numerous treatment sequences have been devised to change various aspects of articulation (see Baker & Ryan, 1971; Delbridge & Larrigan, 1973; Psaltis & Spallato, 1973; McCabe & Bradley, 1975; Weston & Irwin, 1971). Even though there is considerable variation among different treatment sequences, the principles of behavior therapy apply. Deciding which sequence is most effective for a particular child is another matter. It is important that the clinician identify what seem to be the most important elements involved in acquiring a task. Only by clinically testing various aspects of the sequence can we determine which sequence of events results in the most effective treatment.

PROGRAMMED INSTRUCTION

During the late 1960s and early 70s speech clinicians created instructional programs designed to change articulation. These programs were constructed following the format outlined by Fine (1962) as follows:

1. The client responds to a series of instructional items that the programmer has constructed beforehand.
2. The skill to be learned must be thoroughly mastered before the client can advance to the next task.
3. The client is presented with tasks he/she has been prepared to perform.
4. Cues and prompts are provided to help the client respond correctly.
5. The client is reinforced for producing correct responses.

Coolagan (1976) provides a simpler definition of *programmed instruction*. He says it is an interaction between student and instructional material wherein immediate feedback is provided about the adequacy of the student's response.

In order to write an instructional program, one must complete a task analysis. The next step is to decide how antecedent events will be managed.

Management of Antecedent Events

Once the task has been broken into smaller components and behavioral objectives have been written for each component, the activities that will lead to the attainment of each objective must be specified. The clinician will need to show or tell the client what to do. Hence, antecedent events will play an important role in the instructional process. If antecedent events, that is, the instructions for the client, are specified, as well as the consequent events following correct and incorrect responses, the result is an instructional program. The antecedent events may be so specific as to include everything the clinician says to the client. The S-PACK is an example of this type of program (Mowrer, Baker, & Schutz, 1968). On the other hand, the program may be written only to suggest what the clinician should say (see Baker & Ryan, 1971; McCabe & Bradley, 1975).

Usually, cues and prompts are used to introduce learning tasks. For example, a model of the target sound may be presented, followed by a request for the client to repeat the sound. Or the client may be given specific instructions concerning where to place the tongue to produce the sound correctly.

Once the client is able to produce the sound correctly, cues and prompts are faded. For example, the prompt "Stick out your tongue and blow like this, [θ]" might be used early in the program, but several minutes later only cues such as "Say it each time I put my finger up" are provided. As new tasks are introduced, strong cues and prompts are introduced again and then weakened as the client masters task production. The procedure might follow this pattern:

- Task 1
  a. provide both prompts and cues
  b. provide only position cues
  c. provide nonverbal cues such as requesting responses to finger-raising signals

- Task 2
  a. provide both prompts and cues
  b. provide only position cues
  c. provide nonverbal cues

In this manner, supportive cues and prompts are provided when each new task is presented and faded as the client masters the task.

Management of Consequent Events

Usually, every correct response is reinforced when the treatment program is begun and the client is learning to produce a new response. Once the client has practiced saying the correct response many times, the continuous schedule of reinforcement is changed to a variable ratio. The client may be given one token for saying *soap* correctly at the beginning of the program, but later, when asked to say *Sally has some soap*, only one token is given even though four correct responses were produced. As the client attains skill in producing /s/ and is able to use this sound correctly in conversational speech, perhaps 20 correct /s/ sounds must be produced before a token is provided. Soon it is not necessary to provide tokens for correct /s/ responses. The client now has an automatic /s/ response. In a carefully designed program, a changing schedule of reinforcement is included with the aim of eventually eliminating reinforcement altogether.

Criterion Tests

Another feature of instructional programs is the frequent use of criterion tests or behavioral probes. The clinician needs to know how well the client has mastered a task because the succeeding task should not be presented until the prior task has been mastered. Criterion tests may consist of 3 or 4 items or as many as over 30 items. Data from these tests are usually transferred to graphs to provide a quick visual display of the client's performance.

Frequent measures of behavior are taken to provide the clinician with an ongoing account of behavioral change. If samples of behavior are not taken frequently, one is unable to make appropriate changes in the treatment plan that could lead to more effective instruction.

Editing and Validating Instructional Programs

An instructional program, unlike traditional instructional methods, is open to inspection and analysis. An expert, other than the person who wrote the program, should edit the program. This individual may see ways of improving the original program by changing the wording, the sequence of tasks, or schedule of reinforcement. At this stage of program construction, one is still operating from a theoretical framework because it is impossible to know how the client will respond until the program is administered.

After editing the program, the next step is to administer it to a small group of clients. An analysis is made of their responses, which aids in making decisions about changing certain items, rearranging task presentation, breaking tasks into smaller components, and so on. Usually, high error rates in certain parts indicate areas that should be changed. Sections that include a long series of correct responses might indicate that cues could be eliminated gradually or that the task is too easy. It might be decided to omit certain items entirely, resulting in a shortened version of the program.

The revised version of the program is then administered to a similar group of clients and revised again if necessary. This process is continued until a predetermined success rate is reached. If the program writer's intent is to produce a program that is effective with 85% of the target population for whom it was designed, then the testing and validation process is terminated when this criterion level is achieved.

It should be noted that a given instructional program might be validated for use with only one child. If a program is shown to be effective for that client, we can say that it is valid for him, but it is necessary to include more than one individual in the validation process if we want to say that it will be effective with other clients.

Dissemination of the program is the final step. It is published and marketed. An instruction manual should accompany the program so that the user can replicate the findings of the original work.

A large number of instructional programs designed to assist speech clinicians in modifying articulation patterns are currently available (see Chapter 9 in Mowrer, 1982). Some of these programs have been validated through systematic analysis and field testing, whereas others have been placed on the market with little or no previous validation. Some programs provide only general guidelines for administration; others offer explicit directions. Some are designed to modify only one type of articulation response, such as a /θ/ for /s/ substitution (Mowrer, Baker, & Schutz, 1968). Other programs incorporate instructions for the correction of many consonant sounds (McCabe & Bradley, 1975).

The speech clinician has a variety of instructional programs from which to choose. Some are effective procedures for changing articulation patterns and others are less effective. Much depends upon the clinician's ability to follow instructions exactly. Many clinicians choose to use only parts of programs. The following list of criteria for helping speech clinicians choose or devise instructional programs is presented by Mowrer (1982):

1. Clarity of instructions provided for the clinician.
2. Identification of target behavior and target population.

3. Cost of program and time required to administer it.
4. Field test data available.
5. Instructions provided for recording baseline, recording data, use of criterion tests, branching to other steps, rewarding client, and generalizing or maintaining the response.

Costello (1977), Coolagan (1976), and McReynolds (1983) have also provided guidelines to help speech clinicians evaluate instructional programs.

Administering Instructional Programs

Once a program has been edited and field tested, the speech clinician can use it with clients. Some programs are designed for individual instruction; others can be used with small groups of clients.

One of the values of using programmed instructions is that they can be administered by paraprofessionals. Many individuals who have had little or no teaching experience can be taught to administer these programs. For example, Dorothy Bokelmann, a supervisor of speech clinicians of the Clark County School District in Las Vegas, Nevada, organized a project that involved writing instructional programs to be used by paraprofessionals to aid speech clinicians in remediating articulation skills (Lundquist, 1972). Speech clinicians provided treatment for children who misarticulated consonants only until these children could produce the target sounds correctly in several words. Then the children were assigned to paraprofessionals who had been given training in administering the programs and discriminating between correct and incorrect sounds. The purpose of these programs was to help the children use newly learned articulation skills in a variety of contexts and speaking situations.

The programs Bokelmann and her colleagues wrote for the paraprofessionals consisted of a series of speaking activities that were to be practiced by the children. Each aide was provided with a workbook of activities for a specific target sound. The first activity was to name a series of pictures the speech clinician had used in previous treatment sessions. Other activities involved filling in words containing the target sounds in a sentence completion exercise, retelling short stories, asking directions, and so on. Situations were varied from the speech office to hallways, playground, classroom, and principal's office. Frequently, the speech clinician tested the children to monitor their progress. The aides provided the bulk of the instruction using the booklets they were provided.

Carrier (1970) reported results of a similar program in which he provided written instructions for mothers to use with their children who misarticulated /r/. The speech clinician provided a brief treatment program until the children could produce the target sound correctly and then the mothers were given six lessons written in program format. They were instructed to administer this treatment program to their children. Test results following completion of the program revealed that mothers served as effective supportive personnel who could greatly aid the speech clinician in bringing about changes in the articulation of their children.

I have also experienced success in using aides to administer instructional program material designed to correct misarticulation (Mowrer, 1967). Parents, teachers, siblings, and peers have been trained to administer programs designed to correct lisping. One speech clinician used fifth-grade children to administer S-PACK to second- and third-grade children who lisped and found they were as successful in changing lisping as she was. The important point is that other individuals can perform many of the tasks speech clinicians now provide if they have adequate training and instructional materials.

TRANSFER AND MAINTENANCE

Although teaching children to produce sounds correctly in the clinic situation usually is an easy task, many speech clinicians find that children do not produce these sounds correctly while speaking in other situations. It is believed this problem, referred to as *lack of carry-over,* exists because speech clinicians may not plan learning activities that foster generalization of the newly learned response to other speaking situations (Mowrer, 1982). There are several techniques that can be used to help clients articulate correctly in other speaking situations (Griffiths & Craighead, 1972; Gerber, 1973).

Stimulus Generalization

If we wish to improve carry-over, it is important to understand the principle of *stimulus generalization.* Although many factors are involved in vocabulary development, the young child who identifies the mail carrier, the butcher, and the father as "daddy" may be used to illustrate this principle. In this case, the child may have originally been rewarded for saying "daddy" (the response) in the presence of the father (the stimulus). There are many other males who share the same stimulus properties as the father, such as pants, short hair, tall in stature, and so on. These common characteristics, taken together, represent the concept of maleness or "daddyness." Because the child is rewarded for saying "daddy" in the presence of one instance of this concept, the father, other instances sharing the same properties will be responded to in a similar way.

Soon the child learns to differentiate father from other males, namely, the mail carrier, the butcher, the fireman, and the truck driver, by using different verbal labels for each type of male. At first, young children may use only two words, *Daddy* for the father and *man* in the presence of all other males. Later, the child learns to use specific words to name familiar males, such as *Grandpa, Uncle Jim, Mr. Smith, the fireman,* etc. This example illustrates two different processes. First, stimulus generalization occurs when the same response is made to all stimuli that share characteristics with the original stimuli. Later, the process of discrimination is observed when a different response is made to two stimuli that have common characteristics. Sometimes, we want responses to generalize to similar situations, and at other times, we want the client to make accurate discriminations, as in the case of correct and incorrect sounds.

Stimulus Generalization in Phonemic Contexts.   We can take advantage of stimulus generalization when teaching certain sounds. Elbert, Shelton, and Arndt (1967) demonstrated that once /s/ was learned, /z/ was learned even

though clients received no training for /z/. We would expect generalization to occur from /s/ to /z/ because those sounds share many of the same acoustic and motoric characteristics. The clients in this study were also tested for /r/ production. They were unable to produce this sound correctly before treatment of the /s/, and were still unable to produce it correctly after its treatment. Learning /s/ had no effect upon learning /r/. This appeared to be the result of the differences in distinctive features between the /s/ and the /r/ sounds.

Generalization also occurs at the feature level. McReynolds and Bennett (1972) illustrated this fact in their study of three children who were taught specific sounds. They found that generalization occurred in other sounds that shared the same features. For example, if /s/ was taught, then all sounds sharing the [+stridency] feature were learned more quickly once /s/ was learned. I made use of this principle when teaching a young child fricative sounds (Mowrer & Case, 1982). Once the child learned /s/, the other fricatives were learned in less time. Learning to produce one fricative sound facilitated learning /θ/, /ʃ/ and eventually /tʃ/.

There are also instances in which generalization occurs across positions in a word. Weston and Irwin (1971) reported that once the sound was taught in the prevocalic position, the sound was learned more quickly in the postvocalic position. Powell and McReynolds (1969) also found this type of generalization occurring. When they taught sounds in syllables, they found that the child produced sounds correctly in all positions in words. Some investigators have not reported finding interposition generalization of sounds; consequently, more research is needed to verify these findings.

Stimulus Generalization in Situational Contexts.   One of the areas speech clinicians report as their most difficult task is carry-over outside the clinic. The client uses the correct sound while in the treatment situation but not when speaking in other situations, such as in the classroom, at home, or on the playground. In many cases, this problem exists because the speech clinician has no strategy for enhancing transfer of the newly learned speech pattern to other speaking situations. It is possible to facilitate rapid transfer by incorporating procedures that maximize stimulus generalization from one context to another.

It has been demonstrated in numerous studies that positive transfer of training occurs when stimuli contained in the original learning task share features with some of the stimuli in the new situations (McGeoch & Irion, 1952). Holland and Skinner (1961) pointed out that if a subject has been reinforced for making a certain response under a specified stimulus condition, this same response will be produced in the presence of similar stimulus conditions even though the response is not reinforced. By keeping stimuli in the treatment situation similar to stimuli found in other speaking situations, the clinician is more likely to maximize generalization. For example, the words selected for practice should be those the client uses frequently in other speaking situations (McDonald, 1964). A strategy used by Mowrer, Baker, and Schutz (1968) to enhance generalization consisted of teaching the client to respond correctly to a small number of words containing /s/ or /z/. Following training in the clinical setting, parents were asked to provide further speech training in the home. They were given instructional materials containing the same picture stimuli that were used in the clinical training program. Also, many of the instructional items were identical or similar to those used in the original training sessions.

In addition to maintaining similarity of words and pictures, the speech clinician can provide training in other speaking situations, such as in the client's classroom or on the playground. The presence of the speech clinician serves as a reminder for the client to produce the sound correctly. If generalization is to occur, it is important to teach correct articulation in situations where the client frequently talks. It is also wise to involve significant others in the treatment program because the client frequently talks to those persons. Carrier (1970) found that children who were taught sounds by their parents obtained higher scores on an articulation test after treatment than did a similar group who were treated by speech clinicians only.

Teachers also have been asked to play roles in helping their students articulate correctly. One speech clinician conducted three half-hour training sessions for classroom teachers after school (Mowrer, 1967). Her objective was to help elementary classroom teachers (a) discriminate between correct and incorrect /s/ sounds, (b) provide appropriate instructions to children when lisping was observed, and (c) provide some group speaking activities that would foster correct use of the /s/. During the 3 weeks of training sessions, the speech clinician taught the children who lisped how to produce /s/ in words and phrases found in their school reading books.

The children were provided with speech books consisting of pages containing 25 dashes. They were instructed to give their speech books to the teacher as they came to their reading circle. Each time they said /s/ or /z/ correctly while reading aloud, the teacher placed a check above one dash in their speech book. If the child lisped, the teacher placed a zero above the dash and provided an appropriate cue such as, "Remember to close your teeth." At the end of the week, the children brought their speech books to the clinician to redeem points earned by saying /s/ correctly when reading. Small toys were provided as rewards. This is one example of how rapid carry-over can be achieved by using the classroom teacher, daily speaking situations, and familiar materials from reading assignments.

Conley (1966) described a procedure he developed to study the effects of different types of reinforcement paradigms in which peers were used to enhance carry-over. He asked the client to bring four friends to speech class. The client was asked to tell stories containing many /s/ words. Both the client and the peers were rewarded for each of the client's correct productions of /s/. The important point of this activity was that peers, to whom the clients spoke daily, were included as part of the treatment program. Their presence and comments facilitated carry-over.

Speech aides and peers have been used in numerous programs to aid in the generalization process. The program described by Lundquist (1972), and noted previously in this chapter, involved the speech clinician only to a minimal degree. Once the speech clinician had taught the client to produce the target sound correctly in several sentences, an aide was assigned to the client. The aide was provided with a book of exercises the client was asked to practice in a wide variety of speaking situations. These situations included the places the child frequently visited during the day, such as the hallway, the playground, the cafeteria, and the classroom. The purpose of using these situations was to give the client practice in saying target sounds correctly in a number of speaking situations, not just in the clinic setting.

Although teachers, parents, and peers can be helpful in the carry-over phase of therapy, it is important to consider certain factors before deciding to include them. Among these factors are (a) the ability of the helper to discriminate the correct production, (b) the relationship between the child and the teacher, parent, or peer, and (c) the child's feelings about involving a peer in the process.

Carry-over also can be enhanced by teaching the client to produce the target sound correctly in idioms, slang expressions, and rapidly articulated sequences that are used frequently. For example, phrases to be used for clients learning the correct /s/ sound might include short speech sequences, such as *It's a ———, Here's a ———, What's a ———, That's a ———,* and so on. These sequences resemble nonsense syllables. Later, nouns are added to these rapidly articulated sequences to produce sentences, such as *It's a boy, He's a man, There's a bike, It's a car,* etc. The purpose of repeating these sequences is to embed the correct sound in automatic speech responses. This type of speech repetition contrasts sharply with speech sequences found in many game activities that focus upon the child's occasional request to spin a spinner, draw a card, or roll dice. Sentences such as *May I please spin the spinner* or *Please can I take my turn* may provide practice saying the target sound correctly in context, but one cannot expect rapid generalization of /s/ to everyday speaking situations. The child needs to produce /s/ in speech sequences that are often used during daily conversations. In this way, the new response quickly becomes habituated.

Maintaining the Use of the Correct Response.   There has been considerable research conducted by learning theorists regarding factors that enhance retention and use of newly learned responses (McGoech & Irion, 1952). Four factors are associated with increased retention. First, subjects retain information best when *meaningful material* is used. The early work by Ebbinghaus (1913) clearly demonstrated that nonsense material was quickly forgotten when compared with meaningful material. Hence, it seems unwise to use meaningless tongue twisters, nonsense syllables, and poetry as the chief source of words for practice. The clinician is more likely to achieve retention by choosing words that clients use daily than by presenting words chosen randomly from dictionaries. Names of family members, pets, favorite toys, frequently used household objects, and school supplies like a pencil, scissors, eraser, and so on are good choices. Another source of useful words is verbs that are used often. Word lists containing words that children use frequently are available from several commercial publishers.

A second factor found to increase retention is *frequent instruction.* The client who receives practice three times daily is more likely to retain material than the client who receives instruction once a week. Backus and Dunn (1947) studied the effects of providing therapy daily to groups of children as compared with providing therapy twice weekly. They concluded that more progress was made in a 6-week intensive program than was made during the school year when children were seen twice each week.

Studies by Sommers, Leiss, Fundrella, Manning, Johnson, Oerther, Sholly, and Siegel (1970) and Ausenheimer and Irwin (1971) confirm these findings that materials practiced more frequently are learned more effectively than those practiced infrequently. Speech clinicians should examine alternatives for delivery of service that will allow for more frequent instruction. In the public schools, it may be possible to schedule children to be seen several times a day, for example, on their way to the cafeteria, at the playground, during recess, immediately after school, and, in some cases, before school begins.

Overlearning information has been found to improve retention greatly (Lawrence, 1954). But this is true only up to a certain point. Beyond a certain amount of overlearning, little benefit is derived from continued practice. One of the few studies reported in this area was conducted by Diedrich and Bangert (1976). They concluded that clinicians could dismiss children who have been working on /s/ and /r/ sounds when they could produce these sounds correctly 75% of the time. At present, it is not clear what amount of overlearning is needed in the treatment of articulation problems. The proverb "Practice makes perfect" may apply here in that the more one is exposed to saying the response, the better the task is learned. Just how much practice is necessary before further practice is unproductive is not known.

Finally, *motivational state* has been found to be an important factor with respect to retention of a response. The more highly motivated a person, the greater the retention of the material that has been learned. It has been suggested that high motivational states may result in an increased amount of rehearsal time. This, in turn, results in better retention. If this is the case, it would be beneficial to provide incentives for learning. Some speech clinicians argue that their clients do what they are asked to do and require little or no extrinsic motivation. This may be true in the speech class setting, but if increases in motivational states result in improved retention, then it is important that we provide some means of motivating clients to change certain behaviors outside the immediate clinical (speech class) setting.

CONCLUSION

Speech clinicians can follow systematic procedures when adopting a behavior therapy approach to the treatment of articulation problems. Ten rules capture the essence of this approach (Mowrer, 1982):

Rules to Follow Using Behavior Therapy

1. *Immediacy:* In order to help a child learn more efficiently, provide a reward immediately following the child's correct response. It may not be possible or even advisable to give a toy or food item, immediately, so provide a social reward, token, point, or some signal of immediate recognition.

2. *Attention:* Attention is a powerful social reward. Provide attention the way you would use a token, toy, or other form of recognition following a correct response. Be careful that you do not give attention to wrong or undesired behavior. This would only serve to reward the incorrect response. Attention can help children learn correct behaviors but it can also serve to reinforce undesired behavior if used inappropriately.

3. *Pairing Rewards:* Anything paired or associated with a reward also acquires rewarding properties. For example, if we talk to a child while feeding her, talk will become associated with food which is rewarding, and soon talk by itself will serve as a reward. Such a reward is called a secondary reinforcer.

4. *Continuous Reward:* At first when a behavior is being taught, reward each correct response. When the newly learned behavior is easier to produce, provide a reward every other time. Gradually decrease the frequency with which you provide a reward as learning progresses. This reduction in the schedule of reinforcement serves to maintain the behavior better than the continuous reward.

5. *Selective Reward:* Give a reward following the responses that are important for the child to learn. If a child is being taught to say /s/, use the reward for good /s/ productions, not for winning games or activities not related to /s/ production.

6. *Small Steps:* It is important to use small steps in establishing a complex behavior. At first, demand very little from the child. It may be necessary to model the desired behavior several times. By requiring small increases each day, the child can build a series of behaviors into a habit, providing rewards are presented following each bit of correct behavior.

7. *Chaining:* One behavior leads to another in a chain leading to a complex behavior. It is important that the reward follow the behavior that occurs at the end of the chain. Be careful that undesired behaviors are not included in the chain of desired behaviors.

8. *Getting the Child's Attention:* Be sure to get the child's attention (looking, listening or both) when giving directions. Looking and listening are important since children learn better when they are actively attending.

9. *Imitation:* Modeling desired behavior is important as a method of instruction. By rewarding the child for imitating correct models of behavior, we can improve learning.

10. *Relevant Cues:* It is important to use relevant cues when instructing children. For example, the cue "close your teeth when you say /s/" is important to children who lisp. Attention cues like "get ready" and "watch me" are also important. Cues provide children with a preparatory set to help them respond correctly.[1]

SUMMARY

The major purpose of this chapter was to outline a strategy based upon principles of operant conditioning to change behaviors in an effective and efficient manner. The application of these principles frequently has been referred to as behavior modification or, more precisely, behavior therapy. This procedure involves two major elements: (1) effective management of consequent events and (2) careful organization of task sequences to be taught. The application of these two major elements can best be summarized in terms of seven steps that have been outlined below.

First, select a target behavior that is observable and countable. Record the baseline behavior as it exists in the individual's repertoire.

Second, break down the learning tasks into their smallest components or steps.

---

[1]From *Methods of Modifying Speech Behaviors,* 2d ed., pp. 261–262, by Donald Mowrer, 1982, Columbus, Ohio: Charles E. Merrill Publishing Company. Copyright © 1982 by Bell & Howell Company. Reprinted by permission.

Third, devise a set of behavioral objectives that define the learning tasks in terms of what it is you wish the person to do, the conditions under which it is to be done, and how well you want the person to perform. List the criterion the person must meet in order to advance to the next step.

Fourth, deliver the instructional program and include procedures that will maximize transfer and maintenance of the target behavior to environments outside the training setting.

Fifth, manage consequent events to ensure desired behaviors are increased and undesired behaviors are decreased. Use varying schedules of reinforcement to maximize high rates of the desired behavior.

Sixth, keep records of response rates and plot the correct and incorrect behaviors graphically. Make changes in therapy procedures according to results of the data.

Seventh, dismiss the individual from therapy when desired behavior is achieved. Execute a maintenance program if needed to make sure the undesired behavior does not return.

Through careful planning and execution of an instructional program designed to change a specific behavior, one can bring about desired behavioral changes in an efficient and practical manner. As stated at the beginning of this chapter, changing behavior is our principal job. When we learn to do this effectively our job becomes much easier and certainly much more enjoyable. The suggestions in this chapter should help you in planning and executing your instructional materials that are designed to bring about behavioral change.

REFERENCES

Ausenheimer, B., & Irwin, R. B. (1971). Effect of frequencies of speech therapy on several measures of articulatory proficiency. *Language, Speech and Hearing Services in Schools, 2,* 43–51.

Backus, O., & Beasley, J. (1951). *Speech therapy with children.* Boston: Houghton Mifflin.

Backus, O., & Dunn, H. M. (1947). Intensive group therapy in speech rehabilitation. *Journal of Speech and Hearing Disorders, 12,* 39–60.

Baker, R. D., & Ryan, B. P. (1971). *Programmed conditioning for articulation.* Monterey, CA: Monterey Learning Systems.

Boone, D. R., & Prescott, T. E. (1972). Content and sequence analysis of speech and hearing therapy. *Asha, 14,* 58–62.

Carrier, J., Jr. (1970). A program of articulation therapy administered by mothers. *Journal of Speech and Hearing Disorders, 35,* 344–353.

Conley, D. (1966). *The effects of using standardized instructions to evaluate speech correction procedures.* Unpublished masters thesis, Arizona State University, Tempe, AZ.

Coolagan, R. B. (1976). Programming primer. *School, Science and Mathematics, 76,* 381–91.

Costello, J. (1975). The establishment of fluency with time-out procedures: Three case studies. *Journal of Speech and Hearing Disorders, 40,* 216–231.

Costello, J. (1977). Programmed instruction. *Journal of Speech and Hearing Disorders, 42,* 3–28.

Delbridge, L., & Larrigan, L. (1973). *Stimulus shift articulation kit.* Tempe, AZ: Ideas.

Diedrich, W. M. (1971). Procedures for counting and charting a target phoneme. *Language, Speech and Hearing Services in Schools, 55* (2), 18–32.

Diedrich, W. M., & Bangert, C. J. (1976). *Training speech clinicians in recording and analysis* of articulatory behavior. (Grant No. OEG-0-70-1689 and OEG-0-71-18-1689). Washington, D.C.: U.S. Office of Education, Dept. of Health, Education, and Welfare.

Drash, P., Caldwell, L., & Liebowitz, J. (1970). Correct and uncorrect response rates as basic dependent variables in operant conditioning of speech in non-verbal subjects. *Psychological Aspects of Disability, 17,* 16–23.

Ebbinghaus, H. E., (1913). *Memory: A contribution of experimental psychology* (H. A. Ruger & C. E. Bussehius, Trans.). New York: Teachers College Educational Reprint Services. (Original work published 1885).

Elbert, M., Shelton, R. L., & Arndt, W. B. (1967). A task for evaluation of articulation change. *Journal of Speech and Hearing Research, 10,* 281–288.

Fine, B. (1962). *The modern family guide to education.* New York: Doubleday.

Gerber, A. J. (1973). *Carryover.* Philadelphia: Temple University Press.

Graham, C. H. (1951). Visual perception. In S. Stevens (Ed.), *Handbook of experimental psychology.* (pp. 868–920). New York: Wiley.

Griffiths, H., & Craighead, W. E. (1972). Generalization in operant speech therapy for misarticulation. *Journal of Speech and Hearing Disorders, 37,* 485–494.

Harvard Center for Research and Development on Educational Differences. *Newsletter,* Cambridge, Mass: Harvard University, 1964.

Holland, J., & Skinner, B. F. (1961). *The analysis of behavior.* New York: McGraw-Hill.

Lawrence, D. (1954). The evaluation of training and transfer programs in terms of efficiency measures. *Psychology, 38,* 367–383.

Lindsley, O. R. (1964). Direct measurement and prosthesis of retarded children. *Journal of Education, 147,* 62–81.

Lovaas, O. I. (1966). A program for the establishment of speech in psychotic children. In J. K. King (Ed.), *Childhood autism.* Oxford: Pergamon Press.

Lundquist, R. L. (1972). *Speech therapy transfer program.* Las Vegas: Clark County School District.

Mager, R. F. (1962). *Preparing instructional objectives.* Palo Alto, CA: Fearon Publishers.

McCabe, R. B., & Bradley, D. (1975). Systematic multiple phonemic approach to articulation therapy. *Acta Symbolica, 6,* 1–18.

McDonald, E. (1964). *Articulation testing and treatment: A sensory-motor approach.* Pittsburgh, Penn.: Stanwix House.

McGeoch, J. A., & Irion, A. L. (1952). *The psychology of human learning.* New York: Longmans, Green & Co.

McReynolds, L. V. (1983). Evaluation of treatment of children and adults with articulation disorders. In W. H. Perkins (Ed.), *Current therapy of communication disorders: Phonologic-articulatory disorders.* New York: Thiem-Stratton Inc.

McReynolds, L. V., & Bennett, S. (1972). Distinctive feature generalization in articulation training. *Journal of Speech and Hearing Disorders, 37,* 462–470.

McReynolds, L. V., & Huston, K. (1971). A distinctive feature analysis of childrens' misarticulations. *Journal of Speech and Hearing Disorders, 36,* 155–166.

Milisen, R. (1954). A rationale for articulation disorders. [Monograph]. *Journal of Speech and Hearing Disorders, 4,* 5–18.

Mowrer, D. (1964). *An experimental analysis of variables controlling lisping responses of children.* Unpublished doctoral dissertation, Arizona State University, Tempe, AZ.

Mowrer, D. (1967). Programmed speech therapy—a field test. *Asha, 9,* 369.

Mowrer, D. (1969a). *Modification of speech behaviors: Ideas and strategies for students.* Tempe, AZ: Ideas.

Mowrer, D. (1969b). Evaluating speech therapy through precision recording. *Journal of Speech and Hearing Disorders, 34,* 239–244.

Mowrer, D. (1982). *Methods of modifying speech behaviors* (2nd ed.). Columbus: Charles E. Merrill.

Mowrer, D. E., Baker, R. L., & Schutz, R. E. (1968). Operant procedures in the control of speech articulation. In H. Sloane & B. MacAulay (Eds.), *Operant procedures in remedial speech and language training*. Boston: Houghton Mifflin.

Mowrer, D., & Case, J. (1982). *Clinical management of speech disorders*. Rockville, MD: Aspen Publication.

Patterson, G. R., & White, G. D. (1969). It's a small world: The application of "time-out for reinforcement." *Oregon Psychological Association Newsletter, 15*, Supplement No. 2.

Pavlov, I. P. (1927). *Conditional reflexes*. London: Oxford University Press.

Powell, J., & McReynolds, L. (1969). A procedure for testing position generalization from articulation training. *Journal of Speech and Hearing Research, 12*, 629–645.

Psaltis, C. D., & Spallato, S. L. (1973). *Programmed articulation therapy: Time to modify*. Springfield, IL: Charles C. Thomas.

Skinner, B. F. (1953). *Science and human behavior*. New York: Macmillan.

Skinner, B. F. (1956). A case history in scientific methods. *American Psychologist, 11*, 221–233.

Skinner, B. F. (1957). *Verbal behavior*. New York: Appleton-Century-Crofts.

Skinner, B. F. (1959). *Cumulative record*. New York: Appleton-Century-Crofts.

Skinner, B. F., & Ferster, C. (1957). *Schedules of reinforcement*. New York: Appleton-Century-Crofts.

Sommers, R. K., Leiss, R., Fundrella, D., Manning, W., Johnson, R., Oerther, P., Sholly, R., & Siegel, M. (1970). Factors in the effectiveness of articulation therapy with educable retarded children. *Journal of Speech and Hearing Research, 13*, 304–316.

Van Riper, C. (1939). *Speech correction: Principles and methods*. New York: Prentice-Hall.

Weston, A. J., & Irwin, J. V. (1971). Use of paired-stimuli in modification of articulation. *Perceptual Motor Skills, 32*, 947–957.

White, O. R., & Haring, N. G. (1976). *Exceptional teaching*. Columbus: Charles E. Merrill.

7

Linguistic Approaches to Articulation Treatment

The speech-language clinician frequently sees preschool and school-aged children who have so many articulation errors that their speech is very difficult to understand or is completely unintelligible. They are sometimes understood only by their parents, and even parents may fail to understand their more complex sentences. These children often exhibit limited communication characterized by short telegraphic sentences and an inclination to communicate as little information as possible. Children with such severe articulation disorders present many challenges.

GENERAL CONSIDERATIONS IN PHONOLOGICAL DISORDERS

It is likely that children with numerous articulation errors also have difficulty with other aspects of language, including syntax, semantics, and pragmatics (Marquardt & Saxman, 1972; Menyuk, 1964; Panagos, 1974; Paul & Shriberg, 1982; Saxman & Miller, 1973; Smit & Bernthal, 1983). These sets of rules are closely related, and deficits in one area are often accompanied by deficits in another.

This chapter was written by **Nancy A. Creaghead**.

It is also possible that a child's limited language production is a result of the articulation deficit. This can happen in one of several ways. First, a child may reduce linguistic output as a strategy for being understood. Long strings may be more difficult for the listener to interpret than key words accompanied by nonverbal clues. For example, a normal child might say, "We were outside playing kickball, and Billy came up behind me and knocked me down." The child with a severe articulation disorder might produce that sentence as /wi wo aʊtaɪ pei tɪbɔ æ bɪɪ te ʌ biaɪ mi æ nɑ mi daʊ/. The listener would probably not understand that sentence, but might understand /bɪɪ ɪ mi/ to be "Billy hit me," especially if it were accompanied by appropriate gesturing. In other words, there is no point in providing much information that no one will understand.

The second possible reason for a child's use of reduced language is embarrassment or self-consciousness stemming from previous unpleasant speaking experiences. Many children with language and/or articulation problems learn very early that they are not good at talking. Therefore, they may give up trying, or at least restrict their output to essentials. This implies that an important objective of the speech-language pathologist may be to encourage the child to talk more.

The third possible reason for perceived language deficits among articulation-disordered children is that the articulation errors themselves may mask the child's language abilities. The child who omits final consonants will also omit many morphological markers, such as past tense verb endings (*walked, dragged, kissed*), third person present singular verb endings (*drives, hits*), plural markers (*flags, hats*), possessive markers (*John's, the cat's*). The child may know the rules for these grammatical forms but not use them because of the omission of final sounds.

Clinicians and researchers continually seek more effective methods of remediating speech disorders. Traditionally, articulation therapy methods have focused on the correction of one phoneme at a time, often beginning therapy by teaching a sound that usually develops early and moving to those that develop later as earlier ones are mastered. The rationale is that teaching one sound at a time is less likely to confuse a child. However, faced with children who exhibit multiple articulation errors like those described above, the clinician might reasonably look for strategies that would help such children learn several phonemes at one time in order to speed up the remedial process. In such *multiphonemic approaches*, all error phonemes may be targeted for simultaneous correction as described in chapter 11, or the phonemes to be taught may be grouped according to feature similarities as described in chapter 14. Grouping sounds according to the phonological processes involved offers another avenue for multiphonemic correction.

Many multiphonemic therapy approaches are based on phonological theory, as described in chapter 2. They can be described in two major groups: (a) distinctive-feature approaches, and (b) phonological-process approaches. However, there is a great deal of overlap between the two groups. The point of both is to be able to make generalizations about the nature of the child's errors. In order to do this, a sample of the child's speech must be obtained and analyzed as described in chapter 4.

It is important to remember that the task of distinctive-feature analysis or phonological-process analysis is valuable only if it leads to effective remediation techniques. McReynolds and Elbert (1981) emphasize the need to avoid using new procedures or terminology just because they are new. They suggest that without quantitative and qualitative criteria for assigning processes, we are just renaming what had been observed before. For example, we may now use the term *final consonant deletion* rather than *omission of final consonants*, perhaps without attention to the possible subtle differences between the terms.

It is only through careful observation regarding how often and in what contexts an error occurs that the clinician can determine whether an underlying rule or process or a pattern of error is manifest in the child's speech. In their study, McReynolds and Elbert (1981) used the following quantitative criteria for identifying phonological processes: (a) The error had at least four opportunities to occur, and (b) the error occurred in at least 20% of the opportunities. Note that McReynolds and Elbert used only quantitative criteria for evaluation. Other authors (Hodson, 1980; Ingram, 1981; Shriberg & Kwiatkowski, 1980; Weiner, 1979) hold different views regarding the decision-making process. These may include different quantitative and/or qualitative criteria. Other quantitative criteria have been suggested (Hodson & Paden, 1983), and even one instance of a rule may be important, especially if it coincides with an overall pattern of rules. This is an important consideration when only a small sample can be obtained.

The primary advantage of completing a feature or phonological-process analysis and using a multiphonemic approach to therapy is the potential efficiency in teaching a child a rule that may generalize and correct several phonemes at the same time. This of course applies only in instances of multiple misarticulations, so these techniques are not useful for all children.

Examples of clients who are not candidates for these approaches are individuals who exhibit only one or two errors, such as errors on /r/ or /s/, and individuals who exhibit a pattern that is due to a defined physiological/anatomical condition, such as "backing" in children with cleft palate or final consonant omissions and distortions resulting from dysarthria. Multiphonemic approaches seem to be most beneficial for children who exhibit multiple articulation errors in the absence of a definable organic cause. In many cases, the preferred therapy approach for individuals with diagnosed dysarthria, apraxia, or cleft palate may be based more on learning the production of individual sounds with auditory, visual, tactile, and kinesthetic stimulation than on learning phonological rules. In other words, production rather than rule learning may be the primary difficulty with these groups. However, recent attempts to use a phonological approach to describe errors of cleft-palate children (Hodson, Chin, Redmond, & Simpson, 1983; Lynch, Fox, & Brookshire, 1983) and cerebral-palsied children (McMahon, Hodson, & Allen, 1983) have suggested that this approach to therapy may be useful for at least some children in these groups. A third group of children who may not be candidates for a multiphonemic approach is individuals who exhibit errors for which no pattern can be observed. These are usually considered phonetic errors and may be more amenable to a single-phoneme approach.

The remainder of the chapter will describe therapy approaches based on either a distinctive-feature or phonological-process model. It is important to remember that although authors generally describe their procedures according to one or the other model, in actual practice there is a great deal of overlap between the two.

DISTINCTIVE-FEATURE THERAPY APPROACHES

One of two strategies is usually employed for remediating errors from a distinctive-feature base. In the most common approach, one or more target phonemes are used to train the feature (Blache, 1982; Blache & Parsons, 1980; Blache, Parsons, & Humphreys, 1981; Costello & Onstine, 1976; McReynolds & Bennett, 1972). The second approach involves teaching all of the phonemes that have a given target feature at the same time.

In the first approach, phonemes that involve the + and − contrast may be used to illustrate the feature. For example, the phonemes /t/ and /f/ could be used to teach the + and − continuant contrast to a child who does not use continuants. McReynonds and Bennett (1972) and Blache, Parsons, and Humphreys (1981) chose two phonemes that differed by only one feature. For example, /p/ and /b/ or /t/ and /d/ would be recommended for teaching unvoiced/voiced (lax/tense); /t/ and /s/ could be used for teaching continuant/interrupted. This approach is described in detail by Blache in chapter 14.

Costello (1975) recommended training more than one error phoneme in conjunction with the substituted phoneme to demonstrate the contrastive function of distinctive features. Costello and Onstine (1976) trained two phonemes that illustrated the + value of the absent feature, and contrasted those with one phoneme that illustrated the − value of the feature. For example, to teach continuancy, they taught /θ/ and /s/ in contrast with /t/.

Costello (1975, p. 69) outlined the following steps in designing a remediation plan based on distinctive-feature theory:

1. Administer traditional measures of articulation to determine error phonemes and stimulability.
2. Deep-test error phonemes for baseline data.
3. Complete distinctive-feature analysis using Singh and Polen's (1972) system and select target feature and three or four appropriate phonemes as vehicles for instruction.
4. Design a treatment program for these phonemes that includes steps for carry-over in connected speech outside the clinical setting.
5. Following treatment, readminister articulation tests and obtain a spontaneous speech sample.

It has been suggested that features cannot be separated from the phonemes-in-words context (Costello, 1975; Parker, 1976). Parker suggests that features are not a component of speech production, but a component of the language, and hence inseparable from words. Therefore, Blache (chapter 14) recommends teaching the feature contrasts in minimal word-pairs such as *big–pig, bass–bat, first–thirst* (Blache et al., 1981). Further details and advantages of the minimal-word-pair method will be discussed briefly in this chapter and more extensively in chapters 13 and 14.

Generalization

The assumption of distinctive-feature strategies is that the features taught in one contrast will generalize to other sounds carrying the same features. Several studies have tested this hypothesis.

It has been found that generalization does occur from trained to untrained words (Blache & Parsons, 1980; Blache, Parsons, & Humphreys, 1981; Costello & Bosler, 1976; Griffith, Irwin, & Weston, 1980; Pollack & Rees, 1972; Ruscello, 1975; Weiner, 1981b; Weiner & Bankson, 1978; Weston & Irwin, 1971). Blache et al. (1981) found that generalization occurred from one word-pair example of the phonemes to other words. Weiner (1981b) trained two children using the method of meaningful minimal contrasts, which will be described in chapter 13. He found that the suppression of three phonological processes (final consonant deletion, stopping, and fronting) generalized from 4 training words to an untrained list of 20.

In a further test of generalization, McReynolds and Bennett (1972) trained one phoneme example of an absent feature in nonsense syllables to determine if generalization would occur to words and to other phonemes with the same feature. For example, they trained /f/ in nonsense syllables to determine if the child would learn to produce /f/ in words and if he or she would also produce other stridents such as /s/ and /ʃ/. They did obtain generalization to words from nonsense syllables and to other phonemes from the example phoneme. There was, however, variation in degree of generalization based on the target feature and on word position. The findings regarding generalization from syllables to words are supported by Powell and McReynolds (1969).

Generalization across word positions has also received attention (Powell & McReynolds, 1969; Weston & Irwin, 1971; Ruscello, 1975). While generalization has been shown to occur, Dunn (1983, p. 50) suggests that certain factors must be considered in determining whether to train sounds in all positions. These include the particular sound being trained, the individual child's abilities, and the treatment approach.

Other researchers have shown that there is generalization from trained phonemes to other phonemes (Compton, 1970; Costello & Onstine, 1976; Dunn & Till, 1982; Ruder & Bunce, 1981; Weiner, 1981b). As predicted by distinctive-feature theory, generalization seems to occur most effectively across phonemes that share features. Compton (1970) found that for one 4-year-old child, correction of /m/ resulted in correction of other nasals with no effect on any other defective consonants. As might be expected, Elbert, Shelton, and Arndt (1967) and McReynolds and Elbert (1981) found that training /s/ did not improve production of /r/. Further, Dunn and Till (1982) reported that in the training of fricatives, generalization occurred most frequently within place subclasses. For example, generalization occurred within the labiodental class (/f/ and /v/) and within the lingual class (/s/, /z/, /ʃ/), but not as readily between them.

Some researchers question the expectation that generalization will be complete and consistent (Blache et al., 1981; Dunn, 1983; Ingram, 1976; Weiner, 1981b; Weiner & Bankson, 1978; Winitz & Bellerose, 1978). These authors suggest training several examples of a feature or feature contrast rather than only one example in order to promote generalization. Weiner (1981b) stated that although he found training several examples to be effective, further research is needed to determine whether generalization will occur if only one phoneme contrast is used. Ingram (1976) concluded that the evidence for feature generalization is not sufficient to encourage use of a single-phoneme approach. He advocated a conservative view that features are learned in segments, not as features per se, and that all phonemes embodying a given feature should be trained. Hence, he recommended training all relevant phonemes at the same time.

Ruder and Bunce (1981) used a slightly different strategy for training two children with severe articulation disorders that had been classified as phonetic rather than phonemic. These children had very small phonemic repertoires. One child consistently used only /m/, /b/, and /g/. The other used only /g/, /n/, /ŋ/, and /j/. Ruder and Bunce chose phonemes which the children had already produced on occasion to increase their repertoire. In the first case, the child had produced /p/, /s/, and /k/ in addition to the frequent /m/, /b/, and /g/. The authors chose to train /s/ and /k/ to encourage the use of the features +continuant, +strident, +coronal, –voice, +high. A primary research question was: Will training /s/ and /k/, which between them embody all features of /t/, cause /t/ to be produced? Following traditional training through the word level, the child could imitate /t/, /f/, ŋ/, /z/, /tʃ/. On the basis of the generalization theory, /f/, /tʃ/, and /ʃ/ had also been predicted. Ruder and Bunce's research shows that careful selection of phonemes based on features missing from the child's system can encourage the use of new features and thus a larger repertoire of sounds.

Dunn (1983) discussed two kinds of generalization: (a) stimulus generalization, and (b) response generalization. She suggested that it is wise to plan for response generalization by providing diversity of material throughout the therapy program. Attention should be given to generalization across word positions, phonetic contexts, sounds, and linguistic levels, i.e., words, phrases, sentences. If the clinician begins early to measure generalization, it can be encouraged throughout the program. For example, consider the child who is taught one phoneme to represent a distinctive feature class but does not generalize the new production to other phonemes. A useful strategy might be to give the child limited experience with other phonemes in the same class in order to promote generalization.

The studies reviewed here indicate that there is value in examining features that are present and absent in the child's speech and using these features as a basis for expanding the child's repertoire of correctly used phonemes. The potential for feature generalization when target phonemes are carefully chosen seems good, and valuable therapy time may thus be saved.

Limitations

Distinctive-feature approaches have been criticized on the basis of the time required to complete the analysis and the questionable articulatory validity of many feature systems (Parker, 1976; Walsh, 1974). However, Singh, Hayden, and Toombs (1981) showed that the Singh and Singh (1976) distinctive-feature system was useful in establishing a feature hierarchy for the articulation errors of 1,077 children in public-school speech therapy. Further, Toombs, Singh, and Hayden (1981) found that markedness theory provided a better explanation of 801 students' substitutions than did analysis of features per se. Markedness theory, as described in chapter 2, accounts for the relative complexity of phonemes on the basis of the number of features required for production and the physiological complexity of the particular features. However, McReynolds, Engmann, and Dimmitt (1974) found that the articulation errors of the children in their study did not always follow the direction that markedness theory would predict. Grunwell (1982) notes that the theory of markedness is not well developed, and its clinical relevance has not been clearly demonstrated. In regard to use of distinctive features in general, Grunwell states that use of "a formalized distinctive feature analysis procedure" is questionable, but the "concept" of distinctive features is valid and clinically applicable (p. 129).

It is important to remember that the casual application of distinctive-feature therapy without the kind of attention given to choice of target features and phonemes that is evident in research projects may not produce the same progress. Care in choosing therapy goals will be rewarded in efficient use of therapy time.

The advantages of distinctive-feature therapy can be obtained by use of articulatory-based feature systems that relate directly to speech production (see chapter 2). Further, the regularities captured by this approach are largely the same as those determined by phonological-process analysis. A phonological-process approach, however, has the advantage of exposing certain error patterns that are not revealed by distinctive-feature analysis, such as syllable and phoneme deletions and assimilatory processes.

THERAPY APPROACHES BASED ON PROCESS ELIMINATION

A phonological-process approach is based on several assumptions that give direction to the remedial program. First, as in distinctive-feature-based therapy, treatment of phonological processes will result in more efficient therapy than that produced by one-phoneme approaches. Treatment of one or a few processes can effect correction of groups of phonemes at one time. This means that therapy may be directed toward a group of phonemes simultaneously or that one representative phoneme may be taught with the expectation that generalization will occur. Second, this approach assumes that the child's problem is one of rule learning, and therefore the treatment program will entail discovery of rules by the child. Third, the child's problem is proposed to be a phonemic rather than phonetic problem, which suggests that therapy should begin at the word level so that phoneme contrasts are possible, although some work has been carried out at the syllable level, both in research and in clinical practice.

Selection of Processes

Following the identification of phonological processes in the child's speech, the clinician must prioritize the processes for remediation. Ingram (1976) suggested the following three guiding principles from Edwards and Bernhardt (1973) for selection of processes for remediation:

1. Select processes which interfere most with intelligibility. Improvement of intelligibility is the primary goal of articulation therapy. Therefore, selection of target processes directed toward that end is therapeutically sound. The child's own perception of change in intelligibility can be motivating for future therapy.
2. Select less stable processes. It is likely that optional processes will be more amenable to change than those which are stable in the child's speech.
3. Select processes which are most common in young children. If we accept current thinking that phonologically disordered children are not totally unlike normally-developing children, and that earlier learned phonemes or classes of phonemes may be easier than later ones, then it follows that in therapy, the child may have an easier time learning the processes which are characteristic of younger children.

Edwards and Bernhardt (1973) advocated the application of these principles in the above order. In other words, the first process chosen should be the one that will produce the greatest change in intelligibility. If a clear-cut decision cannot be made on this basis, a process that is optional in the child's speech should be chosen. The normal acquisition sequence should be taken into account when the first two principles do not result in a clear choice.

These principles, although stated in linguistic terms, are really very like the criteria used in traditional therapy techniques (Van Riper, 1978). Traditionally, it was said that the target phoneme should be one that (a) interferes with intelligibility, (b) is stimulable, and (c) is early developing.

More recently, Edwards (1983) has given more detail to these principles. She suggests that it is not possible to define an order for remediation of processes because of the variability among children. However, it is important to have guiding principles. The principles are as follows:

1. "Choose processes that should result in early success" (p. 39). These would include processes that are optional in the child's speech (those that do not occur 100% of the time), processes that apply only in certain phonetic environments, and processes that affect sounds that are already in the child's phonetic inventory or sounds for which the child is stimulable. The principle is that the child will more easily and quickly eliminate a process if he has already demonstrated its suppression in some way.
2. "Choose processes that are 'crucial' for the individual child" (p. 39) in that they are especially deviant, call attention to the child's speech, interfere most with intelligibility, create a large number of homonyms, neutralize the distinction between sound contrasts, or apply consistently.
3. "Choose 'early' processes or processes that affect early sounds" (p. 41).

4. "Choose processes that interact" (p. 41) to create substitutions based on more than one rule change. First, work on the process that affects the greatest number of segments. Edward gives the following example: If the child substitutes d/k, b/p, and d/t, work on prevocalic voicing before fronting because it affects all three substitutions.

Edwards suggests basically the same principles as guidelines in selecting phonemes to represent target processes. An additional consideration in selecting phonemes is the position in the word. The sound should be easy to produce in the target position. For example, voiceless sounds might be chosen as final-position targets and voiced as initial because prevocalic voicing and postvocalic devoicing are likely to occur.

Careful study of the principles will reveal some overlap. For example, some "early" processes, like final consonant deletion, are those that create homonymy and interfere most with intelligibility. On the other hand, there is also some contradiction. The clinician needs to choose processes that occur frequently enough to be important in the child's speech, but at the same time select optional processes for immediate success. For a given child, optional processes may not interfere most with intelligibility or be early developing. The important point, then, is that the clinician must have clear guidelines in mind, but apply them thoughtfully to each child. Edwards suggests targeting two processes at the same time in order to speed overall progress toward intelligibility.

The authors of published process analysis procedures have also suggested criteria for selecting target processes after completing the analysis. Through describing case studies, Shriberg and Kwiatkowski (1980) suggest that final consonant deletion would be a priority process for elimination.

Hodson (1982) and Hodson and Paden (1983) first present a formula for determining a composite deviancy score that can be used to determine priority clients for therapy. The formula accounts for pervasiveness of the ten basic deficient patterns (syllable reduction, cluster reduction, prevocalic obstruent singleton omission, postvocalic obstruent singleton omission, stridency deletion, velar deviations, /l/ deviations, /r, ɝ/ deviations, nasal deviations, glide deviations), other deficient patterns, and age. Having determined which children should be seen for therapy, the authors go on to suggest strategies for determining target processes. They state that a target process should occur in at least 40% of the possible test contexts.

In Hodson and Paden's procedure, patterns are prioritized into four levels reflecting intelligibility. Level 0 patterns are characteristic of the most unintelligible children. Basically, these patterns consist of omissions of obstruents and liquids, and less frequently of glides and nasals. Children at this level have the highest priority for therapy. Level I patterns include cluster reduction and omission of syllables, prevocalic singletons, and postvocalic singletons. Substitutions at Level I include fronting of velars, backing, glottal replacement, and voicing alterations. Reduplication of syllables and vowel deviations also characterize Level I. Level II patterns include cluster reduction and omission of stridents as well as stopping, liquid gliding, and vowelization. Level III patterns do not significantly interfere with intelligibility; therefore, Hodson and Paden give them the lowest priority for remediation. They include non-phonemic alterations such as tongue protrusion and lateralization, affrication or deaffrication, minor place shifts, and devoicing of final obstruents. Children at Level I and at Level II will usually exhibit patterns from other levels.

Hodson and Paden suggest that therapy targets should be selected in accordance with the above levels; i.e., Level 0 processes should be selected first and Level III last. This order holds regardless of the percent of occurrence as long as it is above 40%. They focus on one phoneme that represents the pattern, with ease of elicitation the primary criterion for selection of the target phoneme. They recommend probing for a sound that the child can produce successfully, but based on their experience, they also provide a list of suggested target phonemes for each pattern and suggested words for each phoneme. Words are selected to facilitate correct production of the target phoneme. Careful attention should be given to phonetic contexts that will be most helpful. In addition, the words must be representable by objects or pictures.

Weiner (1979, pp. 3–6) recommends selecting a process from each of his three major categories to work on at the same time. He also provides a suggested order for remediation of the processes within each category. These categories and the order of processes are:

1. Syllable Structure Processes
    1. Deletion of final consonants
    2. Glottal replacement
    3. Weak syllable deletion
    4. Cluster reduction
2. Harmony Processes
    1. Prevocalic voicing
    2. Final consonant devoicing
    3. Velar assimilation
    4. Labial assimilation
    5. Alveolar assimilation
3. Feature Contrast Processes
    1. Stopping
    2. Affrication
    3. Gliding of fricatives
    4. Fronting
    5. Denasalization
    6. Gliding of liquids
    7. Vocalization

Compton and Hutton (1978) focus on improving intelligibility as the primary criterion for selecting target patterns. This means that unusual patterns that interfere with intelligibility would receive priority and that patterns and sounds which affect a large number of words would be chosen.

Although the clinician should be aware of and consider certain guiding principles in selecting goals for therapy, the individual child and his or her environment must in the end determine specific goals. In some cases, idiosyncratic factors like the child's name or special concerns of his parents or teacher can influence goal selection. This does not mean that the clinician should teach

/r/ to a 2-year-old because his name is Roger and the parents want him to say it correctly. It is the clinician's responsibility to provide information for parents and to help them to set realistic goals. On the other hand, it is important to remember that therapy should not occur in the absence of interaction with the environment.

REMEDIATION STRATEGIES

Ingram (1976) states that "the acquisition of phonology is concerned with the acquisition of the ability to use sounds contrastively" (p. 141). He outlines three goals for remediation:

1. Elimination of instability in the child's speech. Some children with articulation disorders demonstrate inconsistent production of words. The child who does not have firmly established phonemic contrasts may produce a given word in a variety of ways depending on the exact processes applied. Ingram gives the following example of a hearing-impaired child's productions of *pencil* from Oller and Eilers (1975) (Ingram, p. 142).

1.	bʌ'dɔ	5.	pɛ'ʔtə?	9.	pɛ'tə'
2.	pʌ'bə	6.	pɛd	10.	pʰad
3.	pɪtə	7.	pɛdə	11.	pɪa
4.	ɛ'tə	8.	pɛdza	12.	pɪt
				13.	pʰɛ'ʔtu'

    Ingram states that establishing the form /pɛtə/ as a consistent production would eliminate some minor processes and isolate a stable form for further process elimination. Further, it would help the adults in the child's environment to learn the child's rule system and understand the child better.
2. Elimination of homonyms. The inclusion in a child's speech of many words which have the same phonetic form interferes greatly with intelligibility. For some children, an appropriate therapy strategy may be to teach the child contrastive productions of specific words that are homonyms in his speech. In this case, the selection of target processes will be based on their usefulness in eliminating specific homonyms in the child's speech.
3. Establishing contrasts within the child's system. Ingram explains that the first two methods approach remediation from the basis of specific words in the child's sample. With some children, it may be more appropriate to work on establishing certain contrasts throughout the child's system, which will mean working on a large number of different words. Selection of contrasts would be based on the principles of acquisition outlined in chapter 3 that suggest which consonants and contrasts are learned first. Generally, children learn larger or more general contrasts before finer distinctions.

Weiner (1979) suggests that different remediation strategies may be applicable to different processes. He recommends two procedures for remediating syllable-structure processes. He calls the first a *sorting task* in which the child hears pairs of words like *pool* and *spool* or *pill* and *spill* and sorts them into "cluster" and "noncluster" categories. Weiner states that this auditory sorting will improve production of the cluster.

The second approach is the *lexical approach* in which the child must modify his syllable structure in order to avoid producing homonyms for pairs like *bow* and *boat*. In this approach, also called the *method of meaningful minimal contrasts* (see chapter 13), a game can be played in which the child names one of two pictures and the clinician chooses the picture that the child names (Weiner, 1981b). For example, a child with final consonant deletion will produce *bow* for *boat*, and the clinician will choose the bow picture each time until, on his own or with the help of the clinician, the child modifies his production to include a final sound on *boat*. Fokes (1982) also recommends use of contrast pairs in therapy, but she states that the word pairs do not have to be minimal. She advocates using the pairs in a variety of ways to promote the contrast—dividing them into two categories, imitating them, playing games, and telling stories with them. She suggests using eight to ten different pairs for a given contrast.

For remediation of harmony or assimilation processes, Weiner suggests the paired stimuli approach (Weston & Irwin, 1971), in which a word like *dime* is paired with *dog* or *duck* for a child who shows velar assimilation. *Dime* is a word which will not show velar assimilation. By this pairing, the child may begin to produce *dog* or *duck* correctly. The paired stimuli approach is described in chapter 12. Weiner also recommends the use of facilitating contexts like *mad dog* for eliminating assimilation.

Weiner further suggests a distinctive-feature approach for eliminating feature contrast processes such as stopping, gliding, fronting, vocalization, denasalization, affrication, or neutralization. The use of minimally contrasting pairs of sounds like /t/ and /s/ or /t/ and /k/ may produce generalization to other phonemes. A second approach is to teach awareness of the feature characteristic, like blowing or flowing versus exploding or popping. This awareness can be used in both listening and production. Weiner and Bankson (1978) gave the following outline for teaching frication:

1.   Introduce the stop-fricative concept by describing the fricative as running water and the stop as dripping water.
2.   Present a 20 item probe test for fricatives in the initial position of CVC words. This probe test is repeated after each of the following steps.
3.   Present ten exaggerated fricative and ten stop sounds in words for the child to identify. These words should be different from those used in the probe.
4.   Ask the child to imitate the exaggerated productions and to identify the stop or fricative feature of the clinician's productions. The criterion for moving from this step is 18/20 correct identifications on two successive probes. Productions are not counted.
5.   Repeat Step 4, but omit exaggeration.

6.   Ask the child to name pictures of the ten fricative words used in the above steps and ten additional words. Criterion is 18/20 correct productions on two consecutive trials.

Weiner and Bankson administered this program to four children and concluded that it was most useful with school-age children who had multiple errors and no attentional or behavioral problems.

Hodson and Paden (1983) present a treatment program for unintelligible children based on the following concepts:

1.   "Phonological acquisition is a gradual process" (p. 44).
2.   "Children with normal hearing typically acquire the adult sound system primarily by listening" (p. 46).
3.   "As the child acquires new speech patterns he associates kinesthetic with auditory sensations which enable later self-monitoring" (p. 47).
4.   "Phonetic environment can facilitate correct sound production" (p. 47).
5.   "Children tend to generalize new articulation skills to other targets" (p. 48).

Based on these concepts, Hodson and Paden's program includes (a) intensive auditory stimulation at the beginning and end of each session, (b) the use of auditory, tactual, and visual stimulation for correct production, (c) facilitation of correct production through the above means or through use of facilitating contexts or semantic cues, and (d) a cycle format that targets deficient phonological patterns for a few weeks and then allows time for the pattern to emerge. Not every error phoneme is taught. Target patterns as well as the phonemes to represent the patterns are chosen on the basis of their ease of production for the child. During each session only a few words that can be represented by pictures or objects are used. These words are chosen to facilitate correct production of the target pattern or sequence. Table 7.1 presents suggested target words for facilitating selected patterns (Hodson & Paden, 1983).

Each therapy session begins and ends with 2 minutes of mildly amplified auditory bombardment in which the clinician reads a list of about 15 words. The child only listens and may be engaged in some quiet activity. Production practice consists of incorporating two to five words in play activities. All types of stimulation (auditory, visual, tactile, etc.) are provided to facilitate correct production. Hodson and Paden's rationale is that practice of correct production is important and that use of a few words that the child can produce correctly will result in learning that will later generalize to other words. During each session, probes are used to determine future target patterns, phonemes, and words on the basis of ease of production. It is recommended that parents read the 15-word list to the child at home each day and ask him or her to name the picture cards. Table 7.2 shows a sample time schedule for a 30-minute therapy session based on Hodson and Paden's (1983, p. 68) model for a 50-minute session.

Hodson (1982) reported performance data on 111 children who were seen for therapy using this approach. They were seen once a week for 75-minute

TABLE 7.1
Two Suggested Target Words for Patterns Frequently Targeted in Cycle
One. The Same Words May Serve for Probing.*

Final Obstruents	
Final /p/	rope, soap
Final /t/	hat, boat
Final /k/	lock, bike
Consonant-Vowel-Consonant	
/p/-vowel-/p/	pipe, pop
Syllableness	
Two-syllables	cowboy, baseball
Three-syllables	cowboy hat, baseball bat
Velars	
Final /k/	rock, lock
Initial /k/	car, cow
Final /s/-clusters	
/ts/	boats, hats
/ps/	ropes, cups
/ks/	books, bikes
Initial /s/-cluster	
/sp/	spoon, spot
/st/	star, stop
/sm/	smoke, smile
/sn/	snake, snow
/sk/	sky, school
Liquids	
Initial /l/	lock, log
Initial /r/	rock, rug

*This list does not imply that there are no other words which are appropriate,
nor that all of these words or patterns are routinely targeted, and no others, in
Cycle One.
Source: Targeting Intelligible Speech (p. 65) by B. Hodson and E. Paden,
1983, San Diego: College-Hill Press. Copyright 1983 by College-Hill Press.
Reprinted by permission.

sessions. Some children were also receiving therapy at school. Seventy children
completed the program and were dismissed as intelligible. The average time in
therapy was two semesters, with the longest being 18 months for the children
with the most severe disorders. Thirteen children had progressed substantially,
but were not dismissed by the end of the project. Twenty-three children were
not in the program long enough to be counted.

This program differs from others in its cycle approach, which is based on
the belief that children will progress on their own following a brief experience

TABLE 7.2
Sample Time Schedule for a 30-minute Therapy Session Based on Hodson and Paden's (1983) Model

10:00	Review pictures from preceding lesson
10:02	Auditory bombardment using words with target sound
10:05	Draw 2 to 5 pictures illustrating words with target sound
10:10	Structured play activity using new picture cards
10:17	Second play activity using new cards and cards from previous sessions
10:25	Probing to determine new target for next lesson
10:28	Auditory bombardment
10:30	Give materials to parent and child for work at home

with correct production of the target pattern. In a cycle approach, unlike in traditional methods, a designated number of sessions are spent in training a given pattern. Several patterns may be trained consecutively within a given cycle. At the end of the cycle, probes are used to determine if the same patterns or new ones will be targeted in the next cycle. Each cycle lasts a set number of weeks, which is dependent on the therapy setting.

The procedures discussed thus far have used word-level material for remediation. Elbert (1983) reported using syllables for working on the phonological system of one child with a severely restricted phonetic inventory, consisting of only nine sounds including the glottal stop. The child received token reinforcement for correct imitation of contrasting syllables that illustrated more than one process. For example, the three pairs /a–ab/, /a–at/, and /a–ag/ illustrated final stops, voicing contrast, and a three-way place-of-articulation contrast. Elbert used words as probe items to evaluate generalization. Following 10 months of therapy the child had developed a full phonetic inventory and was highly intelligible. Pollack (1983) also reported using syllables, but found that words worked better for a child with a severe phonological preference for /d/ and /n/ in the initial position. She suggested modifying therapy plans for children with phonological preferences. For example, because of this child's strong preference in the initial position, it was necessary to work in the final position in order to expand his phonetic repertoire.

Grunwell (1983) reported the results of a program that is very different from the ones described above. The program was designed to allow the child to change her phonological system spontaneously through exposure to written English in a special education program, but with no direct articulation therapy. The child attended a preschool program with nine other children who had language-learning problems. The activities that were part of the general reading and writing program for all of the children included systematic exposure to the orthographic system, sound-symbol relationships, discriminating, classifying and sequencing sounds, and sound blending to form words. The child under study followed a normal developmental order for phonological gains, but the changes occurred with much greater rapidity. Grunwell suggests that such a program "facilitates the child's own development of a normal phonological system by providing him or her with direct access to the systematic and structural patterns in the adult system" (p. 75).

Example Therapy Plan

The following example of a therapy program for one child illustrates the kinds of information that the clinician needs to obtain prior to therapy planning. This section also contains a description of therapy goals based on the information gathered and an overview of the remediation process.

Assume that the spontaneous speech sample in Table 7.3 was obtained from a 5-year-old child and analyzed according to the procedures in chapter 4. (This analysis is shown in Table 7.4.) After analyzing the child's speech, the clinician must identify remediation goals. Hodson and Paden (1983) list the following processes as being characteristic of the speech of the most unintelligible children: backing, final consonant deletion, syllable reduction, prevocalic voicing, glottal replacement, and reduplication. Of these, this child exhibits final consonant deletion. Backing consistently occurs for /t/ and /k/, which become /h/. Other major processes are stopping of fricatives, cluster reduction, velar fronting, and liquid simplification. Hodson and Paden (1983) also note these as being characteristic of unintelligible children.

Priority processes for remediation for this child would be:

1. final consonant deletion
2. stopping of fricatives

There are a number of reasons for choosing these two processes as targets for remediation. First, they both have a significant effect on intelligibility. Together, they create many homonymous forms in the child's speech. A few examples are:

man
Max $\longrightarrow$ [mæ]   ball
mask   fox $\Big\rangle$ [bɑ]   six
                                                  this $\Big\rangle$ [dɪ]   it
                                                                            is $\Big\rangle$ [ɪ]

In addition, these processes are widespread in the child's speech. Each of them affects a large number of phonemes. The two phonemes /ʃ/ and /tʃ/ account for a large portion of both the fricatives and final consonants used. Like the two processes targeted, velar fronting creates homonymous forms (/dɑ/ = *got, dog*), but its remediation would change only one phoneme. Another reason for choosing these processes is that developmentally, they take precedence over others that might also increase intelligibility. For example, cluster reduction is widespread in the sample, but its suppression is developmentally more sophisticated. A final rationale for targeting these two processes is the observation that the child does use both fricatives and final consonants on a very limited basis. He uses /ʃ/ correctly and as a substitution for /tʃ/ in the initial and final position. This suggests that remediation of these processes is likely to be successful.

TABLE 7.3
Spontaneous Speech Sample for a 5-year-old Child

zipper	bɪbɚ	feet	bi	cow	hoʊ
baby	bebi	fishing	bɪi	fish	bɪ
blue	bu	five	baɪ	bed	bɛ
feather	bebɚ	birthday	bɝde	fox	bɑ
bathtub	bæə	big	bɪ	finger	bɪdo
ball	bɑ	busy	bɪi	boat	boʊ
soap	bop	pencil	pɛdə	pumpkin	pʌɪ
pretty	pɝni	milk	mɪo	monster	mɑɚ
pipe	paɪ	me	mi	pig	pɪ
P.Mooney	pipume	mouth	maʊ	smoking	moi
Poland	poʊɪ	moon	mu	pants	pæ
Stanley	pæwi	miss	mɪ	Maye	me
picture	pɪpɚ	wagon	weɪ	lamp	wæm
matches	mæʃə	what	wʌ	window	naino
water	wɑdɚ	snowman	nomæ	squirrel	wɝu
one	wə	sit	ni	tooth	hu
witch	wɪʃ	that	dæ	lady	weni
where	wer	scissors	dibɚ	six	dɪ
walking	wɑi	shovel	dʌu	lay	we
lap	wæ	thumb	dʌm	dog	dɑ
seven	dɛbə	carrot	herə	down	daʊ
door	dor	ten	hɪə	tail	heə
get	dɛ	Halloween	hæoʊi	this	dɪ
daddy	dædi	cook	hʊ	Carla	harə
donkey	dɔi	Connie	hɑni	car	har
hammer	hæmɚ	cake	he	help	hɛ
turtle	hɝdə	hill	hi	Terry	heri
taken	heɪ	rabbit	ræbɪ	scratch	ræʃ
homework	hoʊɝ	trip	rɪp	chicken	ʃɪi
shirt	ʃɝ	throw	ro	britches	rɪʃɪ
church	ʃɝʃ	Roundtree	raʊri	yellow	jɛwo
Charlie	ʃari	telephone	ɛwɪbo	vacuum	æu
you	ju	orange	or	airplane	eɪrpe
two	u	stove	o	got	dɑ
eight	eɪ	eating	iə	outside	aʊdaɪ
eleven	ɛbɪ	Santa	ræ	Claus	rɑ
mask	mæ	Christmas	rɪ	ugly	ʌwi
break	re	tree	rɪ	face	be
flag	be	Max	mæ	man	mæ
white	waɪ	wipe	waɪ	have	hæ
cat	hæ	have	hæ	light	waɪ
hat	hæ	knife	naɪ	drum	rʌ
nine	naɪ	brush	rʌ	gun	dʌ
cup	dʌ	floor	bor	four	bor
duck	dʌ	three	ri	go	do
ghost	do	tree	ri	off	ɔ
scare	deɪr	on	ɔ	house	hoʊ
there	deɪr	it	ɪ	is	ɪ

TABLE 7.4
Phonological Analysis of the Speech Sample

Word Structures	Substitutions			Omissions		
	Initial	Medial	Final	Initial	Medial	Final
V	p/m	b/p	ʃ/tʃ	t	m	p
CV	n/w	b/f		v	v	m
VC	b/f	b/v		st	θ	θ
VV	d/ð	b/ð			t	f
CVCV	h/t	n/t			d	v
CVV	n/s	n/d			z	t
VCV	b/z	d/s			n	d
CVCV	w/l	w/l			l	s
VCCV	d/ʃ	p/t			ʃ	z
VCVCV	ʃ/tʃ	ʃ/tʃ			k	n
CVVCV	d/k	d/g			g	l
CVCVCV	h/k	p/pl			mp	ʃ
	d/g	r/tr			st	k
	p/pr				nt	g
	b/bl				nk	ŋ
	r/br				lk	st
	b/fl				kj	sk
	r/θr					ts
	r/tr					ks
	r/dr					nd
	m/sm					
	p/st					
	n/sn					
	w/sl					
	d/sk					
	w/skw					
	r/skr					
	r/kr					
	r/kl					

Phonemic Repertoire:
1. Always used correctly: b, m, w, r, h
2. Used correctly in some context: p, b, m, w, d, n, r, j, h, ʃ
3. Appears, but never correct: none
4. Never appears: f, v, θ, ð, t, s, z, l, ʒ, tʃ, dʒ, k, g, ŋ
5. Not represented in sample words: none

Processes:
1. Final consonant deletion: 93 of 113 opportunities; all phonemes except m, r, tʃ, ʃ
2. Stopping of fricatives: all phonemes except h, final ʃ, tʃ
3. Cluster reduction: all clusters
4. Velar fronting: 6 of 14 opportunities; all opportunites for g
5. Unstressed syllable deletion: 3 of 57 opportunities
6. Liquid simplification: 1 only
7. Backing: h/k, h/t
8. Frication: h/k, h/t
9. Assimilation: 5 examples

The therapy plan might focus on the use of minimal pairs to illustrate the contrast between stops and fricatives and between open and closed syllables. The starting point might be the inclusion of other fricatives besides /ʃ/ in the final position. Words that can be pictured or for which objects are available could be used to illustrate to the child that the target distinctions are important in being understood. One obvious distinction that depends on final fricatives is the singular/plural contrast. The following are examples of appropriate words for minimal pairs:

eye	baby	bee	boy	no	my	two	tea
eyes	babies	bees	boys	nose	mice	tooth	teeth
ice		beef					teach
door	row	car	purr	bear	hoe	night	bow
doors	rose	cars	purse	bears	hose	knife	bows
						nine	boat
							both

A variety of game-like activities involving these pairs could be used. For example, the child could request one of the two objects or pictures, or he could tell the clinician which one to point to or move or find. Inclusion of words ending in /ʃ/ or /tʃ/ would provide an opportunity for immediate success. Procedures of this type are described in greater detail in the chapters in part III.

It is important to remember that therapy planning is not over when initials goals and an initial therapy plan have been established. One of the most crucial and yet most difficult tasks is the continuing modification of goals, target phonemes, and remediation strategies. Suppose that as this child progressed, he began to include final consonants, and did not stop fricatives as he acquired them in the final position. After he had begun to use /f/, /s/, and /z/ in the final position, similar therapeutic strategies might be used to target fricatives in the initial position and additional classes of phonemes in the final. Examples of minimal pairs for the initial position are:

two	bun	bat	toe	passed	bear	tie	tanned
Sue	fun	fat	sew	fast	fair	sigh	sand

It is possible that it would be difficult to eliminate stopping in the initial position, but let us assume that /f/ and /s/ can be elicited through modeling and the minimal-pair method. The next target might be the substitutions of /h/ for /t/ and /k/ because of the bizarre nature of the processes involved. The final process to receive remediation could be cluster reduction. As the child progresses through the remediation program, it is not always necessary to work on the elimination of every process. Some processes may be eliminated without therapy as the child begins to make more sense of the phonological system.

SUMMARY

This chapter has presented an overview of current therapy methods based on phonological theory. The guiding principle is that the child's faulty articulatory patterns may be a result of a phonological system that is different from the standard adult model and that thorough analysis of the child's rule system will lead to efficient management based on remediation of error patterns.

Therapy based on distinctive-feature theory generally involves one of two procedures. The clinician either groups the phonemes that represent a target feature or teaches one or a few phonemes that exemplify that feature in anticipation that correct production will generalize to other phonemes. In therapy based on phonological processes, the clinician helps the child eliminate those processes that cause groups of phonemes to be different from the standard model.

Although procedures based on distinctive features and those based on phonological processes were described separately, they are both directed by the same principles and in that sense cannot be separated. The ingenious clinician will select elements from each and integrate them to deal effectively with each child's problem. In part III of this text, specific therapy techniques are described that are based on these principles or combine them with traditional, behavioral, or communication-centered techniques.

REFERENCES

Blache, S. E. (1982). Minimal word pairs and distinctive feature training. In M. Crary (Ed.), *Phonological intervention: Concepts and procedures.* San Diego: College-Hill Press.

Blache, S. E., & Parsons, C. L. (1980). A linguistic approach to distinctive feature training. *Language, Speech and Hearing Services in Schools, 11,* 203–207.

Blache, S. E., Parsons, C. L., & Humphreys, J. M. (1981). A minimal-word pair model for teaching the linguistic significance of distinctive feature properties. *Journal of Speech and Hearing Disorders, 46,* 291–296.

Compton, A. (1970). Generative studies of children's phonological disorders. *Journal of Speech and Hearing Disorders, 35,* 315–339.

Compton, A. J., & Hutton, J. S. (1978). *Compton-Hutton phonological assessment.* San Francisco: Carousel House.

Costello, J. (1975). Articulation instruction based on distinctive features theory. *Language, Speech and Hearing Services in Schools, 6,* 61–71.

Costello, J., & Bosler, S. (1976). Generalization and articulation instruction. *Journal of Speech and Hearing Disorders, 35,* 344–353.

Costello, J., & Onstine, J. (1976). The modification of multiple articulation errors based on distinctive feature theory. *Journal of Speech and Hearing Disorders, 41,* 199–215.

Dunn, C. (1983). A framework for generalization in disordered phonology. *Journal of Childhood Communication Disorders, 7,* 46–58.

Dunn, C., & Till, J. A. (1982). Morphophonemic rule learning in normal and articulation-disordered children. *Journal of Speech and Hearing Research, 25,* 322–332.

Edwards, M. L. (1983). Selection criteria for developing therapy goals. *Journal of Childhood Communication Disorders, 7,* 36–45.

Edwards, M. L., & Bernhardt, B. (1973). *Phonological analyses of the speech of four children with language disorders.* Unpublished paper, Stanford University, Palo Alto.

Elbert, M. (1983). A case of phonological acquisition. *Topics in Language Disorders, 3,* 1–9.

Elbert, M. A., Shelton, R., & Arndt, W. (1967). A task for evaluation of articulation change: I. Development of methodology. *Journal of Speech and Hearing Research, 10,* 281–288.

Fokes, J. (1982). Problems confronting the theorist and practitioner in child phonology. In M. Crary (Ed.), *Phonological intervention: Concepts and procedures*. San Diego: College-Hill Press.

Griffith, F. A., Irwin, J. V., & Weston, A .J. (1980). A historical overview and critical assessment of the paired-stimuli technique for the modification of articulatory disorders. In W. D. Wolfe & D. J. Goulding (Eds.), *Articulation and learning*. Springfield: Charles C. Thomas.

Grunwell, P. (1982). *Clinical phonology*. Rockville, MD: Aspen Systems Corporation.

Grunwell, P. (1983). Phonological development in phonological disability. *Topics in Language Disorders, 3*, 62–76.

Hodson, B. W. (1980). *The assessment of phonological processes*. Danville, IL: The Interstate Printers and Publishers, Inc.

Hodson, B. W. (1982). Remediation of speech patterns associated with low levels of phonological performance. In M. Crary (Ed.), *Phonological intervention: Concepts and procedures*. San Diego: College-Hill Press.

Hodson, B. W., Chin, L., Redmond, B., & Simpson, R. (1983). Phonological evaluation and remediation of speech deviations of a child with a repaired cleft palate: A case study. *Journal of Speech and Hearing Disorders, 48*, 93–97.

Hodson, B. W., & Paden, E. (1983). *Targeting intelligible speech*. San Diego: College Hill Press.

Ingram, D. (1976). *Phonological disability in children*. New York: Elsevier.

Ingram, D. (1981). *Procedures for the phonological analysis of children's language*. Baltimore: University Park Press.

Lynch, J. I., Fox, D. R., & Brookshire, B. L. (1983). Phonological proficiency of two cleft palate toddlers with school-age follow-up. *Journal of Speech and Hearing Disorders, 48*, 274–285.

Marquardt, T., & Saxman, J. (1972). Language comprehension and auditory discrimination in articulation deficient kindergarten children. *Journal of Speech and Hearing Research, 15*, 382–390.

McMahon, K., Hodson, B. W., & Allen, E. (1983). Phonological analysis of cerebral palsied children's utterances. *Journal of Childhood Communication Disorders, 7*, 28–35.

McReynolds, L. V., & Bennett, S. (1972). Distinctive feature generalization in articulation training. *Journal of Speech and Hearing Disorders, 37*, 462–470.

McReynolds, L. V., & Elbert, M. (1981). Criteria for phonological process analysis. *Journal of Speech and Hearing Disorders, 46*, 197–204.

McReynolds, L. V., Engmann, D., & Dimmitt, K. (1974). Markedness theory and articulation errors. *Journal of Speech and Hearing Disorders, 39*, 93–103.

Menyuk, P. (1964). Comparison of grammar of children with functionally deviant and normal speech. *Journal of Speech and Hearing Research, 7*, 105–108.

Oller, D. K., & Eilers, R.E. (1975). Phonetic expectation and transcription validity. *Phonetica, 31*, 288–304.

Panagos, J. M. (1974). Persistence of the open syllable reinterpreted as a symptom of language disorder. *Journal of Speech and Hearing Disorders, 39*, 23–31.

Parker, F. (1976). Distinctive features in speech pathology: Phonology or phonemics? *Journal of Speech and Hearing Disorders, 41*, 23–29.

Paul, R., & Shriberg, L. D. (1982). Associations between phonology and syntax in speech-delayed children. *Journal of Speech and Hearing Research, 25*, 536–546.

Pollack, K .E. (1983). Individual preferences: Case study of a phonologically delayed child. *Topics in Language Disorders, 3*, 10–23.

Pollack, E., & Rees, N. (1972). Disorders of articulation: Some clinical applications of distinctive feature theory. *Journal of Speech and Hearing Disorders, 37*, 451–461.

Powell, J., & McReynolds, L. (1969). A procedure for testing position generalization from articulation training. *Journal of Speech and Hearing Research, 12*, 629–645.

Ruder, K. F., & Bunce, B. H. (1981). Articulation therapy using distinctive feature analysis to structure the training program: Two case studies. *Journal of Speech and Hearing Disorders, 46*, 59–65.

Ruscello, D. M. (1975). The importance of word position in articulation therapy. *Language, Speech and Hearing Services in Schools, 6*, 190–195.

Saxman, J. H., & Miller, J. F. (1973). Short term memory and language skills in articulation deficient children. *Journal of Speech and Hearing Research, 16*, 721–730.

Shriberg, L. D., & Kwiatkowski, J. (1980). *Natural process analysis.* New York: John Wiley and Sons.

Singh, S., Hayden, M. E., & Toombs, M. S. (1981). The role of distinctive features in articulation errors. *Journal of Speech ad Hearing Disorders, 46*, 174–183.

Singh, S., & Polen, S. (1972). The use of a distinctive feature model in speech pathology. *Acta Symbolica, 3*, 17–25.

Singh, S., & Singh, K. (1976). *Distinctive features: Principles and practices.* Baltimore: University Park Press.

Smit, A. B., & Bernthal, J. E. (1983). Performance of articulation-disordered children on language and perception measures. *Journal of Speech and Hearing Research, 26*, 124–136.

Toombs, M. S., Singh, S., & Hayden, M. E. (1981). Markedness of features in the articulatory substitutions of children. *Journal of Speech and Hearing Disorders, 46*, 184–190.

Van Riper, C. (1978). *Speech correction: Principles and methods* (6th ed.). Englewood Cliffs, NJ: Prentice-Hall.

Walsh, H. H. (1974). On certain practical inadequacies of distinctive feature systems. *Journal of Speech and Hearing Disorders, 39*, 32–43.

Weiner, F. F. (1979). *Phonological process analysis.* Baltimore: University Park Press.

Weiner, F. F. (1981a). Systematic sound preference as a characteristic of phonological disability. *Journal of Speech and Hearing Disorders, 46*, 281–286.

Weiner, F. F. (1981b). Treatment of phonological disability using the method of meaningful minimal contrast: Two case studies. *Journal of Speech and Hearing Disorders, 46*, 97–103.

Weiner, F. F., & Bankson, N. (1978). Teaching features. *Language, Speech and Hearing Services in Schools, 9*, 29–34.

Weston, A., & Irwin, J. (1971). Use of paired stimuli in modification of articulation. *Perceptual and Motor Skills, 32*, 947–957.

Winitz, H., & Bellerose, B. (1978). Interference and the persistence of articulatory responses. *Journal of Speech and Hearing Research, 21*, 715–721.

8

Communication-Centered Articulation Treatment

Communication-centered articulation therapy consists of practicing speech sounds in the verbal utterances of prosocial communicative activities in which correct responses are reinforced by natural consequences. For example, an activity used by one communication-oriented clinician was a plastic bubble basketball game. The player pulled a plunger, which shot the ball into one of several concentric circles to score 2, 4, 6, 8, or 10. To pull the plunger the child said "I want a turn" if he had an /r/ deviation, "I want to shoot" if his problem was /ʃ/, or some other response that gave him a chance to practice his target sound. Keeping score was also an opportunity to use responses that fit individual clients' articulation needs, such as "My score is six" for /s/ or /r/ problems, "Last time my score was five" for /l/, /r/, or /v/ problems.

The clinician made this game a privilege. He used it only briefly in each lesson; thus it continued to be a high-interest activity. On occasion he had the children play with a real ball and backboard. Some also played basketball in their neighborhoods; hence the activity was useful rehearsal for real-life speech and resulted in significant articulation improvement, not only during therapy but in the clients' daily communication as well.

This chapter was written by **Gordon M. Low**, **Parley W. Newman**, and **Mildred T. Ravsten**, assistant professor of educational psychology and member of the core faculty of the Comprehensive Clinic at Brigham Young University, Provo, Utah.

In a relatively early study of a communication-centered approach to articulation therapy, a total of 94 mentally retarded children were studied. Of these, 30 received communication-centered therapy. 26 received traditional therapy, and 38 received no therapy as a control group. The communication-centered group made significantly greater improvement (Lassers & Low, 1960).

Communication-centered instruction (CCI) has been attempted in some form or other for many years. Early efforts to embed articulation improvement in a pragmatic or communication-centered context include those of Backus and Dunn (1947). Backus and Beasley (1951) and Low, Crerar and Lassers (1959). More recently Wulz, Hall and Klein (1983) described similar procedures for home-centered communication training. Increased emphasis on communication pragmatics has given new impetus to CCI not only for the improvement of phonological aspects of language but in the acquisition of all aspects of language and in all other communication-based learning. In the interest of explaining CCI in terms of contemporary principles of learning, a brief rationale is presented for the kind of communication-centered instruction we have been using and refining since 1959.

RATIONALE FOR COMMUNICATION-CENTERED INSTRUCTION

"Communication is the social matrix of psychiatry," according to Ruesch and Bateson (1951). They further suggest that communication is the "one single system for the understanding of the multiple aspects of human behavior" (p. 5).

Validation for these assumptions is found in (a) the interactive conceptions of child development of Piaget (1952a, 1952b) and others (Bruner, 1966, 1975; Aronson, Bridgeman & Geffner, 1978; Sharan, 1980); (b) the coincidence of information theory and communication theory (Berlo, 1960; Cherry, 1978; Garner, 1962; Greeno & Bjork, 1973; Littlejohn, 1978), both of which represent the processes of human learning, including the more simplistic conceptions of learning respresented by operant conditioning, classical conditioning, chaining, and other traditional learning explanations (Gagné, 1977); (c) the coincidence of the problems, instructional approaches, and disciplines of learning disabilities and communication disorders (Lerner, 1981); (d) the logical representation of learning as sign behavior, of which language is the chief example (Osgood, 1957b); (e) the acknowledgment by language specialists that communication, i.e., the pragmatic situation in which language is used and has meaning, is the natural and ideal context for language acquisition (Holland, 1975; Muma, 1978; Rees, 1978), and "the ultimate goal of any language therapy for language disordered children" (Lucas, 1980, p. 223); (f) the apparent relationship of communicative intent and phonological production, as suggested by Leonard's (1971) finding that the speech of a 6-year-old child was characterized by more deviant articulations of /z/ in utterances carrying the least information, and Menyuk's (1980) finding that children with misarticulations, when attempting to communicate information that is important to them, modify their utterance so that it more closely approximates normal speech.

These validations appear to be ample justification for Ruesch and Bateson's conceptions about the place of communication in relation to other aspects of human behavior. We also believe that they justify a companion premise to Ruesch and Bateson's assumption that "communication is the social matrix of psychiatry," namely, that *communication is the matrix of human learning.* We believe that optimum learning takes place only under optimum communicative conditions. It is on this premise that a communication-centered instructional approach for improving speech articulation is based. The principles and procedures are described below.

PRINCIPLES OF COMMUNICATION-CENTERED INSTRUCTION

Communication-centered instruction (CCI) for articulation improvement generally consists of instruction and practice of speech articulation in oral communicative interchange among two or more people. It does not postpone the carry-over or generalization stage of usual speech therapy. Instead, CCI uses procedures of carry-over during each instructional period and thus also during the normal communication experiences the client has between instructional sessions.

Principles of CCI can be stated in various ways. Since a learning formula that includes *stimulus, response,* and *reinforcement* has already been explained (chapter 6), CCI principles are described under these headings, along with explanations of how communication-learning is a system and how CCI takes that fact into account. *System* here refers to the interdependence of all processes and events in the sequence of receiving and sending messages, so that a disturbance at any point can affect other points in the system.

Principles of Communicative Stimulus

The practice situation should be like the performance situation.

The principles regarding stimulus conditions outlined in chapter 6 are important considerations in communication-centered instruction. Stimulus conditions in learning generally include all those elements of the learning situation of which the learner is aware. Hence, these conditions constitute a context or complex of stimuli, not just a single stimulus. As clinicians, we may think that we are offering a client a single stimulus when we ask him or her to imitate a particular speech sound. The fact is that the speech sound presented for imitation is only part of the stimulus complex. Other elements in the stimulus complex are the clinician's dress, grooming, looks, mannerisms, gestures, etc.; the instructions the clinician gives the client; the seating arrangement; the room situation; the expectations both the clinician and client have developed in prior speech-imitation episodes; the generality of client-clinician relationship; and other elements of the situation that may justly be called the *pragmatic elements of interpersonal exchange.*

An important implication of the stimulus-complex conception of the context of learning is that what is learned by the client is not only the speech sound, but its association with all other elements of the stimulus complex.

Herein lies an important explanation of the too-frequent failure of carry-over of new speech learning to the client's daily speech usage. This explanation is found in studies of learning transfer, learning retention, and carry-over.

Some years ago, Osgood concluded that "where stimuli are varied and responses are functionally identical, positive transfer and retroactive facilitation are obtained, the magnitude of both increasing as the similarity among the stimulus members increases" (1949, p. 135). Other similar educational principles are stated by Ellis (1965): (a) "Transfer of training is greatest when the training conditions are highly similar to those of the ultimate testing conditions," and (b) "When a task requires the learner to make the same response to new but similar stimuli, positive transfer increases with increasing stimulus similarity" (pp. 72–73). Hulse, Deese, and Egeth (1975) explain problems of learning carry-over as "cue-dependent forgetting." They suggest that "when we forget something, it does not necessarily mean that the memory trace is lost; it may merely be inaccessible because the current context does not permit retrieval schemes that are congruent with the encoding schemes employed at the time of original learning" (p. 359).

One of the authors of this chapter (GML) recalls a vivid experience as a student clinician with an aphasic client whose speech was unintelligible jargon even after numerous careful attempts at imitation. Together they worked on words that appeared to have some communicative use to the client, including the words "come in." Finally, out of desperation, and with a subsequent insight that has remained primary in this clinician's understanding of remedial instruction, the clinician had the client rehearse the words "come in" in preparation for the daily visits of her friends. She grumbled as she forced herself out of her chair in response to the housekeeper's knock on the door. The clinician asked her to repeat the words "come in" before she crossed the room to the door. She said /ʃembɑ, ʃembɑ/, but when she took hold of the doorknob and pulled the door open, a smile came over her face and she said, /kʌm ɪn/ with perfectly acceptable articulation.

Many clinicians have had this same kind of experience with aphasic and other clients and have realized that clients may demonstrate remarkable success when the stimulus conditions of the testing or performance situation are similar to those of the original learning situation. To use an earlier explanation, these instances of remarkable recall occur because the performance situation permits "retrieval schemes that are congruent with the encoding schemes employed at the time of original learning" (Hulse, Deese, & Egeth, 1975, p. 359).

From this rationale we infer the principle of CCI related to stimulus context that *the practice situation should be similar to the performance situation.* Implied in this principle is the concept of rehearsal in which speech practice simulates daily communication much more than does imitative speech practice. Conditions of clients' daily communication often consist of communicative interaction with other individuals and groups in various activities, including classroom instruction, play at home and school, family activities, encounters with the mail carrier and other community helpers, etc. Practice situations simulate these settings and activities, most often in group instruction. An illustration of the principle as applied to improvement of articulation follows.

Ms. Jones, a speech clinician, engages in a non-communication-centered instructional program for improvement of Gary's /t/k/ substitutions. She has the child practice /k/ in various ways, including repeating a list of /k/-words, such as *car, cake, call, cat, coat, come, pick, tack, talk.* With almost 100% /k/ accuracy in the word list in the clinic, the clinician is pleased to go on to carry-over or generalization activities. She next practices the /k/ in word combinations including such sentences as *Pick a number, Talk to the parrot, Come in, Call the cat,* again achieving a high degree of /k/ accuracy. Then Ms. Jones has occasion to visit Gary's home. She knocks on the door. Gary opens it and says /tʌmɪn/. Ms. Jones is so discouraged she has thoughts of leaving the field of speech-language pathology.

Why has this well-learned correct use of /k/ in the clinic not generalized to the home situation? Figures 8.1 and 8.2 illustrate the stimulus complex explanation of the problem. In Figure 8.1, the stimulus cues include a, b, c, d, e, f, g, whereas in Figure 8.2, the stimulus complex consists of the cues a, b, c, h, i, j, k. To increase the probability of carry-over, the clinician should make the practice situation like the performance situation, which would result in the conditions of Figures 8.3 and 8.4. In Figure 8.3, the stimulus cues are a, b, c, h, i, j, k, and in Figure 8.4, they are essentially the same. On the basis of this similarity of stimulus cues in practice and real life, it is safe to predict that a correct utterance in the clinic will carry over to correct production at home. Of course, making the practice and performance conditions alike is best achieved by making the clinic situation like the client's daily life, not trying to make the client's daily life like the clinic. It is much easier and more effective to ask the family to help the client at home if the help they are expected to give fits the client's daily communication opportunities instead of involving contrived speech practice totally unrelated to family communication activities.

Principles of Communicative Response

The response should be (a) useful to the client—both powerful and frequently occurring in the client's daily communication, and (b) at the client's level of functioning in (c) whole-part-whole practice.

Closely related to the principle of communicative stimulus conditions is the principle of *communicative response.* Deciding what kind of practice material clinicians should use in helping clients improve their articulation brings up two interesting ways of looking at response in the learning formula: (a) the relation of the error speech sound to the rest of the practice word in which it is uttered, and (b) the relation of the practice word to the client's communicative reality.

Words as Contexts of Speech Sounds.   Put simply, more often than not spoken words consist of several speech sounds. The target response in articulation improvement is the correct production, within words, of the client's error sound. The other sounds of the word are part of the stimulus context, and the word itself becomes subject to the principle of communicative stimulus conditions along with all other stimulus elements in the pragmatic communicative situation. For this reason, the word chosen for articulation practice must be one from the client's daily communicative lexicon.

Clinic

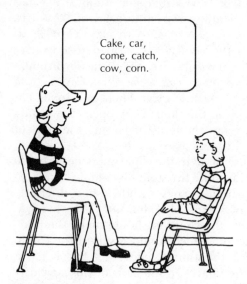

Home

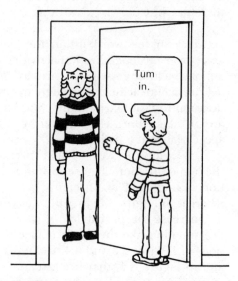

FIGURE 8.1
Stimulus cues in practice situation: (a) clinician, (b) child, (c) come, (d) word list, (e) clinician seated, (f) child seated, (g) chairs.

FIGURE 8.2
Stimulus cues in performance situation: (a) clinician, (b) child, (c) come, (h) clinician standing, (i) child standing, (j) door, (k) reaching for door.

Clinic

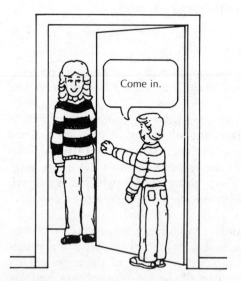

Home

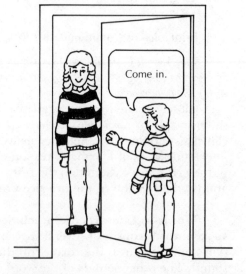

FIGURE 8.3
Stimulus cues in practice situation: (a) clinician, (b) child, (c) come, (h) clinician standing, (i) child standing, (j) door, (k) reaching for door.

FIGURE 8.4
Stimulus cues in performance situation: (a) clinician, (b) child, (c) come, (h) clinician standing, (i) child standing, (j) door, (k) reaching for door.

Words as Communicative Responses.   Because words are the natural contexts of articulated speech sounds, practice words used in articulation improvement should be words that are communicatively useful to the client. This same conclusion is supported by the fact that the practice word is not only part of the stimulus array but is also the response itself. Hence, conditions governing the choice of responses for optimum learning again dictate that responses be communicative in nature (Holland, 1975).

The first important condition of communicative response is that the response should be *useful* to the learner, occurring frequently in his or her daily communication. Obviously, this is not a very different requirement from that of providing natural, real-life learning conditions for response practice. However, in this instance, it is the response, as well as the stimulus, that is drawn from the client's daily life. Coupling real-life responses with real-life communicative stimulus conditions ensures maximum carry-over of the newly acquired speech sound that is embedded in the context of a frequently recurring word. Indeed, it ensures natural reinforcement of the generalized new behavior outside the clinic even though the clinician is not present, thus extending the therapy experience to the daily life of the client.

Another important feature of communicative response is that of *whole-part-whole* practice. Life offers so little opportunity for learning parts of wholes as isolated experiences that clinicians must be careful not to violate natural learning conditions in their well-intentioned practice of isolated speech sounds. However, *part practice* of speech sounds can be very useful as long as it is consistently accompanied by *whole practice*, i.e., the practice of the target sound within the whole context of (a) the communicative response—the practice word or words that contain the target sound, and (b) the communicative situation, in which the client interacts with other people. Under these circumstances, the relation of the part to the whole is realized.

Whole-part-whole learning is an example of *main-task learning*. In main-task learning the student is involved in the ultimate task, which it is his or her goal to achieve, early in training and continuing throughout. In articulation therapy, the main task is effective oral communication, with correct articulation, in daily interpersonal relationships.

In whole-part-whole learning, clients of preschool age may be involved in making requests of others, giving information, offering help, etc., as the communicative activity develops and all children in the group participate in the interaction. Older children may participate in small-group discussion, panel symposia, rehearsal for a classroom presentation, etc. Responses in these situations are often preselected, sometimes spontaneous, and occasionally corrected for articulation improvement. The whole practice of these responses is achieved in a broadly pragmatic sense—with a total communicative context of interpersonal relationships characterized by experience in using presuppositions, i.e., information shared by communicants before communicating (Bates, 1976); non-verbal as well as verbal signs with their semantics, syntactics, and pragmatics (Morris, 1946); speech acts, which communicate intentions to bring about expected response from others (Searle, 1969; Lucas, 1980, 1983; Gallagher & Prutting, 1983); deixis, i.e., use of language that indicates relation of communicators to each other and to other elements in the environment (Clark &

Garnica, 1974; Ingram, 1971); perceptual salience, i.e., emphasis on features of form more than on content or conceptual features (Odom & Corbin, 1973; Parisi, 1974); and whatever else accompanies a meaningful communicative interchange among peers and their adult leader.

The *part* practice in whole-part-whole learning utilizes any useful procedure for achieving correct production of a deviant sound. Any of the many ways of increasing a client's auditory and oral kinesthetic discrimination and appropriate articulatory placement may be used as a brief, necessary diversion from the main task, which is interpersonal communication, usually among members of a group. Although CCI is most often group instruction, clinicians may find it effective to supplement group instruction with individual therapy in which the client may be rehearsed alone in the responses and activities in which he will engage in the group. In individual or in group instruction, part practice for any or all clients may interrupt the activity for a few moments as described by Backus and Beasley (1951) or, if necessary, for more extended periods as described in other chapters of this text. The purpose, of course, is to enable the client to participate in group interaction more effectively and with more accurate speech articulation.

An additional feature of communicative response is that of requiring a response whose difficulty is a challenge to the learner but not so difficult as to be discouraging. In other words, *the response should be at the client's level of functioning.*

Obviously, if a client has deviant articulation, he usually will not be able to produce the sound accurately in conversational speech, even when given a model to imitate. Often, however, after two or three attempts to say the sound correctly in a word, a client may improve his error sound ever so slightly and begin to use the improved sound in communication and communication practice. Gradual improvement may occur as the client uses his or her best daily response until articulation is correct.

One might believe that permitting the client to speak the target sound incorrectly in communication may interfere with the eventual acquisition of the correct sound. Our experience has demonstrated otherwise, as might be expected in light of the process of normal speech-sound development in children. As mentioned in chapter 4 on assessment, Olmsted (1971) analyzed the speech of 100 children ranging in age from 15 to 54 months. He found that children do not acquire individual speech sounds suddenly, but gradually over time, with extended periods during which any particular sound is produced both correctly and incorrectly. There are gradual increases in the percentage of successes and decreases in the relative numbers of errors. Coexistence of success and error, then, is the most frequent pattern of developing use of phones.

Ingram (1976) discusses speech-articulation therapy in which the goal is correct production as compared with the adult model. He refers to this as the "fell-swoop principle" and argues that the transition from the child's utterance to adult pronunciation in one step is based on an unjustified assumption. He gives several reasons why this approach is unsound, and proposes adoption of the "gradualness principle" based on the assumption that a child will progress more rapidly to his next stage of development than to one several stages ahead. He even suggests that the fell swoop principle actually retards development.

An explanation can also be given that is consistent with what is known about learning. First of all, in non-communication-centered articulation therapy the client may continue to use the incorrect sound in his daily communication while he learns to produce the sound correctly. Surely this can be at least as harmful as practicing a gradually improving but not completely accurate speech sound. Secondly, we believe that the conditions of successive approximation are as much at work in this gradual improvement, while the client actually uses his newly developing sound, as they are in those other shaping procedures in which the client must be able to produce the sound correctly before being allowed to use it in communication. Thirdly, in a communication-centered approach it is not necessary for a client to unlearn the association of the response with inappropriate cues that occur in non-communication-centered instruction and which interfere with stimulus generalization: cues such as nonsense syllables as contexts for target sounds or uncommon words or adult-child interactions only. In CCI, carry-over is provided for in each clinical session.

The response that is chosen in CCI should have one other quality. To be appropriately communicative in nature, *the response should be communicatively powerful.* That is, the result of the utterance should in one way or another be satisfying to the person who speaks it. The fact is that most responses used in communication are communicatively powerful, but some are more powerful than others. The literature on infant language is replete with observations and explanations of the kinds of communicative responses children develop. Among these, Antinucci and Parisi suggest that language may be "descriptive" on the one hand and "requestive" on the other (1975) or, as Snyder suggests (1975), "declarative" and "imperative." The implication of these classifications is that declaring and describing are sharing acts and may require less reaction than requesting and commanding. "Manding" (Skinner, 1957) or commanding or requesting may be more powerful than naming and thus more useful in therapy.

The more powerful communicative responses are those that require a reaction from the listener to the speaker's communicative effort. All communicative effort, however, is directed at influencing others and requires some reaction, even though it may appear to be as undemanding as naming, labeling, or describing.

In relation to articulation improvement, the purpose in choosing responses that have power is not only to fulfill the client's need for successful communicative interaction, as important as that may be, but also to establish a condition of learning which no instruction should be without, and that is a meaningful and satisfying consequence of the practice response. Obviously, a powerful response is one that causes something to happen. As we shall see in the next section on communicative reinforcement, the degree of reinforcement of a communicative consequence is directly related to the degree of power of the communicative response.

In communicative activities for children, such responses as "May I have a ____?" "What do you want?" "Ready, aim, fire." "May I look?" "Sit down," "I want to run." "I want the red one." are chosen to provide communicatively powerful responses in which target speech sounds may be practiced. These responses are rehearsed in activities which present the need for the client to say the response in order to obtain the communicative result that the activity calls for.

We recall our efforts to get non-talking Johnny to speak by setting up a ping-pong-ball cannon which required stepping heavily on a rubber bellows to shoot it. Each child in turn became (a) the retriever of the ball, (b) the marksman who aimed the cannon, (c) the one who jumped on the bellows, and finally (d) the commander who said, "Ready, aim, shoot." It was with considerable interest that the clinician and observers waited for Johnny to give the command. What could he do with peer expectations so high? He spoke, right on cue, and, having spoken in the group, continued to do so in subsequent therapy sessions. For the child with /r/ distortion and the one with /ɜ˞/ deviation, the response was also an opportunity for articulation practice in a communicatively powerful activity. This is an example of a single communicative activity serving the different articulation-improvement needs of several clients.

Principles of Communicative Reinforcement

Communicative reinforcement in communication-centered instruction is the fulfillment of the purpose of the communicative response.

Having argued that establishing communicative stimulus conditions and using communicative responses is highly advantageous in improving articulation, we introduce what should be a rather clinching conclusion to our case for communication-centered articulation therapy, i.e., *communicative reinforcement.* We have already referred to "mand"-type communicative language as having particular value as a vehicle in articulation improvement. Among its benefits is the natural, communicative reinforcement that follows mand responses in the home and elsewhere in the absence of the clinician.

In a parent group in our clinic one day, we explained reinforcement in the learning formula. The following account was given to introduce the topic.

Mrs. Smith walked into her kitchen with an armful of laundry. She noticed Jimmy, her mentally retarded child, standing in front of the kitchen sink. Jimmy had never uttered anything that sounded like words. But today, he said, "Wa, wa." Mrs Smith dropped her jaw, and her laundry, and thought very quickly, "This is Jimmy's first word. What can I do to be sure he says it again? I know—reinforcement. I studied that in child psychology."

"Let's see. I could give him a token reinforcer—a tally mark on the bulletin board or a piece of candy. No, maybe I should let him choose from a reinforcement menu—a look at the kaleidoscope, a swing on the top bar of the bunk bed, a chance to feed the fish. Oh, but how about using the probability principle. I could use the high-probability behavior (HPB) to reinforce the low-probability behavior (LPB). Hmm, the low-probability behavior (LPB) is saying "wa, wa"—but what is the HPB? Well, it could be his favorite mealtime activity: smearing peanut butter on the table. Oh, what to do?"

By this time the parents' worst fears were confirmed: These people at the university really are in their ivory tower.

"What would you do as parents to reinforce Jimmy's response?" we asked.

"Give him a drink of water," they replied in unison.

"Yes," we assured them, "the fulfillment of the purpose of Jimmy's communicative effort."

How strange that such a simple concept could be so distorted in the giant step from the shaping of pigeons' behavior to the reinforcement of human learning responses. Let us examine the application of communicative reinforcement to articulation therapy.

Earlier, reference was made to *imperative* language or, as some would call it, *requestive* or *illocutionary* language. It was pointed out that all communicative efforts are intended to influence others, but that some efforts are more demanding than others. Requests and commands have more power than describing or naming, so they are capable of more powerful reinforcement.

Several years ago one of the authors (GML) was visited in his home by relatives who brought with them their non-speaking 3-year-old. David made sounds and many non-verbal communicative efforts, but expressed no intelligible words. That evening it was suggested that everyone go to the movies while David and his uncle, the speech therapist, stayed home.

David took a seated position at one end of a long hallway, his uncle at the other. The uncle said, "Do you want the ball?" David didn't say anything. The uncle-clinician said /pu-pu/ with a high pitched voice, like a cuckoo clock, and rolled the ball to David. When David was ready to return the ball, the clinician said, "Wait, /pu-pu/, okay, roll the ball." Soon David said /pu-pu/ when the clinician asked, "Do you want the ball?' Of course, /pu-pu/ doesn't come up very often in a conversation, so the clinician began encouraging David to say "yes" instead of /pu-pu/. When the movie-goers returned, David was saying /jɛs/, with good articulation, even of /s/, to any of a variety of questions such as "Do you want some candy?" "Are you a little boy?" "Is this your daddy?"

The reinforcement aspects of this situation included controlling an adult, receiving the ball upon requesting it, the approbation of the clinician, and, of vital importance, the reinforcement at home of the same response in the same kinds of activity as practiced with the clinician.

Principles Related to Communication-Learning as a System

A system instructional approach should be used to improve or compensate for dysfunctions of communication processes and physiological dysfunctions that are relevant to the communication disorder.

Communication-centered instruction is based on the premise that processes of communication and learning function as a system that includes both the *interpersonal* exchange among communicants and the *intrapersonal* processing within one individual. The communication-learning system includes the input processes of reception—auditory, visual, and haptic (tactile-kinesthetic) sensation; the integrative processes of perception and conceptualization; the organizational processes of ideation and codification; the output processes of expression—speaking, writing, and other motor production; the pervasive facilitating processes of attention, memory and motivation-affect; and the communicative relationship of the communicants within the system. The learning features of stimulus reception, response emission, and response reinforcement generally coincide, respectively, with the communication processes of reception, expression, and feedback internally from within the individual and externally from the reaction of others. This model of a communication-learning system is similar to other mediational models of human behavior (Gagné, 1977; Osgood, 1957a, 1957b; Wepman, 1960).

In addition to the emphasis in CCI on specific communication dysfunction, CCI is designed to take into account all communication-learning processes and their interdependent function. This is a system approach that may provide for isolation of individual processes for momentary analysis but that also requires that these processes be considered as parts of a whole so that their function can be fully appreciated and realized in relation to the whole. These features of a system approach were described earlier in relation to conditions of communicative stimulus, response, and reinforcement in communication-centered instruction. Learning in a total, real-life context is more of a system approach than learning that involves practice of responses in isolation from the total context.

One of the compelling reasons for a system approach to articulation improvement is the immeasurable complexity of interrelationships among significant part functions of speech articulation. One prominent part is auditory perception. Auditory percepts serve as patterns for motor production of speech sounds, and auditory feedback serves as a monitor in guiding speech production to those patterns (Winitz, 1969). The importance of auditory input is discussed in chapter 9.

As significant as auditory processing is to speech articulation, obviously it is only part of total speech production behavior. Another important component, of course, is movement of the articulatory mechanism. Further, there is tactile-kinesthetic monitoring of articulatory movements which accompanies and helps to guide the neuromotor patterning that determines these movements.

This interrelationship among auditory, haptic, and motor processes in speech articulation appears even more complex when we consider that their interdependence occurs not only during their concurrent functioning, but also during their preresponse and postresponse functioning in feedforward and feedback interactions, e.g, in coarticulation. In addition, there is the further complexity of interrelationships among the many aspects of language of which phonology is but one, namely, the lexical, morphological, syntactic, semantic and pragmatic features of human communication.

The complexity of interrelationships among the various processes involved in speech articulation appears to require a system approach to articulation improvement, which CCI is designed to accomplish. In this connection, CCI addresses a serious problem in remedial instruction: Which of the many part functions in the total complexity of parts should we try to improve and which should we use to compensate for the dysfunction of other parts? In one sense, since all processes are involved during real communication, CCI almost automatically takes care of this problem without the need for the time-consuming and imprecise assessment of the various possible communication dysfunctions.

It is common practice in remedial instruction to (a) improve a client's weak communication processes and skills, and (b) compensate for his weaknesses by utilizing his strong processes and skills (Lerner, 1981). In a system approach, improvement and compensation occur together. For example, in CCI auditory-perceptual training accompanies tactile-kinesthetic-perceptual training during actual speech production, thus training the weak process and capitalizing on the strong processes at the same time. CCI provides for such multisensory remedial instruction with part practice as necessary, but with major emphasis on whole practice in the communication context.

Conditions of Communication-Centered Learning Contexts

Having described the major conditions of stimulus, response, and reinforcement in communication-centered articulation therapy, let us consider the general conditions involved in establishing a communication-centered learning context. We begin with reference again to the premise that communication is the matrix of learning and that the optimum matrix for learning is an optimally effective communication situation.

Communication, as a context for learning, consists of the interaction of two or more people in a meaningful setting. In CCI the communicants are a group of clients and their clinician. The behaviors of clients toward each other, and toward the clinician, and the clinician's behavior toward the clients are important elements in the total communicative context.

For the past several years, we have studied client and clinician communication behaviors, particularly in relation to the communicative context for the improvement of speech and language. Our efforts resulted in the development of two rating scales: the Communication Competence Scale (CCS) for assessing client behavior in CCI, and the Developing Communication Competence Scale (DCCS) for assessing clinician behavior and situation conditions in CCI. In developing the CCS we (a) identified client behaviors important to effective communicative interaction, (b) constructed a scale for assessing client communication competence, (c) used the scale to assess client performance in group CCI, and (d) refined the scale through factor analysis of rating data and use of the scale in training student clinicians in CCI. Similar steps were followed in developing the DCCS.

Contents of the CCS and DCCS are described here to indicate (a) what communication behaviors of children are necessary for an optimum communication learning context, and (b) what instructional behaviors of clinicians are necessary to encourage the desired child behavior. Together these scales are unique in that they (a) describe the teacher behaviors that encourage specific pupil behaviors—pupil behavior is thus the dependent variable in the learning formula, not teacher behavior, as in so many descriptions of effective teaching, and (b) provide an organized system of assessment of pupil and teacher behavior that the clinician can use without paper and pencil in *concurrent diagnostic teaching*, i.e., making immediate adjustments in instruction based on concurrent pupil behavior.

The main attributes of communication competence that were identified through factor analysis and other validation studies and applications are listed in Table 8.1. It will be noted that there are three major attributes of communication competence: communication-learning readiness, communicative relationships, and communicative intentions. These categories factored out in analysis of nearly 2,000 individual CCS rating sheets.

Each of the three main attributes has three subattributes. Communication-learning readiness consists of attending, imitating, and cooperating The category of communicative relationships consists of caring, helping, and sharing. The communicative intentions category consists of self-initiating, trying to cause, and leading.

In each of the nine subattributes there are two predictor items and one criterion item to make up a total of 27 scale items.

TABLE 8.1
Attributes of Communication Competence (CCS)

I. Communication-Learning Readiness

Attending
   1.   Makes eye contact with central person or object
   2.   Maintains interest
   3.   Pays attention

Imitating
   4.   Imitates actions of others
   5.   Imitates words of others
   6.   Imitates others

Cooperating
   7.   Willingly does what others expect
   8.   Accepts help from others
   9.   Cooperates with others

II. Communicative Relationships

Caring
   10.   Acts positively toward others: listens to, directs comments to, touches, smiles, etc.
   11.   Looks out for the interests of others: shows concern for others' well being
   12.   Shows caring behavior toward others

Helping
   13.   Helps others with tasks
   14.   Encourages others to participate
   15.   Helps others

Sharing
   16.   Gives material or information to others
   17.   Accepts material from others
   18.   Shares with others

III. Communicative Intentions

Self-Initiating
   19.   Acts without being prompted
   20.   Expresses ideas spontaneously
   21.   Shows initiative

Trying to Cause
   22.   Makes requests
   23.   Sets example for others to follow
   24.   Tries to make something happen

Leading
   25.   Gets others to follow his or her directions or example
   26.   Influences others to look to him or her for ideas or help
   27.   Leads others

Main attributes of the DCCS are shown in Table 8.2. These are the conditions that clinicians establish to help clients develop communication competence. In the DCCS, previously described principles of CCI are repre-

TABLE 8.2
Attributes of Developing Communication Competence (DCCS)

What Clinician Does in General to Enhance Client's Communication Competence
1. Explains or has child explain expected language and /or action
2. Models or has child model expected language and/or action
3. Structures materials and sequence of events to encourage children to perform expected language and/or action with minimal teacher direction
4. Requires language that is natural for the situation in which it is used
5. Encourages every child to participate
6. Encourages child's best effort to perform expected language and/or action
7. Allows time for children to perform expected language and/or action
8. Has children practice part of the expected language and/or action when whole is difficult
9. Plans situation that provides natural consequences for expected language and/or action
10. Encourages children to perform expected language and/or action willingly
11. Encourages language and/or action by approving that behavior in others

What Clinician Does to Enhance Children's Attending
12. Shows natural enthusiasm through speech and action
13. Creates a feeling of anticipation
14. Plans activities and materials that stimulate and hold children's attention
15. Encourages children to pay attention

What Clinician Does to Enhance Children's Imitating
16. Has children rehearse language and/or action

What Clinician Does to Enhance Children's Cooperating
17. Discourages misbehavior through logical consequences: withholding, firmness, etc.

What Clinician Does to Enhance Children's Caring, Helping, Sharing
18. Demonstrates caring toward children: listens to, directs comments to, gently touches, smiles, shows concern for children's interests
19. Encourages children to look out for the interests of others, to show concern for others' well being
20. Encourages children to help others to participate
21. Plans situation that provides for children to give to and receive from others help, information, and materials
22. Encourages children to give to and receive from others help, information, and materials

What Clinician Does to Enhance Children's Self-Initiating
23. Plans situation that provides for children to act or speak spontaneously
24. Plans situation that provides natural consequences for spontaneous language and/or action

What Clinician Does to Enhance Children's Trying to Cause
25. Plans situation that provides for children to communicate powerfully in a way to make something happen
26. Encourages children to communicate powerfully in a way to make something happen

What Clinician Does to Enhance Children's Leading
27. Structures situation to provide for children to take the lead in activities

sented as general items related to defining, obtaining, and reinforcing responses. Also included are items related to what clinicians do to enhance various CCS behaviors, such as attending and imitating.

These two scales are useful as tests of client and clinician effectiveness in relation to communication competence. Their greatest benefit, however, is in the clinician's use of their defined attributes while actually teaching. If the clinician becomes proficient in evaluating clients' CCS behavior and his own DCCS behavior when using the written scales, he or she can then use those evaluation skills during actual teaching, without using the paper-and-pencil scales. Thus the clinician can concurrently evaluate and adapt instruction to meet the changing needs of the client. The ability to guide one's diagnostic teaching with constructs of CCS and DCCS is essential in communication-centered instruction. Regardless of one's ability to help clients improve the correctness of their articulation, clinicians cannot be competent in communication-centered articulation therapy unless they naturally, or through training, can establish a CCS/DCCS context in their articulation therapy group.

PROCEDURES OF COMMUNICATION-CENTERED ARTICULATION THERAPY

Diagnosis in Communication-Centered Instruction

The usual initial procedure in improving most communication disorders is that of diagnosis with the intent of arriving at a prescription for improvement of the disorder. Diagnosis of articulation disorders may consist of several steps or phases, most of which are universally used by speech clinicians. Some diagnostic procedures, on the other hand, are specifically designed for use with a particular instructional approach. Some of these are described in chapter 4, and in such other reviews as those by Darley (1979). CCI uses many of the usual procedures, but adds some that are necessary for effective communication-centered instruction. Only these additional procedures are described in detail in this chapter.

Case History.   Assessment of conditions relevant to CCI is approached as evaluation of the total communication system. Thus information about both the client and those who communicate with the client is relevant. Besides this information usually assembled from case history interviews and referral reports, information is obtained that is particularly related to the conditions of stimulus, response, and reinforcement as defined in communication-centered articulation therapy. For example, with respect to communicative *stimulus* conditions, making the practice situation like the performance situation requires the clinician to know something about the client's performance situation—home, play, and school activities, particularly communication activities and opportunities. Parents are asked to report on the opportunities their child has for communication. This information may encourage the parents to arrange more communication experiences for the child at home, but it will also be useful to the clinician in planning to simulate the client's daily communication experiences. If the child attends school, similar information can be obtained from the child's teacher so the clinician can plan school-type activities that will be like those the child will experience with his own teacher and classmates.

In reviewing the home and school situations it is useful to obtain names of family members, friends, pets, etc., and information about the kinds of communicative *responses* the child has opportunity to use. There are specific expressions families and teachers use, and it may be far more fruitful for the clinician to rehearse the client in commonly occurring responses expected at home and school than to require the parents and teacher to use responses that the clinician decides might be useful. The clinician's familiarity with curricula and textbooks at various grade levels is a decided advantage in understanding teacher information about daily communication responses used in classroom activities. Whether in group or individual instruction, whether the instruction is communication-centered or not, the client benefits little from the use of words for articulation practice whose probability of occurring in home or school is less than optimal.

Parent and teacher information about the client's communication opportunities may also include information as to the opportunity for powerful *reinforcement*, i.e., for the client to use mand responses that make something happen, that influence someone else with direct observable consequences. There are frequent opportunities for use of such responses at the dinner table, in parent-child discussions, in play, in classroom presentations, etc. The clinician needs to know about these in order to simulate like experiences.

If, in the assessment of communicative stimulus, response, and reinforcement conditions in the home and school, the clinician finds these conditions to be inadequate, he or she may profitably train parents and teachers in arranging better communication circumstances for the client, such as the more effective communication activities that are used in the clinic. We remember the mother who couldn't think of a way to involve her child in communicatively powerful experiences. Another mother said, "You drive all the way to the clinic past many stop lights. Why don't you have Bobby tell you 'red-stop' and 'green-go'?" Subsequent trips to the clinic were probably as beneficial to the mother and child as the daily clinic experience itself, both in mother-child relationships and in language development.

Assessment.   In CCI, assessment may include many traditional procedures for evaluating articulation, auditory processing, language, and other features of the communication system. In addition, since CCI is a system approach, there are assessments that must be made of the various elements of the communication system, and their functioning within that total system, that are not usually included in articulation diagnosis.

From earlier descriptions of the communication-learning context in CCI, it should be apparent that evaluation related to articulation disorders must also include assessment of the communication-learning situation itself, both the client's daily relationships in the home and school and in the instructional situation in the clinic. It is very likely that some of the factors which contribute to a child's articulation deviation are in his relationships with his family. Certainly it is not unusual to find immaturities of speech articulation associated with the client's social-emotional immaturity, much of which may be attributed to the child's communication failures in the home. At the same time, part of the reason for persisting articulation problems may be found in the lack of adequate opportunity for successful communication experiences in the therapy situation itself.

One of the first diagnostic concerns in CCI is the degree of success and failure the client has in daily communication experiences in the home. Parent evaluation of the client's daily communication experiences includes the parents' reporting on the family interactions when the child gets up in the morning, at the breakfast table, when getting off to school, at lunch time, during play with peers or family members, when speaking with father and mother, etc. Parents are helped to understand what constitutes a successful communication experience and also what characterizes a failure experience. They are then asked to report about their child in these terms. Involving the parents in the use of the CCS in assessing their child's communication-learning behavior at home and the DCCS in assessing their own and other family members' interactions with the child is a profitable way to include the daily life communication experiences of the client in the system approach to diagnosis.

Successful communication experiences for children include (a) the child's own performance of the various behaviors described on the CCS, such as being able to speak spontaneously, make requests, help others with tasks, share information or materials with others, and influence others, and (b) their parents' and siblings' performance of the various behaviors described on the DCCS, such as encouraging the child to participate, showing approval, and providing for the child to take the lead.

Parent reports of their child's communication experiences include instances of achievement of the CCS and DCCS behaviors, as well as some negative experiences of communicative interaction. Unfavorable sibling competition is often identified. Parent overindulgence, perfectionistic expectations, and other personally depreciating conditions come to light in this approach. Since the focus is on communication, not on what bad things mothers do or on the emotional status of the family, parents are more apt to acknowledge problems in the communication-learning context and to approach these difficulties as problems rather than as psychological threats to themselves as parents.

But the total communication-learning system includes more than the client and his family. It also includes the clinician and other children with whom the client relates in therapy. Thus the system approach calls for evaluation of the communication-learning context in the clinic as well. This is somewhat unusual in speech therapy—to evaluate the learning situation as well as the learner's behavior. It leads to the peculiar notion that clinicians and what they do may not only not be a solution to the client's problems, but indeed may be part of the problem. We know of junior-high-age children whose years of speech therapy have netted them little improvement of deviant /r/ and /s/ and a seriously negative attitude about their speech, themselves, school, and speech therapy in particular. We are reminded of the observations of Bateman (1974) and Cohen (1971) that poor teaching may be a major cause of poor learning. Bateman suggests that the term *teaching disabilities* be used instead of *learning disabilities* to emphasize the significance of poor teaching in children's learning problems. Since communicative interaction among learners and teachers is the context in which learning takes place, diagnosis in CCI must include assessment of the quality of that communicative interaction.

The companion CCS and DCCS rating scales described earlier are designed particularly as instruments for assessment of communication-learning effectiveness. It was noted that both scales are useful in improving the clinician's ability to respond to client behavior during actual therapy in a kind of diagnostic teaching. However, both scales may also be used in a more formal assessment of client communication-learning behavior and clinician teaching behavior.

The CCS may be used to assess individual client communication competence as well as the degree to which a group of clients is collectively effective in communication, i.e., how well the group provides an optimum communication-learning context. In using the CCS, the clinician designs and conducts a group activity in which there are opportunities for attending, imitating, cooperating, self-initiating, leading, etc. The activity may be videotaped for later analysis or another observer may rate the children's performance on the CCS, to identify communication-learning needs of the individual or the group. The DCCS may be used to assess the clinician's ability to generate effective behaviors in a therapy group. Using the DCCS, the clinician may rate his or her own performance in conducting a group activity by observing a videotaped recording of the therapy session, or another clinician may make the DCCS ratings during the session itself. Results of this assessment, along with CCS data, become the basis for planning therapy.

Other aspects of a system approach to articulation diagnosis include the evaluation of functioning of the various communication processes, particularly during the main task of communication. Assessment of factors such as auditory discrimination, physiological function, and production of specific phonemes will be described in relation to diagnostic teaching.

Concurrent Diagnostic Teaching.   One other aspect of diagnosis that has already been mentioned, but that deserves additional consideration, is concurrent diagnostic teaching: the adjustment of teaching objectives and procedure as information from concurrent, ongoing diagnosis is taken into account.

Diagnosis and teaching follow each other in most instructional approaches: (a) Test data and case history information are analyzed in order to plan instruction, (b) instruction is given based on this diagnostic information, (c) client performance is assessed to see if the client's progress is good, encouraging or poor, (d) instructional plans are changed in light of this new diagnostic information, and (e) the cycle is repeated. This approach follows a paradigm that appears in computer science—e.g., in the TOTE (Test-Operate-Text-Exit) model of Miller, Gallanter and Pribram (1960)—and also in instruction—e.g., in the prescriptive teaching model of Peter (1965) and the clinical teaching model of Lerner (1981). The same model is followed in medical diagnosis and treatment, in scientific searches for problem solutions, in business management, etc. In other words, it is a paradigm that is used universally, apparently because it works.

The reason for combining the terms *diagnosis* and *teaching* is to show that the two processes may occur close to each other in time. A diagnosis could be completed one day and instruction continue for weeks or months without another relevant assessment, as sometimes happens in classroom instruction. When diagnosis and teaching occur this far apart, the term *diagnostic teaching* would not apply. When midterms and other more frequent examinations are given so that the time between test-teach-test-teach is shortened, the process may be more nearly what we would call diagnostic teaching, if the teacher takes account of student performance in his or her teaching. *Precision teaching* (Lindsley, 1974; Kunzelmann, 1970) comes even closer to concurrent-diagnostic-teaching conditions. In precision teaching, a daily probe is made of learner performance to shorten the time between test-teach-test-teach and thus make it possible to guide teaching procedures with more concurrent diagnostic information. These principles are discussed further in chapter 6.

The ideal concurrent-diagnostic-teaching situation is one in which diagnosis and teaching occur simultaneously, where teaching decisions are made from moment to moment depending on the present evaluation of client performance and awareness of the client's present need. Concurrent diagnostic teaching occurs each time a clinician hears a client's target sound and suggests a retrial. Even more concurrent would be the correction by the client of velopharyngeal closure in attempting to overcome excessive nasal sound emission during /b/ and /d/ production while monitoring nasal sound by means of nasal olive and stethoscope. Biofeedback generally has this feature of concurrence.

Diagnostic teaching may be used in articulation remediation in the production of speech sounds, as described above, in ear training, or in improving any other aspect of speech articulation in communication. For example, calling attention to tongue placement in /s/ production heightens the client's haptic awareness of tongue position. How effective this instructional procedure is can be observed in the improved accuracy of /s/. If it works, use it; if it doesn't, try another way. Adjustment can be made in such teaching strategies during the therapy session based on the client's current performance and apparent rate of progress.

Diagnostic teaching in CCI provides not only for monitoring articulation behavior and making appropriate adjustments in teaching the client correct sound production, it also provides for monitoring the learning environment so it can be made optimally conducive to use of correct articulation in the main task of communication. This double-track monitoring provides the necessary data base for guiding instruction toward effective and efficient articulation improvement, the procedures of which will be described later in this chapter.

Exit Evaluation.   The ultimate measure in any instructional program—the dependent variable—is the learner's performance in the main task. In articulation therapy, the dependent variable is the client's correct use of the target sound in daily communication. The place to measure the client's production of corrected articulation thus becomes daily communication. Indexes to permanent improvement include performance on articulation tests, ability to read word lists or paragraphs, and performance in conversation in the clinical setting. A more sure index, however, is the client's performance in clinic activities that are highly similar to communication activities of the home and school. The best test is actual performance communication with family and in classroom and playground activities. Training parents and teachers to evaluate the client's articulation accuracy makes it possible for them to provide useful information about the child's postinstruction articulation competence. Communication-centered articulation therapy would not be complete without confirmation of articulation improvement in the client's real-life communication.

Instructional Procedures in Communication-Centered Articulation Therapy

The several examples of communication-centered articulation therapy procedures sprinkled through earlier sections of this chapter illustrate relatively well the application of principles of CCI in articulation therapy. In this section additional examples are given and specific organizing and therapy techniques are described. The organization is probably presented best in the typical outline of a communication-centered therapy lesson plan.

Lesson Plan for Group Communication-Centered Instruction.   The outline of a typical CCI group lesson plan includes (a) objectives, (b) activities, and (c) recommendations, as represented in Table 8.3. These main features are described here and illustrated with references to a specific lesson theme, namely, *what-is-missing*, an activity that young children may experience at home and play and in pre-reading perceptual training at school.

Objectives.   Consistent with the system nature of CCI, instruction is designed to take account of the various elements of the communication-learning system. Objectives reflect this system orientation, as seen in Table 8.3, where communication competence and the processes of perception, conceptualization, codification (language), and production (speech and other motor) are represented.

TABLE 8.3
Outline of CCI Group Lesson Plan

Categories of Objectives
    Communication competence
    Perception
    Conceptualization
    Language
    Speech production
    Motor production
    Diagnostic

Activities
    Greetings
    Roll call
    Rehearsal
    Activity #1
    Activity #2
    Activity #3

Recommendations

In the communication competence category, establishing an optimum *communication-learning context* is the main objective. This is a learning situation in which (a) the clients pay attention, imitate expected behavior, cooperate with others, care for others, help others, share with others, act and speak spontaneously, try to influence others, and lead others, and (b) the clinician explains, demonstrates, provides opportunity for, encourages and reinforces these behaviors, provides a practice situation and activities like the clients' daily communication activities, and provides for practice of responses in these activities in such a way that natural consequences follow these and other communication efforts of the clients. Before each therapy session, a next-lesson therapy plan is formulated in which each client's performance on the various CCS items is considered, as well as the clinician's performance on each item of the DCCS. The new statement of objectives reflects the CCS needs of each client and the DCCS needs of the clinician. Examples of objectives of communication competence are:

- Activities will be chosen that allow Jimmy, Dawn, and Sue to attend and cooperate for five minutes.
- The clinician will model sharing by relinquishing her toys or materials to each child at least once during the session.
- Given two bottles of glue, the six children will ask for the glue (as modeled by the clinician) and glue a missing piece on the picture.
- The clinician will demonstrate enthusiasm by commenting on the quality of each child's product.
- The clinician will present at least one opportunity for both Jimmy and John to lead others by giving the directions for the activity.

Perceptual objectives have to do with auditory, haptic, and visual perceptual processes, particularly those that are involved in articulation production. Recognizing that perceptual patterns in all three of these input modalities guide speech production as well as speech discrimination, deliberate involvement and client awareness of perceptual processes is a necessary feature of a system approach. Perceptual objectives include the improvement of clients' awareness of differences among speech sounds and among positions of the speech articulators. Examples of perceptual objectives are:

- As the clinician or client produces the word *missing*, Shawn, Jimmy, and Sue will indicate correctly, 80% of the time, whether /s/ is right or wrong.
- During their practice of the word *missing*, Shawn, Jimmy, and Sue will indicate correctly, 80% of the time, whether the tongue position for /s/ is right or wrong.
- As the clinician or client produces the word *little*, Dawn, Sue, and Jimmy will indicate correctly, 80% of the time, whether /l/ is right or wrong.
- During their practice of the word *little*, Dawn, Sue, and Jimmy will indicate correctly, 80% of the time, whether the tongue position for /l/ is right or wrong.

Conceptual objectives have to do with the concepts, ideas, and meaning of communication. The significance of concepts to children depends upon their opportunities and requirements. Preschool children benefit from learning concepts related to play activities, home interactions and perhaps to other concepts at appropriate developmental levels identified by Piaget and his interpreters. School-age children benefit from learning concepts related to play and home and also to their daily experiences in the various curricular areas of their classroom instruction. Problem solving and creative thinking are valid activities for conceptual, i.e., cognitive, development, particularly if they are borrowed from the clients' frequently occurring classroom activities.

Conceptual activities are, like the language that accompanies them, an integral part of the total communication context, and may provide opportunity for practice of specific speech sounds. In planning conceptual activities, the clinician should provide for a degree of spontaneous interaction and for language elaborations beyond the specific planned responses. Muma (1978) and Bloom and Lahey (1978) discuss language elaboration, expatiation, etc., as ways to expand language form and content in communicative interchange. An example of a conceptual objective is:

• Given a display or sequence of items, each child will correctly name the item that is missing and describe it as either *big* or *little*.

Language objectives are frequently as important to clients in an articulation improvement program as are speech production objectives. Significant articulation disorders are often accompanied by language difficulties, as might be expected in light of (a) the interdependent nature of the communication-learning system and (b) the fact that even phonemes by definition have semantic value, as well as direct association with lexical, morphological, and syntactic elements of language. Furthermore, language responses clearly constitute the chief vehicle for articulation improvement.

Language objectives should fit the language needs of the client as determined by appropriate language tests, diagnostic teaching, the types of expressions used in the client's home and school, and the concepts that are objectives of the lesson, and they should fit the articulation needs of the client as well. Thus, if the client has /s/ distortions in his speech, language responses should be chosen that contain /s/. In our clinic, when the phoneme to be remediated is identified, clinicians select four or five words from the child's lexicon that contain the target phoneme, usually in initial position, and a language unit (word category, syntactic form, speech act) containing the same phoneme. This affords practice of the target sound in words useful to the child, and in communicative use from the very beginning of instruction, thus eliminating the need for a separate program of carry-over and maintenance. The preschool lesson being represented here might have the following language objective:

• In the appropriate context, each client will express completely, with or without model: *I want a turn. What is missing? The big one. The little one. That's right. That's wrong.*

Speech production objectives may include improvement of voice, stuttering, articulation, and other speech behaviors. The same communication experiences, the same system procedures, that are beneficial in language improvement may also serve in the improvement of speech. This has been one of the premises of this discussion of CCI. Another basic claim is that procedures for improving specific speech sounds, including speech sounds in isolation, may be incorporated as part practice within the whole context of this system approach. Articulation objectives are, of course, specific for each client and appear much like speech objectives in other instructional approaches. Examples of speech production objectives are:

- Shawn, Jimmy, and Sue will produce improved /s/ 80% of the time as they use the word *missing*.
- Shawn, Jimmy, and Sue will produce improved /s/ 80% of the time as they practice /s/ in isolation.
- Jimmy, Richard, and John will produce improved /r/ 80% of the time as they use the words *turn, right,* and *wrong*.
- Jimmy, Richard, and John will produce improved /r/ 80% of the time as they practice /r/ in isolation.
- Dawn, Sue, and Jimmy will produce improved /l/ 80% of the time as they use the word *little*.
- Dawn, Sue, and Jimmy will produce improved /l/ 80% of the time as they practice /l/ in isolation.

Motor production objectives include improvement of gross and fine perceptual-motor skills where necessary and appropriate. There is some evidence that central nervous system perceptual-motor integration can be strengthened with the kinds of activities described by Kephart and others (Ayres, 1973; Barsch, 1966; Cratty, 1973; Frostig & Horne, 1964; Getman, 1965; Kephart, 1971). Where considerable perceptual-motor abnormality appears, it is not unreasonable to involve young clients in sequential learning activities, laterality discrimination, etc. These same activities may also enhance conceptual growth in the cognitive abilities described by Piaget, such as conservation and spatiality.

The contribution of perceptual-motor learning other than that involved in speech production may not be obvious. However, the integrated performance of body movement in meaningful tasks may well be helpful in strengthening the cues that evoke learned responses. Earlier, for example, we described an adult aphasic client who was unable to produce the words *come in* until she stood at the door, opened it, and addressed the person waiting to come in. This same accompaniment of speech with appropriate body activity in meaningful communication acts has been noticeably effective with mentally retarded clients. An example of a motor production objective is:

- Clients will place the missing piece in a four-part puzzle.

Diagnostic objectives have to do with the ongoing evaluation of client and clinician behavior. As explained earlier, concurrent diagnostic teaching is an essential feature of CCI and consists of continuous observation and evaluation by the clinician and concurrent adjustment of teaching based on these ongoing evaluations. The summary of the clinician's impressions during the therapy session becomes the basis for next-lesson objectives and planning. How well the clients performed in relation to the day's lesson objectives suggests their needs. How well the clients performed and what the clinician did to achieve or fail to achieve good client performance suggests the clinician's needs. As with the objectives already described, diagnostic objectives include many more expected results than are explicitly stated in the lesson plan. Usually diagnostic objectives are stated in terms of most urgent improvements the clients and clinician have been working to achieve.

   Activities.   Most of the guidelines for planning activities of CCI have been described earlier in this chapter as principles of communicative stimulus, communicative response, communicative reinforcement, system-type instruction, and communication-centered learning contexts. These principles suggest that activities be designed that simulate the clients' daily communication experiences. The simulation is not an exact duplication of life experiences for any of the clients. Instead, it is intended to be an ideal representation of the several types of communicative interaction experienced by the clients during their daily life at home, play, and school. They then are able to participate more effectively in these daily experiences as they bring newly learned skills to their daily communication. The ideal communication context is, of course, one in which both CCS client behaviors and DCCS clinician behaviors are optimally achieved.

   Another principle that guides the clinician's planning of CCI is that of diagnostic teaching. Therapy activities in group instruction are designed to achieve the seven objectives that the clinician defines at the end of each therapy session. As described above, these objectives are decided in terms of both client and clinician needs as suggested by the performance of both in previous sessions. To provide the conditions necessary so that all seven objectives can be achieved during the same lesson, the clinician must draw upon his or her knowledge of the different kinds of behavior related to each objective and the kinds of activities that may encourage each of these kinds of behavior. Thus, the activities will be designed (a) to improve the communication competence, perceptual, conceptual, language, speech, and other motor skills of the clients, (b) to improve the clinician's ability to teach these client skills, and (c) to give the clinician opportunity to observe these client behaviors in arriving at that day's diagnostic evaluation.

   Another guideline that is followed in designing CCI activities is that of arranging circumstances more than arranging children. Generally, activities in communication-centered group instruction are arranged to encourage various client behaviors more than to teach them directly. This is a natural feature of communication-centered activities because the communicative interaction of clients with each other, as well as with the clinician, naturally provides opportunity for attending, imitating, self-initiating, cooperating, etc. At the same time, the clinician may explain, demonstrate, wait for, encourage, require, and approve specific client behaviors as well as arrange situations that naturally call for these behaviors.

   Positive group interaction is essential to effective CCI. With it come all the benefits of group work, small-group instruction, and cooperation in education

(Sharan, 1980). Group unity or cohesiveness is a necessary condition of group instruction and often requires emphasis on activities that unify the group by requiring all children to work together to complete a task. For instance, six children may be given two puzzles to assemble rather than providing a separate puzzle for each child. The children then are given opportunities to practice sharing and other social and communicative skills while learning to use language effectively in an interactive environment.

Another important guideline in planning communication-centered activities is based on principles of generalization. Ellis (1965) suggests that in addition to the benefits of making the practice situation like the performance situation, transfer of learning increases (a) with increase in the amount of time spent on learning the original task, and (b) with a few different experiences in tasks that are variations of the original. Similarly, Gagné (1977) suggests that to enhance retention and transfer of learning, "provision needs to be made for encouraging the learner to apply the learning in as great a variety of new situations as can be devised" (p. 296). The activities in CCI are thus designed to follow these recommendations. Practice of target behaviors is repeated in several communication-centered activities, all of which provide for use of the target responses, but all of which are slightly different. For example, activities that provide practice of /s/ in *May I see?* may consist of clients asking the clinician and other clients (a) *May I see the picture?* when the picture is in a book, a Viewmaster, a dime-store viewer, a diorama, a photo album, etc., or (b) *May I see?* when an object is in another person's hand, in a box, out the window, etc.

The activities that constitute the usual communication-centered therapy session are an introduction, a rehearsal, and several practice activities.

The *introduction* usually includes greetings and roll call, in which each child participates in greeting the teacher or teacher's helper and each responds to his name with "I am here," or some other response, such as putting his name tag or picture on the bulletin board.

The *rehearsal* at the beginning of each group lesson introduces (a) the concepts of the lesson, (b) the specific language form or function to be emphasized that day, (c) the speech sounds to be improved, and (d) the kind of communicative interchange in which the language unit may be used. The rehearsal consists of a communication activity, or a story and activity illustrating the story, in which the concepts, language unit, and speech sounds are rehearsed. The rehearsal activity is similar to the rest of the communication activities in the lesson, but with time for whatever practice is necessary to obtain the client's best performance of target behaviors. It is chiefly in the rehearsal that the target speech sound is practiced. In the rehearsal, the target sound in the language response may be isolated for practice in sound discrimination, phonetic placement, or many of the other procedures described in other chapters. This part practice is immediately followed by use of the sound in the target words of the lesson, and finally restored to its whole context of communicative use of the response in the rehearsal activity.

For example, in a what-is-missing activity, the clinician demonstrates the use of *what is missing?* by telling the clients, "Look at the things on the table. Now close your eyes. I took one thing away. Open your eyes. What is missing? Jimmy?"

Jimmy: The big dog.
Clinician: The big dog is there or the big dog is missing, Jimmy?
Jimmy: The big dog is missing.
Clinician: Right. Did you hear how Jimmy said *missing*? Let's all try—*missing*.
                Listen to /s/ and watch where I put my tongue and teeth. Let's try
                /s/. Good. Now, *missing*. Jimmy, you be the leader. Everyone close
                your eyes. Jimmy, take something away. O.K., open your eyes. You
                ask them, Jimmy.
Jimmy: What is missing?

The children respond, and the action is repeated as each child takes the
turn of the leader. Several times a brief moment is spent practicing /s/ in *missing*,
/l/ in *little*, and /r/ in *right* and *wrong*.

Activity #1 is a near-replication of the rehearsal activity, as are the rest of
the activities in the session. They are all designed to provide a communicative
exchange among the group, including the clinician, in which the day's target
responses are used naturally. The activities are different enough to provide
new, but similar stimulus cues in each activity while at the same time repeating
the same responses.

In the sample lesson, Activity #1 may consist of the clinician's displaying a
quarter and a penny in outstretched hand. Then one of the coins is removed
without letting the children see which one, and the clinician's fist is closed
around the remaining coin. The question is then asked, "What is missing?" or
"Which one is missing, Sue, the big one or the little one?"

Sue guesses, "The big one."

The clinician opens her hand and asks, "John, was she right or wrong?"

"Right," says John, "it's the big one."

"All right, Sue, you hold the penny and the quarter. We'll close our eyes
while you take one away."

Each child has a turn guessing which coin is missing and telling whether
the guess was right or wrong.

Activity #2 uses the same responses as the rehearsal and Activity #1 in a
different setting. For example, the clinician has prepared a picture of a carnival
in which there are two clowns, one selling balloons of different sizes and one
juggling some balls of different sizes. Colored paper discs are lightly stuck on
the balloon and ball outlines in the picture. The children close their eyes while
another child removes a ball or a balloon and then asks what is is missing;
appropriate responses are given.

Activity #3 uses the same responses as in the other activities. This time a
cloth or paper bag is used to conceal big and little paired objects, such as toys,
coins, and balls. The children take turns removing one of the paired objects
and asking another child to feel in the bag and tell what is missing.

Several other activities may follow, in each of which the target responses
are practiced in relation to what-is-missing situations.

Recommendations are the last feature of the lesson plan; these are not
formulated until the day's lesson is over. Then, having been aware throughout
the lesson of the behaviors of the individual clients in relation to the lesson
objectives and of her own effectiveness as a clinician, the clinician may summarize progress and present needs. These needs, along with the long-term com-

munication goals of each client, provide the basis for objectives of the next
therapy session. Recommendations may be summarized, as illustrated here, or
they may be stated as new objectives for the next group or individual therapy
session.

- Shawn and Jimmy need more practice on /s/ discrimination and placement in both individual and group therapy.
- Jimmy, Richard, and John are more nearly approximating /r/. John
  and Richard should have more /r/ discrimination and placement during individual therapy. Jimmy has enough to do with /s/ practice.
- Dawn, Sue, and Jimmy are beginning to produce a good /l/. The
  inclusion of /l/ in whole responses in group and individual lessons will
  likely be sufficient to remediate /l/.
- CCS strengths were the increased cooperation of Jimmy, Dawn, and
  Sue and Jimmy's willingness to take the lead. CCS weaknesses were
  John's frequent lack of attention and reluctance to be the leader in an
  activity.
- DCCS strengths were the involvement of all clients in the various roles
  of each activity, including their making something happen with the
  language they used to practice their specific target articulation. DCCS
  weaknesses were too many failures to commend John for his occasional
  spontaneous behavior and not introducing the language response in a
  clear way so the children would use it naturally.

Lesson Plan for Individual Communication-Centered Instruction.   Except
for the extensive CCS and DCCS provisions of group communication-centered
articulation therapy, the objectives and activities of individual instruction are
much the same as those for group instruction. The key to planning individual
therapy is the performance of the client in group therapy as well as in home,
school, and play activity. In fact, if we follow the resource model of education,
we find an optimum relationship of individual therapy to group therapy. In
the resource model, school experience is a supplement to and rehearsal for the
client's daily-life activities. So, also, remedial instruction, i.e., group therapy, is
a supplement to and rehearsal for both the client's school and daily life.
Individual instruction, then, as a resource to group instruction, becomes a
supplement to and rehearsal for the client's group, school, and life activities.

As the clinician rehearses the individual client in the responses that have
been or will be used in the group, there is more opportunity than in the group
for isolating the target sound from the whole response for phonemic and
phonetic discrimination and for practice in articulatory placement and movement.
Further contextual testing (chapter 4), distinctive-feature analysis (chapter 14),
paired-stimulus practice (chapter 12), phonologically based procedures (chapter
7), and other useful articulation evaluation and therapy procedures may be
pursued as part of the individual lesson, always accompanied by whole practice
of the target sound in communicative responses and communicative activities,
some of which are rehearsal for subsequent group lessons.

Communication between clinician and client in individual instruction may
still be a meaningful and powerful communication experience, although not

usually as effective, in our experience, as such communication among peers. Having the client use communicative mand responses that direct the adult to act in various ways, such as *throw the ball, drop the ring, give me the little one,* is a communicatively reinforcing use of language. To enhance the communicative value of individual therapy, another client may be involved in the communicative interchange. We recall a clinician's efforts to involve a mentally retarded child who was listless and unresponsive until the clinician brought a little girl into the activity. Little boys, of course, will stand on their heads for little girls. Immediately the activity came alive as the interaction included three instead of two people, peer-peer-clinician relationships instead of child-clinician only.

Individual therapy is considered a supplement to group therapy in a communication-centered articulation therapy program. The influence of the group on individual clients is so essential in establishing communication-learning conditions that it may be assumed that instruction without client interaction achieved in small groups is not optimally communication-centered. At best, individual instruction provides an opportunity for a child to rehearse behaviors that can be used effectively in group activities.

Home Instruction. As indicated throughout the description of CCI, simulation in the clinic of communication activities from clients' daily lives involves awareness on the part of the clinician of the clients' home, school, and play situations. This simulation is generally the best guarantee of carry-over of clinic learning to daily life. However, parents, teachers, and even friends can hasten a client's articulation improvement if they are given some understanding of the instruction the client receives and specific instruction as to how they can create situations in which the client may be expected to use newly acquired speech behavior. An important feature of communication-centered articulation therapy is sharing with parents and teachers information that allows and expects them to encourage the use of their child's new articulation skills, particularly in language units practiced in the clinic.

SUMMARY

In this chapter, we have described what we believe to be a logical, integrated approach to articulation therapy. The eclectic nature of this approach allows the integration of many new and used techniques within its whole-part-whole learning contexts. CCI is applicable not only to articulation therapy, but also to stuttering, voice problems, and language disorders in particular. In general, CCI is effective in improving the communication and learning of the mentally retarded, learning disabled, aphasic, autistic, and other handicapped children and adults. CCI provides an optimal learning context for most kinds of learning, helps clients learn behaviors of significance among their peers, and improves clients' interpersonal skills and feelings of worth, not only among those in the clinic but with those at home, at school, and at play.

The ability to adjust to new interpersonal communicative situations generalizes from CCI to the clients' daily lives along with their improved communication and learning skills, and in that process many of the unfavorable learning and psychogenic conditions contributing to the communication disorder are greatly reduced. As a child's confidence in his speech and language skills increases, he interacts more with others, which provides more opportunity for practice and improvement in speech-language and social-emotional relations.

As a closing comment, let us consider an often-repeated concern of clinicians who are unsure of using CCI. "But I only have 15 minutes with each client," the clinician says. "I can't have the client repeat the response enough times for adequate practice if I make the activity communication-centered." Usually this observation changes when consideration is given to the relative importance in learning of repetition, on the one hand, and communicativeness of the learning situation, on the other.

Clinicians should approach remediation of communication disorders, including articulation deviations, as problems in communication that need communication solutions. CCI, as described here, may be one way for clinicians to center their instruction in communication.

REFERENCES

Antinucci, F., & Parisi, D. (1975). Early semantic development in child language. In E. H. Lennenberg & E. Lenneberg (Eds.), *Foundations of language development: A multidisciplinary approach* (Vol. 1). New York: Academic Press.

Aronson, E., Bridgeman, D., & Geffner, R. (1978). Interdependent interactions and prosocial behavior. *Journal of Research and Development in Education, 12*, 16–29.

Ayres, A. J. (1973). Sensory integration and learning disorders. Los Angeles: Western Psychological Services.

Backus, O., & Beasley, J. (1951). *Journal of speech therapy with children.* Cambridge, MA: Houghton Mifflin Co.

Backus, O., & Dunn, H. (1947). Use of conversational speech patterns to promote speed and retention of learning. *Journal of Speech and Hearing Disorders, 12*, 135–142.

Barsch, R. (1966). Teacher needs—motor training. In W. Cruickshank (Ed.), *The teacher of brain-injured children.* Syracuse, NY: Syracuse University Press.

Bateman, B. (1974). Educational implications of minimal brain dysfunction. *Reading Teacher, 27*, 662–668.

Bates, E. (1976). Pragmatics and sociolinguistics in child language. In D. M. Morehead & A. E. Morehead (Eds.), *Normal and deficient child language.* Baltimore: University Park Press.

Berlo, D. K. (1960). *The process of communication.* New York: Holt, Rinehart and Winston.

Bloom, L., & Lahey, M. (1978). *Language development and language disorders.* New York: John Wiley & Sons.

Bruner, J. S. (1966). On cognitive growth: II. In J. S. Bruner, R. R. Olver, & P. M. Greenfield (Eds.), *Studies in cognitive growth.* New York: John Wiley & Sons.

Bruner, J. S. (1975). The ontogenesis of speech acts. *Journal of Child Language, 2*, 1–19.

Cherry, C. (1978). *On human communication.* Cambridge, MA: MIT Press.

Clark, E., & Garnica, O. (1974). Is he coming or going? On the acquisition of deictic verbs. *Journal of Verbal Learning and Verbal Behavior, 13*, 559–572.

Cohen, S. A. (1971). Dyspedagogia as a cause of reading retardation in learning disorders. In B. Bateman (Ed.), *Learning disorders—reading* (Vol. 4). Seattle: Special Child Publications.

Cratty, B. (1973). *Intelligence in action.* Englewood Cliffs, NJ: Prentice-Hall.

Darley, F. L. (1979). *Evaluation of appraisal techniques in speech and language pathology.* Reading, MA: Addison-Wesley Publishing Co.

Ellis. H. C. (1965). *The transfer of learning.* New York: Macmillan Co.,

Frostig, M., & Horne, D. (1964). *The Frostig program for the development of visual perception.* Chicago: Follett.

Gagné, R. M. (1977). *The conditions of learning* (3rd ed.). New York: Holt, Rinehart & Winston.

Gallagher, T., & Prutting, C. (Eds.). (1983). *Pragmatic assessment and intervention issues in language.* San Diego: College-Hill Press.

Garner, W. R. (1962). *Uncertainty and structure as psychological concepts.* New York: John Wiley and Sons.

Getman, G. (1965). The visuomotor complex in the acquisition of learning skills. In J. Hellmuth (Ed.), *Learning disorders* (Vol. I). Seattle: Special Child Publications.

Greeno, J. G., & Bjork, R. A. (1973). Mathematical learning theory and the new "mental forestry." *Annual Review of Psychology, 24,* 81–116.

Holland, A. R. (1975). Language therapy for children: Some thoughts on context and content. *Journal of Speech and Hearing Disorders, 40,* 514–523.

Hulse, S. H., Deese, J., & Egeth, H. (1975). *The psychology of learning* (4th ed.). New York: McGraw-Hill.

Ingram, D. (1971). Toward a theory of person deixis. *Papers in Linguistics, 4,* 37–53.

Ingram, D. (1976). *Phonological disability in children.* New York: Elsevier Publishing Company, Inc.

Kephart, N. (1971). *The slow learner in the classroom.* Columbus: Charles E. Merrill.

Kunzelmann, H.P. (Ed.). (1970). *Precision teaching: An initial training reference.* Seattle: Special Child Publications.

Lassers, L., & Low, G.M. (1960). *A study of the relative effectiveness of different approaches to speech training of mentally retarded children.* San Francisco: San Francisco State College.

Leonard, L.B. (1971). A preliminary review of information theory on articulatory omissions. *Journal of Speech and Hearing Disorders, 36* (4), 511–517.

Lerner, J.W. (1981). *Learning disabilities* (3rd ed.). Boston: Houghton Mifflin Co.

Lindsley, O. (1974). Precision teaching in perspective. In S. Kirk & F. Lord (Eds.), *Exceptional children: Educational resources and perspectives.* Boston: Houghton Mifflin.

Littlejohn. S. W. (1978). *Theories of human communication.* Columbus: Charles E. Merrill Publishing Co.

Low, G. M., Crerar, M., & Lassers, L. (1954). Communication-centered speech therapy. *Journal of Speech and Hearing Disorders, 24,* 361–368.

Lucas, E. V. (1980). *Semantic and pragmatic language disorders.* Rockville, MD: Aspen Systems Corporation

Lucas, E. V. (1983) *Pragmaticism: theory and application.* Rockville, MD: Aspen Systems Corporation

Menyuk, P. (1980). The role of context in misarticulations. In G. H. Yeni-Komshian, J. F. Kavanagh, & C. A. Ferguson (Eds.). *Child phonology: Vol. I. Production* (pp. 211–226). New York: Academic Press.

Miller, G. A., Gallanter, E., & Pribram, K. H. (1960). *Plans and the structure of behavior.* New York: Holt, Rinehart & Winston.

Morris, C. W. (1946). *Signs, language and behavior.* Englewood Cliffs, NJ: Prentice-Hall.

Muma, J. R. (1978). *Language handbook: Concepts, assessment, intervention.* Englewood Cliffs, NJ: Prentice Hall, Inc.

Odom, R., & Corbin, D. (1973). Perceptual salience and children's multidimensional problem solving. *Child Development, 44,* 425–432.

Olmsted, D. L. (1971). *Out of the mouth of babes: Earliest stages in language learning.* The Hague: Mouton.

Osgood, C. E. (1957a). Motivational dynamics of language behavior. In M. R. Jones (Ed.), *Nebraska symposium on motivation*. Lincoln, NE: University of Nebraska Press.

Osgood, C. E. (1957b). A behavioristic analysis of perception and language as cognitive phenomena. In C. E. Osgood (Ed.), *Contemporary approaches to cognition*. Cambridge, MA: Harvard University Press.

Osgood, C. E. (1949). The similarity paradox in human learning: A resolution. *Psychology Review, 56,* 132–143.

Parisi, D. (1974). What is behind child utterances? *Journal of Child Language, 1,* 97–105.

Peter, L. J. (1965). *Prescriptive teaching.* New York: McGraw-Hill Book Co.

Piaget, J. (1952a). *The origins of intelligence in children.* New York: International Universities Press. (Originally published 1936)

Piaget, J. (1952b). *The construction of reality in the child.* New York: Basic Books. (Originally published 1937)

Rees, N. S. (1978). Pragmatics of language. In R. L. Schiefelbusch (Ed.), *Basis of language intervention.* Baltimore: University Park Press.

Ruesch, J., & Bateson, G. (1951). *Communication: The social matrix of psychiatry.* New York: W. W. Norton and Company, Inc.

Searle, J. R. (1969). *Speech acts.* London: Cambridge University Press.

Sharan, S. (1980). Cooperative learning in small groups: A review of recent methods and effects on achievement, attitudes, and ethnic relations. *Review in Educational Research, 50,* 241–271.

Skinner, B. F. (1957). *Verbal behavior.* New York: Appleton-Century Crofts, Inc.

Snyder, L. S. (1975). *Pragmatics in language disabled children: Their prelinguistics and early verbal performatives and presuppositions.* Unpublished doctoral dissertation. Denver: University of Colorado.

Wepman, J., Jones, L. V., Beck, R. D., & Van Pelt, D. (1960). Studies in aphasia: Background and theoretical formulations. *Journal of Speech and Hearing Disorders, 25,* 323–332.

Winitz, H. (1969). *Articulatory acquisition and behavior.* New York: Appleton-Century-Crofts.

Wulz, S. V., Hall, M. K., & Klein, M. D. (1983). A home-centered instructional communication strategy for severely handicapped children. *Journal of Speech and Hearing Disorders, 48,* 2–10.

9

Auditory Considerations in Articulation Treatment

Articulation errors cannot be treated easily by a single approach. Generally, the developers of treatment methods for articulation disorders do not intend their methods to apply to all circumstances. Rather, a treatment approach is recommended for application to a restricted set of conditions, because articulatory acquisition involves several different albeit interrelated processes.

The recognition that several process levels are relevant was reflected in Van Riper's (1939) insightful and comprehensive presentation on articulation disorders. As described in chapter five of this volume, Van Riper outlined three primary process levels in articulation learning: (a) auditory practice, (b) articulatory production, and (c) carry-over.

Van Riper held that the first step in articulation treatment should involve extensive auditory experience with the sound the child is to acquire. Not all clinicians endorse the principle that auditory experience is to be emphasized in articulation training. However, there has been reconsideration of the usefulness of auditory experience with the increased use of phonological theory in descriptions of articulation disorders. A phonological approach is particularly useful because it provides a method for describing systematically patterns of articulation errors. Treatment methods based on phonological theory are dis-

Harris Winitz, Ph.D., is a professor of speech science and psychology at the University of Missouri–Kansas City.

249

cussed in chapters 7, 13, and 14. In this chapter the role of auditory discrimination in relation to these and other approaches will be considered.

LEVELS OF ARTICULATION BREAKDOWN

Until recent years, functional articulation disorders were generally thought to be caused by an inability to execute motor movements even when there was no evidence of an underlying organic pathology. As more has become known about the many dimensions of articulation performance, several additional areas of potential breakdown have been posited.

Five potential sites at which a breakdown can occur in the articulation acquisition process have been identified. First, the source of difficulty may lie at the level of auditory input. Children with articulation errors may have difficulty hearing differences between sounds. Perhaps they have had limited experience hearing speech sounds or their auditory system is defective (Weiner, 1967; Winitz, 1969, 1975, 1981, 1984; Monin, 1984). Another possible reason for difficulty at this level is that the phonological system of children has fossilized at a certain point in development, and, therefore, the development of speech perception is inhibited (Winitz, 1969) in a way similar to that of individuals acquiring a foreign language. Individuals acquiring a second language often find that the phonology of their first language creates certain expectations, and these expectations seem to interfere with the perception of phonetic differences and phonetic variations in the second language (Brown & Hildum, 1956). For example, in the Hawaiian language the /ŋ/ sound occurs in the initial word position, but in English this sound is not permitted in this position, often causing English speakers to perceive the initial /ŋ/ in Hawaiian as /n/.

A second type of breakdown in articulation acquisition can take place, regardless of the quality of the auditory input, at the phonological level (Haas, 1963; Winitz, 1969; Compton, 1970; Ingram, 1976). Auditory factors may contribute to this impairment, but there is the possibility that an impairment in reasoning, memory, or motivation may be responsible for the delay in phonological development. It is also possible that individual children, as they are acquiring language, may minimize their attention to the phonological system in order to concentrate on other language components, such as syntax or semantics (Panagos, 1982; Edwards & Shriberg, 1983).

A third site of breakdown is the link between the phonological system and the articulatory system (Smith, 1973; Macken, 1980), originally defined by Chomsky and Halle (1968) as the systematic phonetic level. In contrast to the phonological component, which contains abstract phonological units, the systematic phonetic level contains the phonetic specifications, somewhat abstract in form, of the sounds of a language. For example, at this level are represented the many phonetic forms of the English /t/ phoneme and the contexts in which they appear. As described in chapter 2, the abstract phonological units are the underlying representation, and the phonetic specifications determine the surface representation. In English the /t/ may have one or more phonetic features such as dentalization, aspiration, and rounding.

Conceivably, a child could acquire correct phonological forms, but be unable to learn the corresponding systematic phonetic units. An example might be a child who produces fricatives appropriately, but systematically alters place of articulation so that the fricatives are distorted. Speakers of a foreign language sometimes show distortion of phonetic units, even though they have acquired complete knowledge of the underlying phonological system. Perhaps one way to identify children with a deficit at the systematic phonetic level would be to devise discrimination tests that evaluate both phonetic and phonemic differences. An investigation of this type was conducted by Hoffman, Stager, and Daniloff (1983), and their results seem to provide evidence that some children with errors of /r/ do not have auditory knowledge of the phonetic parameters of /r/, although they have acquired auditory distinctions that indicate that /r/ has been acquired as a phonological unit, i.e., they can distinguish among /r/, /l/, and /w/.

A fourth possible type of breakdown is at the level that involves the planning of articulatory acts. In this case, the phonetic instructions to the articulatory system may be correct, but there may be difficulty in establishing articulatory programs or schemata. A motor scheme starts with knowledge of articulatory targets and the context in which these targets occur. From this information, an articulatory plan is formulated that serves as the input to the speech motor system. It is possible that some children have difficulty in formulating articulation programs. This difficulty is called *apraxia* (to be considered in chapter 10).

The fifth and final source of difficulty is the inability to execute an intended motor schema. Here sensory, tactile, and auditory systems are involved. The breakdown may occur because damage to the peripheral nervous system impairs the initiation of speech motor movements or causes feedback systems, which provide information after an articulatory movement has been initiated, to operate poorly. This type of breakdown may result in *dysarthria* (see chapter 10). When neurological tests do not confirm the presence of apraxia or dysarthria, a breakdown at the fourth and fifth levels cannot be confirmed by using traditional tests of the speech peripheral mechanism (Winitz, 1975; Williams, Ingham, & Rosenthal, 1981). As pointed out by Kent and Lybolt (1982), levels four and five are inextricably woven together in that the formation of articulatory plans rests, in part, on the development and use of feedback systems that are involved in the execution of speech motor movements.

Table 9.1 summarizes the five levels of articulatory breakdown. Although the levels were presented as a "top" to "bottom" system, it should not be assumed that, in development and in usage, the process of articulation is one that begins at the top with auditory discrimination and proceeds through each step until the bottom is reached. The levels interact with each other in complex but as yet unknown ways as children acquire and use the phonological and articulatory patterns of their language. In addition, current diagnostic procedures do not reliably distinguish among these five potential levels of breakdown in articulation acquisition. Nevertheless, it is possible that a particular child may have more difficulty at one level of articulatory functioning than at another level.

The focus of this chapter is on the auditory component as it contributes to each of these five potential areas of breakdown in the acquisition of articulation.

TABLE 9.1
Five Levels for Potential Breakdown in Articulatory Acquisition

---

1. Level of auditory input—Child may not discriminate among sounds.
2. Level of phonological system—Child may fail to learn the rules of the system.
3. Level of systematic phonetics—Child may be unable to link the phonological system to the phonetic specifications.
4. Level of articulatory planning—Child may be unable to plan the motor acts to produce sounds or sound sequences.
5. Level of articulatory production—Child may be unable to execute the motor movements to produce sounds or sound sequences.

Auditory processing will be discussed with regard to the discrimination, production, and carry-over of speech sounds, often regarded as three fundamental phases of articulation acquisition, and the relationship of each to the five areas of potential breakdown.

TESTING AUDITORY DISCRIMINATION

In its most narrow sense, *auditory discrimination* involves distinctions between sounds. This definition does not restrict this process to phonological distinctions, although it is often used in this specific way. A phonological distinction or phonological contrast refers to differences between the sounds of a language that signal semantic intent. For example, in English the /p/ and /b/ distinguish between the words *pat* and *bat*. A third word, namely *sat*, is indicated by placing /s/ within this same context. These words are called *minimal pairs* because the distinction among these three words in each case is due to a difference of one sound. The difference between the words *pat* and *bad*, however, is not a minimal-pair distinction because the word difference is signalled by the contrast between /p/ and /b/ in the initial word position and /t/ and /d/ in the final word position.

In standardized tests of auditory discrimination, phonological distinctions generally are tested. However, when children produce nonstandard errors or distortions it is often useful to determine their ability to distinguish between each nonstandard error and the corresponding target sound, as, for example, when a child produces an /r/ sound whose production is intermediate between /r/ and /w/.

A common procedure in discrimination testing is to ask the child to indicate whether two sounds are the same or different. For example, the traditional format for testing the distinction between /r/ and /w/ is illustrated as follows:

> *Clinician:* Tell me whether these two sounds are the same or different: /ru/ /wu/.
> *Child:* Responds by saying either "same" or "different."
> *Clinician:* /ri/ /wi/.
> *Child:* Responds by saying either "same" or "different."

There are other approaches (Locke, 1980a, 1980b) that can be used to assess auditory discrimination, but it is not presently clear that these alternate methods assess different processes or produce different results in testing (Winitz, 1984).

The overriding question that usually surfaces when the auditory discrimination of children with articulation errors is considered is: Does the performance of articulatory-defective children on auditory discrimination tests differ from that of normal-speaking children? The answer to this question has been mixed. Some investigators have concluded from their research that children with articulation errors are not different from normal-speaking children on tests of auditory discrimination (McReynolds, Kohn, & Williams, 1975; Locke, 1980a, 1980b). Other investigators take the opposite position by citing evidence that indicates a positive relationship between articulation performance and auditory discrimination. In 1967, Weiner provided a comprehensive summary of the major research efforts to that date, and concluded that a strong relationship exists between auditory discrimination skills and articulation performance when certain testing constraints, to be described, are met. Subsequent investigations, as reviewed by Winitz (1969, 1975, 1981, 1984), have supported Weiner's position.

Selection of Contrastive Items

Two testing constraints Weiner and others have discussed pertain to the composition of the test items. First, the auditory discrimination items should be relevant, that is, they should involve the specific sounds that each child misarticulates. Second, the paired items of the auditory discrimination tests should contain the child's specific error response. For example, consider a child who misarticulates /r/ with a [w] substitution. Relevant discrimination items are those that examine the auditory discrimination of /r/ in contexts in which it is misarticulated, such as a particular word position, blend, or the preceding or following vowel. Paired items that contain /w/ to form contrasts, such as /ra/–/wa/ and /drim/–/dwim/, utilize the specific error response of the child. Similarly, when a child substitutes [θ] for /s/, the /s/ should be examined in the contexts in which it is misarticulated. Furthermore, /θ/, not other typically observed errors, such as /t/, a lateralized /s̺/ or an omission of /s/, is regarded as the appropriate contrast for /s/ in the paired items of the auditory discrimination test.

Several writers (Weiner, 1967; Winitz, 1969, 1975, 1981, 1984; Locke, 1980a) have commented that most auditory discriminaton tests are designed to measure general sound-discrimination ability. These tests, of which the Wepman (1960) test is the most widely used, are called *general auditory discrimination tests* (Winitz, 1969, 1981, 1984; Monnin, 1984). The paired items of a general discrimination test contain a wide range of paired sound contrasts, such as /s/–/θ/, /r/–/l/, and /p/–/b/; however, only one example of each type is generally included. The reason this test format is used is that auditory discrimination is considered to be a general underlying ability that is assessed by administering to each child a large number of auditory contrasts. This procedure, however, does not take into account the sounds that each child misarticulates or the type of errors that he or she makes.

A *specific auditory discrimination test* is a test that is individualized for each child. There are no standardized specific discrimination tests. The clinician selects items that are relevant and contain the appropriate error response, taking into account the contexts in which each sound is misarticulated.

Context is important in the design of specific discrimination tests. Often children are able to distinguish between two sounds in one context and not in another, or in one word and not in another (Spriestersbach & Curtis, 1951). Examples of four contexts for a /θ/ substitution are (a) vowel contexts (/θi/–/si/ and /θɑ/–/sɑ/), (b) word position (*think–sink, pathway–passway* and *bath–bass*), (c) consonantal context (*tenth-tense* and *frothed-frost*), and (d) morphological environment (*eighths-eights*). Additionally, there is a degree of variability or test error that cannot be avoided when testing individuals, especially children. For this reason a large number of contexts should be included for each target sound that is misarticulated.

When auditory discrimination tests containing a limited number of contexts and few item-pairs for each sound have been used to assess the auditory discrimination of articulatory-defective children, a small or nonexistent relationship is found between auditory discrimination and articulation (McReynolds, Kohn, & Williams, 1975; Locke, 1980b). However, in investigations in which the test protocols contained a sufficient number of relevant contrasts in which each child's errors were reflected in the paired items in a number of contexts, a strong relationship was found between articulation performance and auditory discrimination (Weiner, 1967; Winitz, 1969; Monnin & Huntington, 1974; Strange & Broen, 1981; Broen, Strange, Doyle, & Heller, 1983).

Weiner (1967) made another interesting observation regarding the use of general discrimination tests. He commented that children with few articulation errors are unlikely to show a deficit in auditory discrimination when general discrimination tests are used. However, he noted that the auditory discrimination performance of children with moderate and severe articulation disorders or general discrimination tests often is below that of children who do not have articulation errors. Weiner recognized that when children have a large number of articulation errors, the chances are increased that at least some of the items of the discrimination test are relevant to the sounds which they misarticulate, their specific errors, and the contexts in which the errors occur. For this reason, a positive relationship between articulation and discrimination often is found for children with multiple articulation errors when general discrimination tests are used.

Developmental Considerations

Another important consideration in the testing of auditory discrimination involves the complex relationship between the development of auditory discrimination and the development of articulation. Recent investigations indicate that the development of auditory discrimination precedes the acquisition of articulation (Edwards, 1974; Eilers & Oller, 1976; Winitz, Sanders, & Kort, 1981). An interpretation of this finding is that the process of learning how to articulate the sounds of a given language involves learning the correspondence between auditory input and the mechanisms involved in the production of speech sounds. It is believed that children first acquire an auditory concept of a speech sound. This concept then provides the perceptual framework for the formation of the phonological and articulatory systems. As we know, however, there are many dimensions to each of these processes. Therefore, although auditory learning may precede a particular aspect of speech-sound learning, it is not implied that all phases of auditory learning must precede each developmental step in phonology and articulation (see chapter 3).

Partial and interactive learning is exemplified by instances in which children have been found to produce error sounds that are variations or distortions of standard sounds (Kornfield, 1971). For example, a child may substitute a sound for [r] that is intermediate between /r/ and /w/. The production of intermediate or distorted sounds may be the result of articulation acquisition that takes place without full development of each auditory contrast (Greenlee, 1980; Hoffman, Stager, & Daniloff, 1983).

Although it is recognized that auditory input is the primary source through which information about the phonological system and its phonetic properties is acquired, there are, no doubt, complex interactions among auditory perception, phonology, and articulation, such that the development of each influences the development of the other. For example, articulation learning may provide certain sources of feedback to the auditory system to cause it to attend in a certain way to incoming signals. Similarly, one's implicit knowledge about the phonological system and other dimensions of language no doubt influences the perception of the speech signal. These considerations notwithstanding, the developmental constraint of discrimination first, articulation second must be taken into account when analyzing the results of studies on the relationship between auditory discrimination and articulation.

This developmental process may be identified as having three acquisitional stages:

1. Neither auditory discrimination nor articulation has developed.
2. Auditory discrimination has developed, but articulation has not developed.
3. Both auditory discrimination and articulation have developed.

When articulatory-defective children are selected as subjects, they may fall into either Category 1 or 2 as some investigators have observed (Eilers & Oller, 1976; Winitz, Sanders, & Kort, 1981; Broen, Strange, Doyle, & Heller, 1983). If an overwhelming number of subjects in a given study fall into Category 2, no difference in auditory discrimination between the articulatory-defective and the normal-speaking children will be found. The conclusion that there is no relationship between articulation performance and auditory discrimination is correct when the majority of articulatory-defective children fall into Category 2. However, it does not necessarily follow that auditory discrimination is unimportant in the development of articulation. In those investigations in which no relationship was found, this particular developmental constraint may have been a consideration.

In summary, we have identified three conditions that may be responsible for the observation that in some investigations a positive correlation between articulation performance and auditory discrimination was not found. These conditions are inadequate sampling of the relevant auditory contrasts, paired contrasts that do not take into account the type of articulation error the individual child makes, and developmental constraints. When these considerations are taken into account, the experimental evidence indicates that a certain proportion of children with functional articulation errors show a deficit in auditory discrimination. Furthermore, it is recognized that the auditory discrimination deficit is restricted to the individual articulation errors of each child. There is no evidence to indicate that the auditory discrimination deficit is caused by an underlying auditory disability of general origin. We conclude from these findings that auditory discrimination training is an important component in the rehabilitation of children with misarticulations.

TEACHING AUDITORY DISCRIMINATION

The procedures of training that are described in this section place almost exclusive emphasis on an extended period of auditory discrimination training prior to productive practice. As indicated earlier, this approach does not ignore the relationship that may exist between the perceptual system and other systems of articulation development. It does, however, consider auditory input to be a fundamental skill in that its development, for the most part, precedes that of other systems that contribute to the development of articulation.

A number of procedures can be used to teach children to attend to the relevant phonetic cues of sounds that they misarticulate after it has been determined that they do not discriminate between a target sound and its respective error sound. Discrimination testing should be thorough. It should involve a variety of phonetic and linguistic contexts, and, if possible, the target sounds and the child's substitutions should be tested in full sentences as well as in single words. For example, the difference between the syllables /sɑ/ and /θɑ/ can be assessed in short sentences, as in *He put the /sɑ/ on the table–He put the /θɑ/ on the table*, or in meaningful units, as in the following pair of sentences: *The artist sketched the mouth with a pen–The artist sketched the mouse with a pen*. Children are to indicate whether the sentences are the same or different. Sentences should be said at a moderately fast pace to determine whether or not accurate discriminations can be made when the test items approximate normal conversational speech rate. It is well known that some speech sounds are reduced or altered in significant ways in the normal flow of speech. If a child discriminates well when the test items involve isolated words, but does poorly when the test items are sentences, there is a strong possibility that accurate discriminations are not being made in conversational speech.

Formal Approach

When children do not discriminate well in isolated word contexts and/or in sentence contexts, the primary goal is to teach them to hear the relevant differences. Both a formal approach and an informal approach can be used. In the *formal approach* the child is drilled on sound pairs. The training method is essentially the same as the testing format just described. The training should be fairly extensive and should include sentence contexts that are said at a rapid rate. Production practice is not introduced at this point.

Informal Approach

Informal practice involves training in communicative contexts. Goal-oriented activities, tasks, and situations that involve completion of an activity or the accomplishment of a goal are used by the clinician to provide meaningful and realistic listening situations. Activities such as arts and crafts, games, and minor work situations are used to focus the child's attention on speech for communicative purposes. The clinician selects objects and activities in which the target sound will appear often. Through these activities the child is motivated to request items, ask questions, and listen attentively so as to be able to participate.

When listening skills are trained through informal practice, the communicative activities serve as the focus of training. Children are never directly aware that listening is being trained because formal exercises are not used. Nor are they directly aware that their performance is being evaluated because all evaluations are part of the communicative process. For example, the paired contrast between /r/ and /w/ can be presented by devising a game about "witch people" and "rich people." The clinician can say, "Pick up the witch people and we will play that game." If the child responds inappropriately by picking up the objects that go with the rich people, the clinician might say, "No, I said the witch people. These are the witch people and these are the rich people. Let's play the witch game." At another training session the clinician might ask, "Which game would you like to play?" If the child responds "witch people" the clinician would pick up the objects for the "witch people" game. The child might respond, "No, I meant the witch people," and then immediately point to the "rich people." The clinician may respond, "These are the rich people, and these are the witch people," in order to emphasize again the contrast. Although in this latter example the child is engaged in conversation, the purpose of the activity is to teach auditory discrimination in meaningful contexts.

It is particularly difficult to find /r/–/w/ minimal pairs for the frequently misarticulated /r/ because /w/ and /r/ show few contrasts for the same part of speech. For example, *wag* is a verb, and *rag* is a noun. Also, *red* is an adjective and *wed* is a verb. Additionally, there are many other /r/ words for which there is no /r/–/w/ contrast, such as *rabbit, road,* and *reach,* or the contrast is an infrequent word. For /r/, artificial minimal-pair contrasts need to be devised within the context of activities and games. One activity is to line pictures whose labels or names are in minimal contrast up against a wall and place an object in front of each picture. Then ask the child to find the object in front of a particular picture, and to place it somewhere else to win the game (e.g., "Put the pencil in front of the *wag* (or *rag*) on the table.") In this way, minimal contrasts can be utilized in a context that is meaningful for children. Pictures that represent words might be used, such as *wag* (a dog wagging his tail) and *rag, run* and *one,* and *rent* and *went.* Other suggestions regarding the use of minimal pairs can be found in chapter 13.

The informal approach has two primary objectives. One is to provide meaningful input in which the target sound and the respective error sound are in contrast frequently. A second objective is to use the communicative process to indicate to the child in an indirect way that a correct discrimination is important for effective communcation. As a consequence, it is expected that a substantial amount of phonological restructuring will take place.

Informal teaching is preferred for reasons described in the preceding chapter. Nevertheless, there are instances in which formal instruction seems appropriate. Usually formal instruction is provided when discrimination training must be direct and highly focused. It is used as a last resort when informal training has failed to teach auditory discrimination.

Amount and Timing of Auditory Discrimination Training

Whether a formal approach or an informal approach is used, two frequent questions that surface pertain to the amount of time to be spent on auditory training, and whether the auditory training is to precede or coincide with articulation training. Some clinicians take the position that no direct training in auditory discrimination should be provided prior to articulation training. Others take intermediate positions.

The approach we recommend is that auditory discrimination training should be *intensive* and should precede all levels of articulation production training. It should extend over several weeks and perhaps months of training. No production should be insisted upon during this period, although in an informal training situation children will make spontaneous attempts to produce the target sound because communicative, goal-oriented activities most generally stimulate children to talk. There is no easy solution as to when to begin articulation production practice. This decision is largely subjective. However, regardless of the position one holds, the child should not be asked to produce sounds at each succeeding production level (e.g., sound, syllable, sentence, and conversational utterance) until it has been determined that the appropriate speech sound discrimination for that level can be made easily and rapidly.

CONSIDERATIONS REGARDING LEVEL OF BREAKDOWN

Thus far, this chapter has considered primarily Level 1 of the five levels of potential breakdown (Table 9.1). One goal of auditory training is to alter a child's underlying phonological system in the direction of the adult phonological code. Discrimination training is a necessary first step. However, improving auditory discrimination will not necessarily cause a child's underlying system of phonemes to change; conceivably, children may be able to hear phonetic distinctions, but be unable to apply this knowledge at the phonological level (Level 2). It is also possible that the underlying phonological system can be correct, but for some reason, this information is not provided to or cannot be utilized at the phonetic and articulatory levels (Levels 3, 4, and 5). Each of these possible sources of breakdown will be discussed.

Correct Sound Discrimination with Incorrect Underlying Phonological System: Level 2 Breakdown

Some children with misarticulations have normal auditory discrimination. The source of their difficulty apparently lies along other dimensions. One area of difficulty may be in the organizational processes that are involved in learning complex rule systems like phonology. However, the source of this difficulty cannot be easily explained. Generally, children who are unable to learn concepts are thought to show a retardation in intellectual ability. However, intelligence is not related to articulation performance for children whose IQs are above 70 (Winitz, 1964). Children with IQs below 70 will often show a greater number of articulation errors than normally intelligent children, but this observation does not explain phonological retardation for normally intelligent children. Possibly, some children acquire phonological concepts slowly because of specific language deficits, or because their language experience or language acquisitional strategies have in some way inhibited the development of phonological competence.

One procedure for determining whether the breakdown occurs at the phonological level involves the use of context-free sentences in which both the target sound and the respective error sound are appropriate. According to a procedure we have developed recently, children hear three sentences, all of which contain the target sound or the error sound. After hearing these three sentences, the children signify their understanding by selecting the appropriate picture from a set of two pictures. For example, a child listens to three context-free sentences in which the same /w/ or /r/ word is used in all three sentences, and then is immediately asked to point to one of two pictures, choosing the one that represents the meaning of the three sentences. Two sets of three sentences are as follows:

A. 1. I was to wake it up.
    2. I didn't want to wake it up.
    3. Finally I was told to wake it up.
B. 1. I was to rake it up.
    2. I didn't want to rake it up.
    3. Finally I was told to rake it up.

After these three sentences from set A or B are presented, the child is shown the two pictures in Figure 9.1, and is asked to point to the picture that correctly describes the sentences.

This procedure, termed the *phonological performance test*, is currently being tested with children who substitute /w/ for /r/. We are interested in determining whether children who are able to discriminate between /w/ and /r/ in single words and sentences perform poorly on the test. If they do, a reasonable interpretation is that they can *hear* the difference between /w/ and /r/, but they do not *utilize* this distinction in their phonological system when words occur in context.

A second procedure is to determine whether the children can detect mispronounced words (Cole, 1981). For example, a story is read and some of

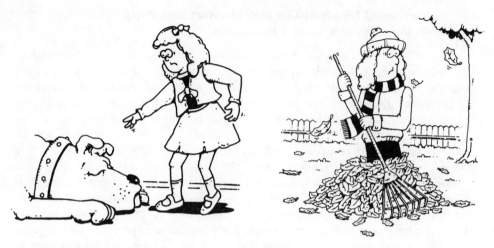

FIGURE 9.1
Example of picture test items used to assess phonological performance. One of
the following two sets is read to the child prior to the simultaneous presentation
of these two pictures:

I was to rake it up.
I didn't want to rake it up.
Finally I was told to rake it up.

I was to wake it up.
I didn't want to wake it up.
Finally I was told to wake it up.

the words beginning with /r/ and /w/ are purposefully mispronounced. The
substitution of [w] for /r/ and [r] for /w/ provides a way to determine whether
children who can discriminate between /w/ and /r/ readily detect mispronunciations of these sounds. If they fail to detect these mispronunciations, we may
infer that the /r/–/w/ distinction is not part of their phonological system because the mispronunciations of /r/ and /w/ are considered to be correct. It
should be noted, however, that this is a metalinguistic task in that the child is
asked to make a judgment about the phonological system. It may thus be
influenced by metalinguistic as well as discrimination abilities.

The focus of treatment for children who *can* discriminate between the
target sound and the error sound, but who do not *utilize* this distinction in their
phonological system, centers on instructing the child to make changes in his or
her underlying phonological system. The same goal-oriented communicative
activities that are used to teach speech discrimination can be applied here
without the need to focus exclusively on the teaching of minimal-pair distinctions.

Informal Training in Phonological Restructuring.   Training in phonological restructuring is regarded as somewhat different from training in speech
sound discrimination. In auditory discrimination training there is concentra-
tion on teaching the paired difference between two contrasting sounds. In
phonological training all error sounds that are presumed to be governed by a
particular phonological rule are treated simultaneously. Children are taught to

alter the underlying phonological rules that govern their sound errors without at first being required to produce the target sound.

Of primary importance is the way the clinician responds to the child's verbal and nonverbal remarks. When a child does not respond appropriately, either through nonverbal expression or through verbal expression, the clinician should not show understanding of the child's communicative intent. For example, when a child substitutes a [w] for /r/ in conversation or selects a /w/ item when the clinician says an /r/ item, the clinician should respond only to what the child says or does.

If the child requests a toy by saying, "I want the 'wabbit,'" the clinician may respond, "I don't know what you mean. There is a rock, radio, ring, and rabbit on the shelf. Which one do you want?" At this point the child may signify through gestures that the intended word is *rabbit*. The clinician may respond by saying. "Oh you mean the rabbit, the toy rabbit. At first I didn't understand you." In this instance the error sound does not produce a linguistic contrast; therefore, it is not recommended that the clinician say, "Oh you meant the rabbit, but you said the wabbit." Possibly, in communicative situations, the use of the error sound may reinforce its incorrect pronunciation. In formal auditory discrimination training the error sound is often presented as a non-linguistic contrast, but here the child is advised that one production is correct and the other is incorrect, and usually nonsense items are used so that words are not mispronounced.

An important aspect of informal training in phonological restructuring is to teach children with articulation errors to realize that errors often cause the clinician, and, by generalization, peers, teachers, and parents, to misunderstand them. As a result children may attend carefully to the communicative process and may modify their articulatory errors without conscious attention to their speech. The purpose of the informal approach, then, is to convey to the child, in an indirect way, that communicative responses must be accurate if appropriate communication is to take place.

Formal Methods in Phonological Restructuring.   When informal procedures do not work well, formal methods may be used. A number of formal procedures have been used to teach children to change the underlying set of phonological rules that govern their misarticulations. Although these procedures vary in approach, they all include production practice. One approach is to present the error sound and the target sound to the child and ask him or her to imitate both (Ingram, 1976). A second approach (Weiner, 1981) is to point to objects or pictures that the child names. If the names of these items are in minimal contrast, and the child uses the same sound in both words of a minimal pair (e.g., [wæg] for *rag* and *wag*), the clinician will point to the incorrect picture or object when the target sound is misarticulated. This procedure will indicate to the child that his or her articulation errors contribute to a failure to convey the correct meaning. As a consequence, the child may be motivated to correct his or her articulation errors by paying close attention to phonological distinctions that are important for communication (see chapters 7, 13, and 14 for further discussion). These two approaches are not always successful because, although children may understand the purpose of each of the two training procedures, they may require initially standard procedures of auditory training and articulation correction in order for them to learn the production of the target sound so that they can participate effectively (Shelton, 1982).

A third approach to altering underlying phonological structure is to use standard procedures of articulation correction (Compton, 1970). Investigators who stress articulation procedures as a means of changing underlying phonological structure assume that production practice is an essential component in the restructuring process. However, the use of articulation practice *only* is somewhat problematic in that it does not necessarily follow that correct understanding of a phonological pattern results from practice in correct articulation.

We recommend another strategy to begin the teaching of phonological restructuring. In this approach, children are taught to identify categories of sounds prior to and independently of articulation practice (LaRiviere, Winitz, Reeds, & Herriman, 1974). The target sound and the error sound are presented in groups. For example, consider the pattern of stopping. In this case the clinician would tell the child to listen to a series of sounds and to notice that each sound in the series is similar. The child hears the first series (the target sounds, or in this illustration fricatives) followed by a pause, and then hears the second series of sounds (the error sounds, or stops). The child is then told that each series is to be identified by a number and to try to learn that number. The clinician then presents in random order each group of sounds followed by the number 1 or 2, e.g., all the fricatives followed by the number 1, and all the stops followed by the number 2. After several trials, the clinician no longer says the numbers. At this point the child is to say the correct number after the clinician says the sounds of each group and the clinician immediately tells the child whether the number was correct or incorrect. The objective here is to teach the child that stops and fricatives are categories of sounds and that stopping is an inappropriate category for fricatives.

Correct Underlying Phonological System with Incorrect Underlying Phonetic System: Level 3 Breakdown

Currently, precise diagnostic procedures do not exist that distinguish between errors of underlying phonology and underlying phonetics. Auditory discrimination tests might be used for this purpose if the error sound is a nonstandard sound. For example, if children distinguish well between contrasts of English, and also do well on the phonological performance test, but have difficulty distinguishing between a target sound and its corresponding nonstandard error sound, there is the possibility that the error sound has been internalized as an underlying phonetic unit. On the other hand, if auditory discrimination is normal, then the problem may lie at the articulatory level.

If the formation of underlying phonetic units is incorrect, our recommendation is to postpone production practice until an individual child can discriminate reliably between the target sound and the corresponding nonstandard error sound. Previous research has indicated that intensive auditory discrimination training is a satisfactory method for achieving this objective (Winitz & Bellerose, 1967).

Correct Underlying Systems with Incorrect Articulatory Programming/Execution: Level 4/5 Breakdown

When no apparent difficulty exists at the auditory, phonological, or phonetic level, training in articulation production should be started immediately. Perhaps one final check of auditory coding should be made. It would be useful to know whether discrimination can be made between sequences of phonemes such as *tan–nat* and *books–boosk*. It is possible that some children with functional articulation errors perceive strings of sounds incorrectly. A disorder of this type may be evident from their performance on specific discrimination tests. If this disorder is present, auditory discrimination training should be evaluated and, if necessary, given careful attention prior to training in articulation production.

MOTIVATIONAL CONSIDERATIONS

Some children may have the capability for learning all of the component levels of articulation that have been discussed, but fail to want to alter their articulatory patterns beyond a certain point. In second-language learning, stabilizing grammatical usage at a certain point in the acquisition of a foreign language prior to full mastery is called *fossilization* (Selinker & Lamendella, 1978). Fossilization in second-language learning and in native-language learning is not well explained at this time. Social factors, especially the motivation to talk and communicate, are important considerations in the treatment process, as we have indicated above. Children who discriminate between sounds well and who imitate the target sound correctly on stimulation or who show in other ways by their "inconsistent" production of sounds or features that they can articulate the sounds they misarticulate should receive training that is geared to motivate them to listen and to communicate.

One question that often arises when the intervention strategies of communication and intensive listening are recommended is: Why do these procedures, administered by a professional in a professional setting, provide greater motivation than the everyday communicative experiences of children, as they seem to resemble the kinds of communicative and listening experiences that children receive in the classroom or in the home, where apparently they have failed to be effective? The answer to this question lies in how the communicative listening experiences provided in the speech and language clinic differ from those already taking place in the natural environment of the child. First, the clinic experiences are focused to provide practice with specific sounds and speech contexts. Second, the communicative contexts that are set up to make the child a better listener involve strategies of responding, as discussed above, that indicate directly or indirectly to the child that correct articulation usage leads to clarity and understanding in communication. Third, the clinician responds within the communicative context, but does not cause children to have anxiety about their speech difficulty. Children with few articulation errors will benefit especially from planned communicative experiences because they are usually intelligible, and therefore often communicate well with their peers, teachers and parents. Planned communication experiences will place them in a setting in which their articulatory errors will be the focal point of the communicative process.

AUDITORY DISCRIMINATION TRAINING AND ARTICULATION TRAINING

Auditory training should not be limited to pretraining phases of articulation training. There are three reasons for continuing auditory discrimination training during articulation production training. The first pertains to the degree of auditory perception that is required to achieve the standard articulatory productions of the community language. The second pertains to the type of monitoring that may be necessary in order to learn new articulatory productions. The third concerns the number of different phonetic and speech contexts that must be taken into account when learning speech sounds.

Degree Of Auditory Perception

Speech sounds contrast on a number of phonetic dimensions, and usually not all of these are critical in learning to hear differences between sounds. For example, English /l/ and /r/ can be distinguished on the basis of the lateral or nonlateral place feature. No other differences need to be considered when making a discrimination between them. Yet this limited information about the differences between these two sounds will *not* enable one to articulate these sounds correctly. Learning to articulate correctly often requires a greater degree of discrimination training than is involved in learning to hear differences between two sounds.

It may be that full attention is not given to the auditory cues that mark a speech sound unless an imitative response is required. For this reason, partial learning of auditory contrasts may represent a legitimate stage in the perceptual development of sounds. As children acquire the sounds of their language, they continue to refine their auditory discrimination as they improve their articulation. This reciprocal relationship between articulation and discrimination in the normally developing child may come about because children attend to phonetic cues closely when they are required to imitate them correctly. Children with articulation errors who also show a deficit in auditory discrimination initially may show little progress in the development of articulation unless auditory discrimination training is given special emphasis in articulation training. Not only may such children require special attention before articulation practice is begun, but this special attention may need to be carried out throughout all stages of articulation training.

Monitoring

The acquisition of articulatory responses requires continuous monitoring on the part of the child. In most training procedures the auditory channel is used by the child to evaluate the accuracy of a newly learned articulatory production. A typical articulation training paradigm begins with the clinician's production, followed almost immediately by the child's production, and concluded by an evaluation of performance that the clinician conveys to the child. In effect, the child's articulatory productions are monitored with reference to the clinician's productions in that judgments of self-performance involve a comparison between self-produced responses and those of the clinician.

Later, when the production of a sound is acquired, children judge auditory output with reference to an abstract, internally derived conceptualization of the sound. Similarly, adult listeners judge a sound as right or wrong by comparing it with an internally generated concept of the sound held in memory. In this regard, successful learning in articulation training relies heavily on the auditory channel to monitor the acquisition of articulation productions. As more is learned about how auditory feedback is used as a monitor in articulation learning and usage, clinicians will be better able to use auditory feedback in treatment.

Phonetic and Speech Contexts

Articulation training, as practiced by most speech-language pathologists, usually involves the training of sounds in isolation or in syllable contexts. As the sound is acquired, the complexity of the context is increased. However, auditory training is usually ignored when the shift is made from isolation and syllables to words, and finally to sentences. Earlier we recommended intensive discrimination training prior to articulation training. As training in articulation production is implemented, we recommend continuing discrimination training so as to provide auditory experience for the target sounds in contexts that closely approximate those of conversational speech.

Carry-over

Clinicians often report that carry-over is the most difficult area of articulation treatment. A number of procedures are often used to provide for effective carry-over in settings outside the clinical environment. All of these approaches have one common purpose in mind: to "remind" the child to continue to use the newly acquired sounds in conversational contexts when not in the clinic.

Our recommendation is not to begin carry-over training until children can detect errors in the speech of others and in their own speech. Detection of errors of other speakers can be trained effectively by reading children stories in which some of the words are purposively mispronounced when uttered at a conversational rate. Children can learn to monitor their own speech errors by reading a story and reporting after each sentence whether any words were said incorrectly. These procedures do not assure that children will consistently monitor their speech in settings outside the clinic, but they do provide a beginning in this direction.

SUMMARY

Intensive auditory training prior to articulation production practice is regarded as an important component in articulation treatment along several dimensions. Auditory discrimination training directed to the differences between the target sound and the error sound provides the special kind of listening that children with articulation disorders need in order to acquire phonological distinctions. It was recommended that children with articulation disorders be given auditory discrimination training in communicative situations in order to utilize newly acquired phonetic distinctions as part of their developing phonological system. It was also recommended that auditory training be continued throughout all later stages of articulation treatment to provide the kinds of experiences that are essential in learning to monitor speech, and in the acquisition of carry-over.

REFERENCES

Broen, P. A., Strange, W., Doyle, S. S., & Heller, J. H. (1983). Perception and production of approximant consonants by normal and articulation-delayed preschool children. *Journal of Speech and Hearing Disorders, 26*, 601–608.

Brown, R. W., & Hildum, D. C. (1956). Expectancy and the identification of syllables. *Language, 32*, 411–419.

Chomsky, N., & Halle, M. (1968). *The sound pattern of English.* New York: Harper and Row.

Cole, R. A. (1981). Perception of fluent speech by children and adults. In H. Winitz (Ed.), *Native language and foreign language acquisition, Annals of the New York Academy of Sciences, 379*, 92–109.

Compton, A. J. (1970). Generative studies of children's phonological disorders. *Journal of Speech and Hearing Disorders, 35*, 315–339.

Edwards, M. L. (1974). Perception and production in child phonology: The testing of four hypotheses. *Journal of Child Language, 1*, 205–220.

Edwards, M. L., & Shriberg, L. D. (1983). *Phonology: Applications in communicative disorders.* San Diego: College Hill Press.

Eilers, R. E., & Oller, D. K. (1976). The role of speech discrimination in developmental sound substitutions. *Journal of Child Language, 3*, 319–329.

Greenlee, M. (1980). Learning the phonetic cues to the voiced-voiceless distinction: A comparison of child and adult speech perception. *Journal of Child Language, 7*, 459–468.

Hass, W. (1983). Phonological analysis of a case of dyslalia. *Journal of Speech and Hearing Disorders, 28*, 239–246.

Hoffman, P. R., Stager, S., & Daniloff, R. G. (1983). Perception and production of misarticulated /r/. *Journal of Speech and Hearing Disorders, 48*, 210–215.

Ingram, D. (1976). *Phonological disability in children.* New York: American Elsevier.

Kent, R. D., & Lybolt, J. T. (1982). Techniques of therapy based on motor learning theory. In W. H. Perkins (Ed.), *Current therapy of communication disorders: General principles of therapy.* New York: Thieme-Stratton.

Kornfield, J. (1971). What initial clusters tell us about a child's speech code. Massachusetts Institute of Technology Research Laboratory of Electronics, *Quarterly Progress Report*, 218–221.

LaRiviere, C., Winitz, H., Reeds, J., & Herriman, E. (1974). The conceptual reality of selected distinctive features. *Journal of Speech and Hearing Research, 17*, 122–133.

Locke, J. L. (1980a). The inference of speech perception in the phonologically disordered child. Part 1: A rationale, some criteria, the conventional tests. *Journal of Speech and Hearing Disorders, 45*, 431–444.

Locke, J. L. (1980b). The inference of speech perception in the phonologically disordered child. Part II: Some clinically novel procedures, their use, some findings. *Journal of Speech and Hearing Disorders, 45,* 445–468.

McReynolds, L. V., Kohn, J., & Williams, G. C. (1975). Articulatory-defective children's discrimination of their production errors. *Journal of Speech and Hearing Disorders, 40,* 327–338.

Monnin, L. M. (1984). Speech sound discrimination testing and training: Why? Why Not? In H. Winitz (Ed.), *Treating articulation disorders: For clinicians by clinicians.* Baltimore:University Park Press.

Monnin, L. M., & Huntington, D. A. (1974). Relationship of articulatory defects to speech-sound identification. *Journal of Speech and Hearing Research, 17,* 352–366.

Netsell, R., & Kent, R. (1976). Paroxysmal ataxic dysarthria. *Journal of Speech and Hearing Disorders, 41,* 93–109.

Panagos, J. M. (1982). The case against the autonomy of phonological disorders in children. *Seminars in Speech, Language and Hearing, 3,* 172–181.

Selinker, L., & Lamendella, J. T. (1978). Fossilization in interlanguage learning. In C. E. Blatchford & J. Schacter (Eds.), *On Tesol '78, EFL policies, programs, practices.*Washington, D.C.: Teachers of English to Speakers of Other Languages.

Shelton, R. (1982). Response to Weiner. *Journal of Speech and Hearing Disorders, 47,* 336.

Smith, N. V. (1973). *The acquisition of phonology: A case study.* London: Cambridge University Press.

Spriestersbach, D. C., & Curtis, J. F. (1951). Misarticulation and discrimination of speech sounds. *Quarterly Journal of Speech, 37,* 483–491.

Strange, W., & Broen, P. A. (1981). The relationship between perception and production of /w/, /r/, and /l/ by three-year-old children. *Journal of Experimental Child Psychology, 31,* 81–102.

Van Riper, C. (1939). *Speech correction, principles and methods.* New York: Prentice Hall.

Weiner, F. (1981). Treatment of phonological disability using the method of meaningful minimal contrast: Two case studies. *Journal of Speech and Hearing Disorders, 45,* 97–103.

Weiner, P. S. (1967). Auditory discrimination and articulation. *Journal of Speech and Hearing Disorders, 32,* 19–28.

Wepman, J. M. (1960). Auditory discrimination, speech, and reading. *Elementary School Journal, 58,* 259–268.

Williams, R., Ingham, R. J., & Rosenthal, J. (1981). A further analysis for developmental apraxia of speech in children with defective articulation. *Journal of Speech and Hearing Research, 24,* 496–505.

Winitz, H. (1964). Research in articulation and intelligence. *Child Development, 35,* 287–297.

Winitz, H. (1969). *Articulatory acquisition and behavior.* New York: Appleton-Century Crofts.

Winitz, H. (1975). *From syllable to conversation.* Baltimore: University Park Press.

Winitz, H. (1981). Considerations in the treatment of articulation disorders. In R. Rieber (Ed.), *Communication disorders.* New York: Plenum Press.

Winitz, H. (1984). Auditory considerations in articulation training. In H. Winitz (Ed.), *Treating articulation disorders: For clinicians by clinicians.* Baltimore: University Park Press.

Winitz, H., & Bellerose, B. (1967). Relation between sound discrimination and sound learning. *Journal of Communication Disorders, 1,* 215–235.

Winitz, H., Sanders, R., & Kort, J. (1981). Comprehension and production of the /-əz/ plural allomorph. *Journal of Psycholinguistic Research, 10,* 259–271.

10 Considerations for Organic Disorders

Thus far, the focus of this book has been on functional articulation problems, i.e., those problems for which no organic cause has been determined. However, there are certain disorders of articulation that are quite different in nature from functional articulation problems, although they often share similar perceptual characteristics. This group of disorders is referred to as *organic articulation disorders*.

Organic articulation disorders can be defined as those disorders that arise from physical anomalies affecting structure or function of the mechanisms of speech. The damage may be to the structures of the oral mechanism as well as to the central and/or peripheral nervous systems.

The etiological or causal differences between organic and functional articulation disorders lead to a number of points of special consideration. First of all, the umbrella term *organic disorders* should not be interpreted as meaning a single disorder. Within the category of organic disorders are a number of types of disorders, each with its own specific causes, speech and language characteristics, and associated problems. This, of course, has implications for diagnostic procedures, treatment, and prognosis.

Dorothy H. Air, Ph.D., is the associate director of audiology and speech pathology at the University of Cincinnati Medical Center. **Ann Stace Wood**, Ph.D., is a clinical speech and language pathologist in private practice in Cincinnati.

269

Treatment for organic problems tends to be multidisciplinary, since rarely is speech the only affected area. For example, in cerebral palsy, the same motor dysfunction that affects speech affects more generalized motor function as well. Therefore, both evaluation and treatment will involve several disciplines working together. Another example of a multidisciplinary problem is cleft palate, where the total treatment program may require the efforts of the surgeon, orthodontist, prosthodontist (the specialist who provides artificial oral devices), speech pathologist, and audiologist, to name but a few. Although in some cases a team approach may be necessary in the treatment of a functional articulation problem, frequently the speech pathologist is the only professional involved due to the more narrow scope of the problem.

Another major difference between organic disorders and functional disorders is that of prognosis. Prognosis has a direct relationship to the degree of organicity. Therefore, the success which can ultimately be achieved is related to the degree of physical damage. This has important ramifications for goals, treatment planning, and counseling.

Because of these physiologic limitations, success for the organic problem may be defined differently than for the functional problem. Rather than in maximum potential for *speech*, success in treating the organic problem lies in maximum potential for *communication*. In some cases, it may be possible to achieve normal, or at least a useful, articulation level. This may be done by using standard approaches to articulation therapy to improve articulatory accuracy, or it may involve teaching compensatory methods to more closely approximate normal articulation. In severe disorders, such as degenerative neurological disease, or severely involved static neurological problems, prognosis for oral communication may be quite poor. For individuals with these disorders, non-oral communication strategies may be necessary either as an augmentative measure or as a total approach.

Working with severely involved organic disorders requires that the speech pathologist be knowledgeable enough to plan realistic goals. While it may seem obvious that an individual cannot progress beyond his/her physiologic limits, the speech pathologist must be able to recognize those limits and respond accordingly. It has not been unheard of to find patients who have spent years in speech therapy working on very limited goals and making minimal progress, when some of that energy might have been more productively directed toward non-oral communication. On the other side of the coin, all clinicians have seen patients who were never referred because the referral source felt there was no potential for improvement. When, in fact, these patients finally did make their way to the clinic, there was indeed some potential present. If a realistic appraisal is made, the most effective management can follow.

Counseling for organic communication disorders may be a difficult task, as many sensitive issues must be considered. Issues such as changing roles, acceptance of limited skills, deteriorating conditions, etc., are critical issues to patients. How they ultimately handle these crises affects the course of therapy. Counseling should always be honest, yet maintain a balance between the positive and the negative factors. For the individual with a poor prognosis, consideration of negative factors alone may destroy motivation and limit progress beyond the physiologic constraints. Emphasizing positive factors alone is misleading and may result in the patient setting very unrealistic goals for himself. One must always remember that recognizing the potential of the individual and communicating information to the family and patient in an honest and realistic way are as essential to the treatment process as are the specific treatment techniques used.

One final reminder should be mentioned concerning articulation problems. The population with organic disorders may also have functional problems; it cannot be assumed that all symptoms reflect organicity. Those who have organic disorders are subject to maturational lags and environmental influences just as everyone else is.

As has been mentioned, there are a number of types of organic disorders that can affect articulation. Each of these will be considered in some detail.

APRAXIA OF SPEECH

Before developing this section on apraxia of speech, it is appropriate to discuss the controversy over the concept among members of the profession. There are some who insist that the articulatory manifestations labeled *apraxia* should be considered a linguistic impairment (Martin, 1974) and others who maintain that an isolated apraxia of speech almost never exists (Geschwind, 1975). However, Darley, Aronson, and Brown (1975) note that for 100 years, observers of the speech and language of the left-brain-damaged person have identified the same characteristics over and over again, although each observer gave the symptom complex a different name—*expressive aphasia, aphemia,* and *cortical dysarthria,* to name a few. Darley, Aronson, and Brown (1975) maintain that the term *apraxia of speech* is an all-inclusive label for the motor speech disorder that often accompanies aphasia.

We believe that there is an apraxia of speech and that it can be differentiated from other types of speech sound disorders. Clinical experience shows that it can be resolved via a method of treatment that does not produce results with other speech or language problems.

Definition

Apraxia of speech is defined as a sensorimotor speech disorder. It is manifested as an impairment of the central motor programming for the voluntary production of phonemes and the sequencing of muscle movements for the production of words (Darley, Aronson, & Brown, 1975; Wertz, 1978). In simpler terms, it might be said that the person cannot call up the commands for the motor programming necessary to produce individual or sequenced speech sounds. In the last chapter, Winitz outlined five levels of articulatory breakdown. Apraxia of speech results from breakdown at the fourth level, which is the level of articulatory planning. The most salient characteristics are errors in articulation of consonants and changes in the normal patterns of prosody. The articulatory programming problem, apraxia of speech, may appear alone in a left-brain-damaged person. However, the symptoms are most commonly seen in conjunction with aphasia, which refers to language disorders resulting from brain injury, and sometimes with dysarthria, the other motor speech disorder to be described later in this chapter. The point to be remembered is that aphasia and dysarthria are not the causes of apraxia; they are coexisting disorders.

Etiologies

Apraxia of speech is caused by the same insults to the brain that cause aphasia, namely, stroke, trauma, tumors, and infection. The probable site of lesion is the third frontal convolution of the left hemisphere, which is also called Broca's area. There is controversy regarding the exact site of damage causing apraxia; however, it is important to remember that a lesion causing apraxia of speech is not discrete. It nearly always results in the coexistence of aphasia and apraxia.

Speech Characteristics

Darley, Aronson, and Brown, in the classic book *Motor Speech Disorders* (1975), provide a detailed description of the characteristics of apraxia of speech. The following is a summary of their findings.

Apraxia of speech is most easily identified by difficulties in articulation. However, inability to coordinate phonation, rate, and/or stress may be observed. The manifestations of articulatory involvement are as follows:

1. Articulatory struggle occurs, during which the patient many times shows awareness of his difficulty. Some patients will get disgusted and give up with a gesture of "forget it."
2. Errors increase as the length of the word increases.
3. The articulation errors are inconsistent and vary among substitutions, repetitions, prolongations, and additions.
4. Sometimes the error will be perseverative with rearticulation of an already completed phoneme (bottle-bobble). Other times, the error seems to be anticipatory (hospital-hostital).
5. Consonants are more difficult than vowels.
6. Initial consonants are more troublesome than final consonants.
7. Articulation errors increase as the complexity of the motor pattern increases. Therefore, vowels are easier than single consonants. Of single consonants, fricative and affricate phonemes evoke the most errors.
8. The most difficulty is manifested on consonant clusters, which may be simplified by the insertion of the schwa (*scrap*–/skəræp/).
9. To confound the clinician, the patient, and the patient's family, there are often islands of perfectly articulated speech, particularly when these are automatic or highly practiced utterances (Hi! How are you? Fine. What's going on? Where have you been?).
10. Patients articulate more easily when they can watch a highly visible word being pronounced by a clinician.

Associated Problems

Other impairments may or may not appear with apraxia of speech. Some patients present an oral apraxia, which is the inability to perform oral vegetative movements such as blowing, chewing, protruding the tongue, or licking the lips voluntarily upon request. Other apraxic patients may present an oral-sensory perceptual deficit (Rosenbek, Wertz, & Darley, 1973), which is the inability to recognize the form of an object placed in the mouth.

A great number of apraxic patients also manifest an accompanying aphasia, an inability to understand and use symbolic aspects of communication. They may have problems with auditory memory, sequencing, and discrimination. They may have difficulty with reading and reading comprehension. Writing and speaking may be marked with reduction of available language and difficulty in sentence formulation, use of correct syntax, and organization of material.

Furthermore, all of the physical, social, and emotional problems associated with brain damage are likely to be present. The physical problems may include hemiplegia, or weakness of the arm or leg, on the right side of the body. Patients with these symptoms are easily fatigued and sometimes unable to withstand frustration. When their frustration tolerance has been exceeded, they may experience such physical symptoms as hyperventilation, fainting, and rapid heartbeat. Apraxic patients may experience reduced sensation in the mouth and extremities and visual problems such as hemianopsia (loss of vision in one half of the visual field) and diplopia (double vision).

Emotional problems may include emotional lability, which is defined as inappropriate laughing and crying. Depression may set in earlier with apraxic patients than with aphasic patients, because apraxic patients are usually more aware of the loss of their speech ability than are aphasics. When it can be demonstrated to a patient that relearning can take place, the depression begins to lift. Anger and low self-esteem are often present due to the patient's loss of abilities and changes in relationships at home and at work.

The apraxic patient sometimes has even greater problems with adjustment to the condition than do the aphasics. Because the individual with apraxia of speech can self-monitor production so well, and because there is more language available, frustration with the inadequate production, the inconsistency of production, and the necessary slowness is at a high level.

Assessment of Apraxia of Speech

Although oral assessment has been covered in chapter 4, the following additional measures are especially important.

Because there is a high probability of the presence of both apraxia and aphasia in the same left-hemisphere-damaged patient, test batteries used for aphasia are appropriate for helping the clinician to ascertain the presence of apraxia. In addition, there are informal methods of assessing the motor and sensory involvement of the articulators in both vegetative and verbal performance. These informal measures are often among the first tasks the clinician requests of the patient. By knowing the extent of the motor programming deficit, the clinician can better judge the oral language responses.

Assessing oral apraxia can be accomplished by making the following requests (La Pointe & Wertz, 1974):

1.	Show me how you blow.	
2.	Show me how you kiss.	*Lip function*
3.	Show me your teeth.	
4.	Show me how you chew.	
5.	Show me how to bite.	*Jaw function*
6.	Show me how your teeth chatter.	
7.	Stick out your tongue.	
8.	Put your tongue on your teeth.	*Tongue function*
9.	Lick your lips.	

Observation of verbal apraxia can be facilitated by remembering the characteristics of the disorder and requesting tasks to elicit the presence or absence of the characteristics. The following checklist is adapted from Wertz (1978):

1. Vowel production is least likely to be affected. Ask the patient to produce all vowels in isolation.
2. Consonant blends, affricates, or fricatives are likely to be most difficult. Ask the patient to repeat words beginning and ending with /f, s, ʃ, tʃ, dʒ, z/. Also ask for production of a representative sample of blends of /l, r, st/.
3. Because no sequencing is involved, sometimes the repetition of single phonemes will be intact. Ask the patient to repeat single consonant phonemes, such as /b, p, t, d, g, k/.
4. Repetition of multisyllable sequences should show error. Ask the patient to say [pʌ–tʌ–kʌ]. Ask the patient to produce multisyllabic words (*snowflake, considerable, synchronization*). Ask the patient to produce words of increasing length (*funny, funnier, funniest, seem, seeming, seemingly*).
5. Words with the same initial and final phoneme should show a greater number of errors in the initial position (*cake, tot, church, judge, fife, peep*, etc.).
6. Repetition of sentences and descriptions of action pictures will be very difficult. Sometimes the patient will refuse the task.

Additional oral evaluative instruments are oral sensory measures, such as those used by Rosenbek, Wertz, & Darley (1973), and the articulation tests listed at the end of chapter 4. The oral sensory measures aid in determining the severity of the inability to recognize forms in the mouth, and the articulation test provides data on the hierarchy of difficulty of speech sounds and selected clusters.

One of the most common clinical questions and one of the most difficult to answer unequivocally is how to differentiate paraphasia from apraxia-of-speech errors, since speech resulting from either condition may sound the same to the inexperienced clinician. Paraphasic errors are articulatory errors resulting from difficulty with grammatical and phonological rules, whereas apraxia results from difficulty in motor programming of the articulators. Some attempts to document the differences between apraxia and paraphasia have

been made. Trost and Canter (1974) suggested that apraxic patients are phonetically logical in their errors. For example, they may substitute p/f, w/r, d/dʒ and
often show only one-feature errors. Clinically, we have observed that apraxic
errors tend to occur within the framework of a speech struggle, whereas
paraphasic errors occur in a run of fluently articulated and prosodically normal
speech. Unless the patient is mute, performance will improve vastly if there is
instruction to watch the mouth of the clinician. Patients making paraphasic
errors do not benefit from visual cues or repetition; in fact, they seem to get
more confused. Often, apraxic patients are very aware of their errors. On the
other hand, patients exhibiting paraphasic errors usually go blithely on, making no effort to self-correct, although there are exceptions to this in mild cases.
Vowels tend to be involved in paraphasic errors, whereas in apraxia of speech,
the vowel is sometimes involved, but the distortion of it seems to be related to
the consonant struggle before it.

One of the classic examples of a paraphasic error occurred when a patient
was ordering a steak. He first told the waitress he wanted it "medium rear,"
then he changed to "medium roar," and finally settled on "medium rare." In
contrast, the apraxic patient might have said, "bedium mare, no—medium
mare, no—redium rare, no—porget it."

Prognosis and Remediation

Prognosis.   Because the lesion that produces apraxia is the same one that
produces aphasia, the prognostic variables relevant to aphasia—such as type and
interaction of the size and location of the lesion—are also applicable to apraxia.
In addition, there are some other behavioral characteristics associated with
apraxia of speech that are prognostic. A coexisting oral apraxia is a negative
prognostic indicator for recovery from verbal apraxia (Rosenbek, Wertz, &
Darley, 1973; Vignolo, 1964). The more severe the accompanying aphasia,
the poorer the prognosis. When a patient with a moderate to mild apraxia
demonstrates awareness of the errors and attempts self-correction, the prognosis can be considered more positive (Wepman, 1958). Other factors, such as
age, physical health, family environment, motivation, and early therapeutic
intervention affect recovery from apraxia, as they do recovery from aphasia.

Therefore, a young, motivated, healthy patient with a supportive family,
who has only a verbal apraxia resulting from trauma, will recover better than
the older, depressed, physically debilitated patient, with an accompanying oral
apraxia from vascular etiology (stroke), who lives alone.

Remediation.   Depending on the severity of the oral and/or verbal apraxia
and the presence or absence of an accompanying aphasia, therapy will vary.
Many times, the first move is to help the speechless patient work through the
accompanying oral apraxia. Often in a moderate to severe apraxia (with relatively good auditory comprehension), the motor speech problem will need to be
improved first. After some improvement is observed, expressive language tasks
can be incorporated into the apraxia drill. Sometimes very mild verbal apraxics
learn quite soon that if they slow their rate of presentation, they experience
fewer difficulties.

Severe apraxics may have no speech in the early days of their recovery. However, they should not be confused with severe aphasics, who are also often speechless, but in addition, have a severe auditory comprehension deficit, which the apraxic patient does not. It is frustrating to the patient and the therapist to begin only apraxia therapy with a severe aphasic. The key to differentiation between the two, which must be accomplished in order to plan the appropriate therapeutic task, is the degree of auditory comprehension difficulty.

When the diagnosis of apraxia of speech has been made, there are several possible avenues of therapeutic intervention. However, they all include the concepts of imitation, auditory-visual stimulation, motor repetition, and phonetic placement. Darley et al. (1975) state that the goal of apraxia therapy is to regain voluntary control over articulation, and that the articulation therapy should therefore be direct. There will be no need to work on auditory discrimination, respiration, phonation, or resonation. The essentials of their therapeutic approach are as follows:

1. Choose a phoneme that is typically easy for the patient and one that is easily visible (/w, m, b, f/). Phonemes worked on in succession should be as dissimilar as possible so that the patient is not confused.
2. Begin with phonemes in isolation and then move to consonant-vowel combinations. The instructions might be, "You watch my mouth, and say what I say. We will say each sound three times together. Let's say *buh*. Ready—buh, buh, buh. Good. Now let's try *bah*. Bah, bah, bah. Good."
3. Then add consonant-vowel-consonant combinations to be repeated three times (*bab, bub, beeb*, etc.).
4. Then string these syllables together (*bab-bub-beeb, bab-bub-beeb*).
5. Next work on words with the phoneme in initial, then medial, then final position (*bat, rubber, cob*).
6. Provide repetition of 2-word phrases using the phoneme (*big boy, Bob bites babies*).
7. Then ask questions and provide sentence frames which require answers using the practice words the patient has learned (*What do you do to the candles on your cake? What color is the sky on a sunny day? The day you were born is called your ____. The opposite of white is ____.*).

The patient should watch the clinician's mouth during production. Some patients are also helped by using a mirror, but this must be an individual decision. Some patients are upset by the change in their appearance since the onset of the illness and find the mirror distracting. Other patients will need phonetic placement instructions and sometimes actual manipulation of the articulators.

Rosenbek, Lemme, Ahern, Harris, and Wertz (1973) have developed an eight-step program, which emphasizes the transfer from imitative to volitional purposive utterances. This program also incorporates other language modalities. A summary of this technique follows.

1. The clinician encourages the patient to watch and listen while they make the utterance together.
2. The patient imitates the clinician after a slight delay. At this point, the auditory cue is faded and the visual cue remains.
3. The patient is asked to repeat after the clinician in the absence of any cues.
4. The patient is asked to repeat after the clinician several times without any intervening visual or auditory cues.
5. The clinician presents a written stimulus and the patient reads it aloud.
6. The written stimulus is shown and then removed so that the patient gives a delayed response.
7. The imitative model is replaced with experiences that provide the opportunity for spontaneous and meaningful utterances. The appropriate utterance is elicited by asking a question.
8. Appropriate spontaneous responses are stimulated through role playing.

A third variant of therapy for apraxia of speech is melodic intonation therapy (MIT) described by Sparks, Helm, and Albert (1974) and Sparks and Holland (1976). These authors have used some of the results of current research concerning the roles of the right and left hemispheres in language to create a therapy model. Although the final integration of language function occurs in the dominant left hemisphere, the right hemisphere possesses an auditory vocabulary and seems to be the area in which the suprasegmental aspects of language (stress and intonational contours) are processed. Because the right hemisphere is also dominant for music, Sparks, Helm, and Albert (1974) theorize that by combining basic language with musical form, they can facilitate cooperation between the two hemispheres and tap the latent language abilities of the right hemisphere. The entire method must be learned under supervision. However, a summary of the philosophy and the techniques are provided here.

Melodic intonation therapy should be used on patients with relatively good auditory comprehension, but severely restricted verbal output. Essentially, the patient is asked to "intone" or sing phrases in a very restricted melodic pattern that resembles the true pitch varieties of speech. It is not true singing, and overlearned and popular melodies must be avoided because the patient will often sing the words to the popular song rather than the language being practiced.

Melodic intonation therapy consists of several levels, each of which has several substeps. Progression through the levels occurs only after the patient has had 10 successful therapy sessions at the previous level. The four steps of the first level are

1. The clinician intones a phrase such as *salt and pepper* or *apple pie* and helps the patient to tap his hand to the rhythm and stress of the sentence. Hand tapping accompanies all four steps of the first level.

2. The patient is asked to join the clinician in intoning the sentence.
3. This step is like step 2, except that the clinician begins to fade his participation so that the patient continues independently.
4. The clinician intones a sentence and the patient repeats it solo.

If the patient progresses to the second level, there are five steps. The goal of this level is to move the patient from the intoning of phrases to speaking the phrases. Patient selection, criteria for moving from one step to another, scoring of responses, and what to do if a patient fails are all incorporated into the program (Sparks, Helm, & Albert, 1974; Sparks & Holland, 1976).

There is some evidence that gestural language can be offered as a facilitating, supplementary, and/or alternative form of communication for some severely apraxic patients. The gestural program presented by Skelly, Schinsky, Smith, and Fust (1974) used an adaptation of Amerind, American Indian Sign Language, as a facilitator of speech. Gestural communication is not a language in that it has no grammatical structure and uses a logical associative order. Although gestural communication has limitations, it is in daily use by most people. Putting the finger to the lips means "be quiet," and crooking the finger means "come here." Any gesture or group of gestures that adequately conveys the idea is acceptable. Skelly et al. reported improved and expanded oral communication after the improvement of manual gesturing. As they suggest, more systematic clinical reasearch is required. Indeed, this is an avenue of communication that must not be underestimated. This approach is further supported by Kimura (1976), who presented material indicating that speaking and manual activities are closely associated in the left hemisphere.

While the patient is working to develop usable speech, writing, gestures, and augmentative communication aids may be considered, if the patient is an appropriate candidate and desires this kind of intervention.

Conclusion

Apraxia of speech is a disturbance of the volitional motor programming of the articulators. Although it coexists with both aphasia and dysarthria, it must not be confused with them. Its correct diagnosis terminates in a unique type of therapy that is based on imitation, auditory-visual stimulation, oral motor repetition, and phonetic placement. This therapeutic approach is not effective with any other expressive disorder.

DEVELOPMENTAL APRAXIA OF SPEECH

The subject of apraxia of speech cannot be concluded without a discussion of apraxia of speech in children. There is controversy over the existence of this disorder, as well as its manifestations (Williams, Ingham, & Rosenthal, 1981), just as in apraxia of speech in adults. We believe that there is a developmental apraxia of speech, and we have also observed that speech-language pathologists who work with adult brain-damaged patients seem more likely to accept and use the classification as it pertains to children. However, it is clear that more definitive research is necessary to resolve the controversy.

The recent work of Yoss and Darley (1974a), Rosenbek and Wertz (1972), and Chappell (1973) has helped to begin to clarify this diagnostic category and to separate developmental apraxia of speech from functional articulation disorders. Three characteristics found in all the studies were: (a) a high incidence of an accompanying oral apraxia, (b) efforts at imitation marked by struggle and groping responses from the articulators, and (c) unusual substitutions and distortions, which indicated confusion of features and/or two- and three-features errors, such as m/s or t/f.

Children diagnosed as presenting apraxia of speech often demonstrate other associated problems. They may display a number of "soft" neurological signs, such as difficulty in fine motor skills and/or difficulty in coordination of the extremities, particulary in alternating movements (Haynes, 1978; Yoss, 1974a). Oral sensory deficits may also be observed in some children when they are tested on oral form identification and two-point discrimination (Haynes, 1978). To further complicate diagnosis (just as in adults), these children may or may not present a concomitant language problem. Often their receptive skills are normal and/or may appear quite accelerated in relation to their speech. When the apraxia has begun to clear, some children will clearly demonstrate an expressive language problem. Others do not, and will just as easily use the newly acquired phoneme /s/ to mark plurals, possessives, and third person singular forms of the verb as they use it in the initial, medial, and final position of words. Some children with a developmental apraxia of speech do not demonstrate language problems until they reach the third or fourth grade, where they begin to manifest difficulty in the higher language processes such as categorizing, organizing, and abstracting. Yoss and Darley (1974a) reported that some of the children in their study were classed as learning disabled.

Assessment

Diagnosing developmental apraxia of speech should begin with a thorough articulation test. Some apraxic children do fairly well in a single-word articulation test. However, in connected conversation, they become completely unintelligible, with numerous inconsistent substitutions, distortions, and omissions that were not present at the one-word level. Therefore, it is imperative to engage the child in conversation and picture-description activities also.

Yoss and Darley (1974a), Rosenbek and Wertz (1972), and Chappell (1973) all noted the high incidence of an accompanying oral apraxia. Consequently, testing for this condition is diagnostically significant. Yoss and Darley (1974a) noted that some children produce isolated oral movements quite well. (The movements requested are the same as those requested of adults.) However, when the children were asked to sequence oral movements—coughing, sticking out the tongue, and showing how they kiss, for example—they were unable to perform. This difficulty in sequencing can be demonstrated by asking the child to do the following:

1.   As quickly as you can, say puh-puh-puh.
2.   As quickly as you can, say tuh-tuh-tuh.
3.   As quickly as you can, say kuh-kuh-kuh.
4.   As quickly as you can, say puh-tuh-kuh.

The child will probably be unable to perform *puh-tuh-kuh* correctly if developmental apraxia of speech is present. In addition to testing oral motor function, the clinician should examine oral sensory function. Ringel, House, Burk, and Dolinsky (1970) constructed a test of oral form discrimination for children. The results of their testing indicated that the more severe the articulation problem, the poorer the performance on tasks of oral discrimination.

Because developmental apraxia of speech can appear in concert with expressive and sometimes receptive language disorders, no diagnostic evaluation is complete without in-depth testing of language abilities.

Remediation

Therapy for developmental apraxia of speech follows the same principles of visual cuing and motor repetition used for adult apraxic patients (Darley, Aronson, & Brown, 1975; Rosenbek, Lemme, Ahern, Harris, & Wertz, 1973; Haynes, 1978; Yoss & Darley, 1974b; Rosenbek, Hensen, Baughman, & Lemme, 1974). Variations for children may include extensive work on vowels and introduction of age-appropriate syntactic and semantic rules. Children with developmental apraxia must always be cautioned to slow their speech. Carry-over to conversational skills is based on their being able to produce the phonemes they have learned at a slower rate than is usual in conversation. Yoss and Darley (1974b) made further suggestions for the treatment of developmental apraxia of speech. Because some degree of oral apraxia is present, oral imitation and sequencing tasks of the tongue, lips, and jaw can be initiated early. In addition to having the child imitate sustained vowels and visible consonants, the clinician can help the child imitate CVC syllables (just as in adult therapy) by using some type of body movement, such as arm swinging, to accent stress patterns. The children should be taught self-monitoring skills early in therapy. Some children will spontaneously begin to produce phonemes that have not been directly practiced in therapy. However, even if this does happen, apraxia therapy for children is a long process, because usually each phoneme and consonant blend must be taught individually. Nightly parental drill with the child is a necessity.

Because there may be language and learning problems associated with developmental apraxia of speech, it is wise to carefully evaluate these children, as well as children with other speech sound disorders, as they enter school. They should be evaluated for reading competence in the first and second grades and then evaluated for higher language functions upon entering the fourth grade. By monitoring and ultimately treating the possible associated problems, the speech pathologist can contribute significantly to the child's successful education.

Conclusion

Developmental apraxia of speech is a sensorimotor speech disorder that interferes with the voluntary motor programming of the articulators. In children, this disorder is often accompanied by an oral apraxia (the inability to perform oral vegetative movements upon request), articulatory struggle, and unusual substitutions and distortions that involve confusion of features and/or two- and three-feature errors. Developmental apraxia of speech may be a more prevalent disorder than we have been led to believe (Haynes, 1978). Careful testing by the speech-language pathologist, who recognizes that disordered communication can take place at the sensorimotor level as well as the symbolic level, will lead to the appropriate therapeutic strategies.

DYSARTHRIA

The subject of dysarthria is a complex one. Only recently have standardized dysarthria tests been developed, and treatment approaches are still evolving.

The course of treatment undertaken will be greatly affected by the cause of the dysarthria, the severity of the problem, and the stage of the disease process. Etiological factors weigh heavily in determining realistic achievement. The speech pathologist must decide whether the best communicative success will be accomplished through increased speech skills, maximized speech skills accompanied by augmentative measures, or augmentative measures alone.

Definition

Dworkin (1984), drawing on the work of Darley, defines *dysarthria* as "disorders of phonation, articulation, resonation, and prosody which occur either singly or in combination as a result of weakness, paresis, incoordination, and/or abnormalities in the tone of the muscles of the speech mechanism . . . and are due to impairment of the central nervous system, peripheral nervous system or both . . ." (p. 264). In contrast to apraxia, which results from difficulty in programming speech sounds, dysarthria results from difficulty in the actual production of them. This is a disorder at the fifth level of articulatory breakdown according to chapter 9.

As indicated by the definition, dysarthria cannot be strictly equated with faulty articulation, since articulation represents only one of the processes of speech. The muscles of respiration, phonation, and resonation may also be involved and therefore their function affected as well.

It has been established that dysarthria is not a single entity, but a group of related problems. The specific symptoms depend upon the cause and location of the damage within the nervous system. The most detailed and classic contribution on the classification of dysarthria comes from Darley, Aronson, and Brown (1975). They described the motor system as being organized into six hierarchical levels of function, and they identified clusters of symptoms that are related to different levels of nervous system impairment.

Speech Characteristics

Typical speech characteristics of dysarthria fall into the areas of phonation, resonation, respiration, articulation, and prosody. A summary of the types of symptoms that might occur are found in Table 10.1. The specific symptoms that appear depend on the level of motor system impairment. Darley, Aronson, and Brown (1975) describe six types of dysarthria in terms of the following primary characteristics.

TABLE 10.1
Dimensions of Dysarthria

I.   *Phonation*
  A.   Pitch
    1.   Pitch level
    2.   Pitch breaks
    3.   Monopitch
    4.   Voice tremor
  B.   Intensity
    1.   Monoloudness
    2.   Excess loudness variation
    3.   Loudness decay
    4.   Alternating loudness
    5.   Loudness (overall)
  C.   Quality
    1.   Harsh voice
    2.   Hoarse (wet) voice
    3.   Breathy voice (continuous)
    4.   Breathy voice (transient)
    5.   Strained/strangled voice
    6.   Voice stoppages
 	
II. *Resonation*
  A.   Hypernasality
  B.   Hyponasality
  C.   Nasal emission
 	
III. *Respiration*
  A.   Forced inspiration/expiration
	B. Audible inspiration
	  C. Grunt at end of expiration
	
	IV. *Articulation*
	  A. Imprecise consonants
	  B. Phonemes prolonged
	  C. Irregular articulatory breakdown
	  D. Phonemes repeated
	  E. Vowels distorted
	  F. Intelligibility
	  G. Bizarreness
	
	V. *Prosody*
	  A. Rate
	  B. Phrases short
	  C. Increase of rate in segments
	  D. Increase in rate overall
	  E. Reduced stress
	  F. Variable rate
	  G. Intervals prolonged
	  H. Inappropriate silences
	  I. Short rushes of speech
	  J. Excess and equal stress
	
	VI. *Other*

Note. The specific characteristics (e.g., pitch level, pitch breaks, monoloudness) are from *Motor Speech Disorders* by F. Darley, A. Aronson, and J. Brown, Philadelphia: W. B. Saunders & Co., 1975.

Flaccid Dysarthria.   The two major characteristics of this type of dysarthria are weakness and lack of muscle tone. Enervation of the muscles of all of the speech processes can be affected. The speech characteristics most often associated with flaccid dysarthria are hypernasality, imprecise consonants, monopitch, nasal emission, breathiness, and audible inspiration.

Spastic Dysarthria.   The four major problems of this type are spasticity, weakness, limited range of movement, and reduced diadochokinetic rate. The most typical speech characteristics include imprecise articulation, reduced rate, low pitch, harsh voice and strained-strangled phonation. Prosody may also be affected, in the form of reduced stress, limited pitch, and loudness changes.

Ataxic Dysarthria.   Patients with this type of involvement experience movements that are slow, inaccurate, and irregular. There is reduced muscle tone and tremor. The speech characteristics, as described by Yorkston and Beukelman (1981b), in concurrence with Darley, Aronson, and Brown, include imprecise articulation, often with irregular articulatory breakdowns, prosodic abnormality with slow rate, excess and equal stress, monoloudness, monopitch, and prolonged syllables.

Hypokinetic Dysarthria.   In hypokinesia, muscle functions for speech and other motor movements are generally slow and limited in range and mobility. Speech is characterized by monotone and monoloudness, reduced stress, and imprecise articulation. Rapid, short bursts of speech, inappropriate silences, and a tendency to "trail off" and run speech together are other typical characteristics.

Hyperkinetic Dysarthria.   Within this category two distict types can be identified. In the quick form, movements are quick, random, and include involuntary movements. The speech pattern includes imprecise consonants, prolonged intervals, voice stoppages, limited pitch variation, harshness, vowel distortion, and hypernasality.

In the slow form, movements are slow and sustained. By contrast to the quick form, characteristics include harsh voice, strained-strangled voice, monopitch, monoloudness, and unplanned variations in loudness.

Mixed Dysarthria.   The dysarthrias already discussed occur when only one part of the motor system is involved. However, frequently more than one part of the motor system is impaired, and when this occurs a combination of problems occurs.

Associated Problems

The type of motor system impairment that affects speech affects other motor function in a similar manner. Patients, depending upon the level of motor impairment, might experience difficulty with gait, balance, fine motor coordination, and gross motor coordination.

Etiologies

There are numerous problems that can affect the central or peripheral nervous system and result in dysarthria. Among the causes which have been identified are cerebrovascular insult (stroke), head trauma, degenerative diseases, and tumors. Cerebral infections and toxic conditions are also potential threats to speech integrity. Specific incidence figures for dysarthria are difficult to find because dysarthria is associated with so many different causes. However, the highest incidence results from stroke and certain degenerative neurological diseases. Studies indicate that the occurrence of some neurological and congenital problems is influenced by geographic, racial, and age factors, so incidence figures may also vary according to the population being studied (Rosenbek & LaPointe, 1981).

Assessment of Dysarthria

Although this chapter focuses on evaluation of the speech processes, a complete diagnosis of dysarthria is based not only on speech involvement, but also on other motor involvement. The evaluation process, therefore, involves an interdisciplinary approach.

Numerous assessment approaches are described in the literature, each having its own philosophical basis. Peterson and Marquardt (1981), however, state that a complete evaluation should include the structural and functional integrity of the five processes of speech (i.e., respiration, phonation, articulation, resonation, and prosody). *Structural integrity* refers to the size, shape, and relationship of the speech structures to each other. *Functional integrity* refers to the adequacy of these structures to perform speech movements.

Assessment of structural and functional integrity can be accomplished through the use of instrumentation, such as biofeedback equipment, manometers to measure airflow, cinefluorography to observe structure and function through X-ray photography, and others, as well as through a perceptual approach. Instrumentation will not be considered in this chapter. While instrumentation can produce information that might be considered more scientific and exact, it can be very costly and is not accessible to all speech pathologists. Even when instrumentation is possible, it must be used in combination with other traditional evaluative procedures.

Although specific evaluative procedures may vary from patient to patient, a general evaluation procedure would include an oral-facial examination and evaluation of function for nonspeech movements and speech movements.

Oral-Facial Examination.   Examination of the structures involved in articulation is described in some detail in chapter 4. Of specific interest to the dysarthria evaluation are the following:

1.   Symmetry of the articulatory structures: One should observe whether the structures are equal in appearance and movement on both sides of the midline.
2.   Other neurological symptoms: The examiner should note any evidence of tremor, signs of atrophy (wasting away of tissue structure) or ridging of the tongue, weakness, and the occurrence of involuntary contractions. Drooling or the presence of food in the oral cavity after a meal should also be noted.

Gross Motor Function.   The procedures described in chapter 4 for evaluation and function of the mandible, lips, velum, pharynx, and tongue are appropriate for the evaluation of dysarthria. Specific observations of function should include the following:

1.   Smoothness: Movement should be smooth and even, without groping, tremor, or jerkiness.
2.   Range: Movement should have full excursion and be equal on both sides of the midline.
3.   Strength and duration: Position should be maintained against mild resistance, and movements should be sustained over time with no evidence of deterioration.
4.   Rate: Diadochokinetic rates should fall into normal range.

5. Coordination: Alternating sequential movements should be accurately produced.

Since the focus of this book is on articulation, the evaluation procedures discussed so far have been limited specifically to articulation. However, in dysarthria, the other processes of speech (respiration, phonation, resonation, and prosody) are also often significantly altered and have an influence on articulation. Although evaluation of these processes will not be detailed in this chapter, the following basic observations should be included in the complete evaluation:

1. Respiration: adequate breath support and coordination of respiration with speech. Adequate loudness should be demonstrated.
2. Resonation: evidence of hypernasality, nasal emission, or hyponasality.
3. Phonation: evidence of abnormalities of pitch or voice quality, such as high pitch, monopitch, uncontrolled pitch fluctuations, pitch breaks, voice tremor, breathiness, hoarseness, and strained-strangled quality.
4. Prosody: abnormalities of timing, melody pattern, and stress.

Speech Function.   Evaluation of nonspeech performance is only one level of function. Adequate performance at this level does not mean that function will be adequate for the more complex demands of speech. Therefore, standardized articulation tests as well as a speech sample should be included in the evaluation of all dysarthric patients unless the patient is so impaired that this is impossible. Deep testing of articulation is more useful than testing individual phonemes or testing phonemes in a limited context, because errors may vary according to different coarticulatory combinations. It is important that a speech sample be long enough to determine the individual's consistency over time. In some types of problems the patient may do well initially but break down when performance must be maintained for a period of time. Error patterns are as important as specific phoneme errors, and stimulability for improved production should also be tested.

According to Yorkston and Beukelman (1981a), measures of general intelligibility in relation to rate are as important as assessing specific articulation performance. These authors state that although symptoms vary, intelligibility is a constant factor. It can also serve as a measure of severity and provide an understandable scale to patients and families. Since in many cases normal articulation will not be achievable, improved intelligibility may be a more practical and realistic goal.

Prognosis and Remediation

There are special considerations for dysarthric patients not only in the assessment process, but in the treatment process as well. As mentioned earlier, the emphasis of treatment will be on *communication*, which may mean speech, augmented speech, or alternative communication methods.

Determining realistic goals is critical to the success of the treatment program. The speech pathologist does not want to set the patient up for failure or lead him or her to expect unrealistic levels of accomplishment. Unlike most functional problems, the ultimate goal for the dysarthric patient is generally compensated rather than normal speech (Rosenbek & LaPointe, 1979). One must also recognize that goals may fluctuate and have to be revised downward, depending on the course of the disease. When a patient's condition is a deteriorating one, goal planning must consider this, and utilize approaches and augmentative or alternative systems that are flexible enough to accommodate changing status. One would not want to recommend an expensive augmentative communication system that seemed practical now but would not be usable by the patient later when the disease process is more advanced.

Improving communication skills may require interdisciplinary cooperation. For example, a given case may require the expertise of a physical therapist for positioning the patient for better muscle tone during speech activities or providing girdling for support when significant muscle weakness is present; a physician for supervising girdling recommendations or for administering medication; and a prosthodontist for assistive devices.

With these preliminary considerations in mind, we can discuss more specific aspects of treatment.

General Principles of Therapy. According to Darley, Aronson, and Brown (1975), five principles form the foundation of dysarthria therapy: (a) compensation, (b) purposeful activity, (c) monitoring, (d) an early start, and (e) motivation.

No one knows how actual improvement of function occurs; however, it is suggested that the system compensates for impaired areas and develops the ability to make maximum use of the potential that remains. Speech, once an automatic process, must be brought under intentional control. This involves developing an awareness of the activity of the articulators and producing these activities in a deliberate manner. Self-monitoring is, with dysarthria as with all other disorders, an important element. If the patient is unable to identify errors, he or she cannot make the necessary adjustments and corrections for improvement. Therapy should begin early, before faulty speech patterns have had an opportunity to become too firmly established. If the disease process is progressive, patients may be able to learn in the early stages to conserve or maximize skills they presently have. The importance of motivation in any disorder cannot be overemphasized. There are no passive exercises to which a patient can be subjected. Improvement relies heavily on active participation of the patient. Only a motivated patient will be vigilant in the monitoring and practicing that is so necessary.

Goals and Techniques of Therapy. The importance of establishing realistic goals for ultimate level of accomplishment has already been mentioned. Now let us consider more specific goals. Rosenbek and LaPointe (1979), recognizing the many differences among dysarthric patients, suggest eight treatment goals as a model for therapy. These include

1. assisting the patient to develop a productive attitude, i.e., a willingness to cooperative with the therapeutic process and to assume an active role

2. increasing physiological support for speech by modifying abnormalities of posture, tone, and strength

3. modifying the five processes of speech production, i.e., respiration, phonation, resonation, articulation, and prosody, for improved function

4. assisting in the use of augmentative communication when functional speech is limited

Therapy for dysarthria is very structured and very repetitive. Building muscle strength, increasing rate of movement, increasing range of movement, and improving muscle tone for speech are like building any other muscle functions. They require appropriate techniques to stimulate development and they require practice. The improvement that occurs will probably be in the form of progressive approximation. When adequate return does not result, therapy may turn to initiating compensatory strategies.

Articulation is affected by an interaction of all of the processes of speech, and improvement in articulation may occur in conjunction with improvement in other areas. Accordingly, LaPointe (1982) states that "lately there seems to be less primary emphasis on treating articulation in motor speech disorders. In both apraxia of speech and the dysarthrias, attention to the interaction of rate, stress and durational factors in the accuracy of speech sound production is gaining favor" (p. 395).

To elaborate on this point, articulation can often be improved through indirect approaches or through methods that have generalizing effects on articulation. For example, slowing rate has been shown to have a significant effect on intelligibility (Yorkston & Beukelman, 1981b). This can be accomplished by tapping out rhythms or using a metronome. The Delayed Auditory Feedback Unit has been suggested as a possible technique to slow rate and increase loudness (Hanson & Metter, 1980). Exaggeration of consonant production can increase accuracy and slow rate.

Articulation therapy may involve techniques similar to those used for other types of articulation problems when working on specific articulation goals (see chapter 5). However, because in dysarthria the speech pathologist is dealing with an impaired motor system, therapy must be directed to those specific problems as well. Proper positioning is important so that the patient's energy can be directed toward speech goals rather than trying to maintain head or trunk control. Poor positioning may create negative force on muscles and make speech postures more difficult to achieve. Exercises designed to extend range of movement, to increase strength and speed, and to improve coordination of movements may be necessary preliminary steps before specific articulation therapy can begin. Examples of such exercises might be:

- Range of Movement: After stabilizing the mandible, have the patient elevate the tongue tip to the alveolar ridge. Patient may accomplish this in gradual stages.
- Increase Strength: Protrude tongue and see if the patient can maintain position against resistance applied by tongue depressor.
- Increase Speed: Have the patient perform alternating movement such

as lateral tongue movement or protrusion/retraction at gradually increasing speeds.
• Coordination: Produce alternating movement patterns in controlled fashion. Examiner may have patient perform movement according to a pattern tapped out or spoken by therapist. Exercises with increasing difficulty levels for alternating or sequential movements can also be used.

When the patient can perform these types of exercises on gross motor movement tasks, he or she can move on to incorporating phoneme production into the exercises. Following that, syllable, word, and sentence production may be undertaken, assuming that each of these stages is potentially feasible. In addition to traditional articulation approaches, electrical stimulation techniques, described by Netsell and Cleeland (1973) have been used. Biofeedback techniques have been applied to assist the patient in monitoring movement and accuracy.

When the process just described is not feasible, alternative goals must be established. According to Logemann (1984), these alternative goals fall into three areas:

1. compensatory speech production (e.g., substituting a perceptually similar phoneme for a phoneme which cannot be produced normally)
2. surgical compensation (such as teflon injection or pharyngeal flap when velar movement is inadequate)
3. prosthetic devices (such as a palatal lift for reduced velar function)

The speech pathologist should be familiar with all of the compensating strategies and be able to recognize when such measures are appropriate.

Again, the importance of the other speech processes to articulation and intelligibility cannot be ignored. Although discussion has been limited to direct and indirect articulation strategies, when problems of respiration, phonation, resonation, and prosody exist, these must also be addressed in therapy. In some cases, treatment in these areas may precede articulation goals and at other times occur concomitantly.

Conclusion

The study of dysarthria is still in an early stage. Dysarthria affects all speech processes, and specific symptoms vary according to the level of neurological involvement. It is generally agreed that many patients can benefit from direct therapy even though they will not achieve normal speech. When prognosis is poor, the emphasis of therapy must be upon facilitation of communication rather than speech.

CEREBRAL PALSY

Cerebral palsy is a developmental disability often accompanied by speech and/or language disorders. It is not a diagnostic label for a unique speech or language disorder. In fact, the most common motor speech disorder in children who are diagnosed as having cerebral palsy is dysarthria.

Why, then, is cerebral palsy singled out for individual discussion if the speech manifestations are not unique? Cerebral palsy must be studied separately because diagnosis and treatment begin much earlier than in discrete speech and language problems in children. Furthermore, cerebral palsy must be differentiated from pure articulation disorders because, as a developmental disorder, it encompasses so many other problems that the speech pathologist cannot treat the individual without being a member of a "cerebral palsy team" that includes the physical therapist, the occupational therapist, the physiatrist, the psychologist, the social worker, and the teacher. In cerebral palsy the articulation disorder can be best understood by understanding the entire disability.

Definition

Cerebral palsy is a developmental disability characterized, mainly, by abnormal muscle activity and disorders of movement and/or posture, but usually accompanied by sensory, cognitive, and behavior problems (Denhoff, 1976). Although parents of cerebral-palsied children, and sometimes the involved individuals themselves, have avoided the term *disease,* Cruickshank (1976) has written that as a neurophysical and neuropsychological deviation, cerebral palsy is basically a disease, although it is not progressive, contagious, or epidemic in form. Crothers and Paine (1959), on the other hand, state that cerebral palsy is not a disease in any usual medical sense. However, it is a useful term for designating individuals who are handicapped by motor disorders due to non-progressive abnormalities of the brain.

Minear (1956), on behalf of the American Academy for Cerebral Palsy, defined *cerebral palsy* in a manner reflective of many professions: "Cerebral palsy comprises those motor and other symptom complexes caused by a non-progressive brain lesion or lesions. The characteristic thing about cerebral palsy is that it is a well defined entity with a variety of etiologies and pathologies" (p. 842). This definition indicates that there is now a better appreciation of the complexity of problems categorized under the name *cerebral palsy*. Professionals will do well to think of cerebral palsy as a spectrum of disabilities including aberrant motor function, sensory and perceptual dysfunction, intellectual and cognitive deficits, and difficulties in hearing, speech, language, adjustment, learning, and vision.

More recently, proponents of neuro-developmental treatment (NDT) have put forth another definition of *cerebral palsy*. NDT, which was developed by Berta Bobath (1967), involves early team intervention for the treatment of cerebral palsy. In this approach, cerebral palsy is seen as a problem of abnormal coordination of muscle action rather than paralysis or weakness of muscles. The brain lesion interferes with normal maturation of the brain, which then interferes with normal motor development. Adherents of the neuro-developmental approach consider the accompanying intellectual, cognitive, sensory, and perceptual deficits secondary to the cerebral palsy. In other words, the primary inability to coordinate muscle movement has deprived the child of the ability to explore the environment and develop other abilities. The Bobaths consider "movement" to be the foundation of learning.

The insult causing the symptom complex of cerebral palsy must occur in utero, at birth, or early in life. Early in life means up to the age of 2 years (Myzak, 1980) for some authors, and up to the age of 6 for others (Boone, 1972). According to neuro-developmental treatment theory, cerebral palsy caused postnatally, after a certain degree of motor development has already occurred, will require different assessment procedures and treatment planning.

Etiology

Cerebral palsy is caused by damage to, or malformations of, the brain. There are many factors that can contribute to these brain anomalies. The causes of cerebral palsy are often classified according to three vulnerable periods in the life of the fetus-infant-child: prenatal, perinatal, and postnatal or early infancy.

Some prenatal factors (those that occur during pregnancy) include infection, RH factor, hemorrhage, and anoxia (lack of oxygen to the fetal brain), which is the most common.

Perinatal factors, or those that occur from the onset of labor until the baby is visible, include anoxia as the main contributor, and trauma as the second most common. Denhoff (1976) reported that "small for date" babies and those involved in labor and delivery complications constitute the majority of the cases of cerebral palsy.

Postnatal factors account for only 10 to 15% of the cases of cerebral palsy. Some of those factors are traumatic injury such as auto accident, falls, and blows to the head; and infectious diseases such as meningitis and encephalitis.

Associated Problems

Cerebral palsy presents itself in many forms. There are so many variations of these forms that problems other than the actual neuromotor handicap may cause more difficulty than the condition itself. Newton (1977) mentions that the degree to which the child's disability handicaps him or her increases proportionately to the number and severity of related problems. Therefore, it is necessary to attend to the problems related to cerebral palsy in order to understand their nature and effects. The three major categories of problems that must be conquered by the cerebral palsy child and, of course, the family, are physical problems, psychological problems, and learning difficulties.

The physical problems of children with cerebral palsy include difficulty in ambulation and learning self-care activities. They also have impaired ability in chewing, sucking, and swallowing, which interferes with one of the most important early relationships of the child—feeding. Between 35 and 60% of cerebral-palsied children will have a seizure in their life (Perlstein, Gibbs, & Gibbs, 1947). Although anti-convulsive drugs, such as Dilantin, control seizures, they have side effects that impair attention and learning. Visual defects are found in 50% of cerebral-palsied children (Pearlstone, 1969) and about 20% have hearing loss (Nober, 1976). Dental problems may also result from the oral motor difficulties of cerebral palsy.

Emotional disorders experienced by those with cerebral palsy are not necessarily typical of the cerebral palsy population, but are the kinds of problems that are common to people in trouble. It is easy to understand why low self-esteem, immaturity, and dependency are fostered in the child with cerebral palsy.

Mental retardation is estimated to affect 50 to 75% of the cerebral-palsied population (Cruickshank, 1976). Thus, educational problems are common in this group, yet vary with the abilities of each individual child. Perceptual problems are not as obvious as physical disabilities, but nevertheless are a significant contributor to learning disabilities and educational failure. Some of these children are hyperactive and/or easily distracted, which adds to the burden of learning.

About 68% of cerebral-palsied children have speech and/or language disorders (Cruickshank, 1976). The diversity of these problems is wide. The disorders include all varieties of dysarthrias, articulation problems, and language disorders, such as difficulty in abstracting, organizing, and drawing conclusions.

The remainder of this section will be devoted to the articulation problems of the cerebral-palsied child, and will address the characteristics, assessment, and remediation of these problems.

Speech Characteristics

The articulation problems in the cerebral-palsied child are usually the most obvious component of the speech problem. These disorders are often referred to as *developmental dysarthria*. However, the articulation of a cerebral-palsied child cannot be separated from the other motor processes of speech, which include respiration, phonation, and resonation. These processes need to operate at fundamental levels before useful articulation patterns can be taught. In addition, the posture of a cerebral-palsied child needs to be considered. If it is inadequate, then it should be established before working with the speech. Some of the articulation problems in children with cerebral palsy are caused by persistence of feeding reflexes, such as rooting, lip-mouth opening, and sucking. Another cause of articulation problems is paralytic involvement of some of the articulators. Articulation of the cerebral-palsied child can also be hampered by involuntary movements or by inconsistency or limitations in the range, strength, and direction of movements. Apraxia may also be present in cerebral-palsied children, creating difficulty in making voluntary movements. In general, there is no typical articulation pattern for the cerebral-palsied child.

Assessment

Twenty years ago, this section on assessment would have begun directly with the traditional methods of evaluating the oral musculature as described in chapter 4. However, the concept of early intervention in the treatment of cerebral palsy has significantly changed the content of the speech assessment of cerebral-palsied children. What was thought to be early intervention at ages 3 and 4 is now not considered early. Early intervention in the comprehensive treatment of cerebral palsy is some time before the end of the first year, and the earlier the better.

In 1966, Kong reported the results of an early intervention program based on the neuro-developmental approach developed by the Bobaths (1972). The rationale was that early intervention in cerebral palsy could improve the long-term prognosis of the children. The program initiated intervention in the first 6 months of the infant's life. The goals were inhibition of the abnormal movements and reflexes and facilitation of normal automatic movements, so that more normal sensorimotor patterns of development could be acquired. The program provided for active participation of the parents, so that the program's goals were incorporated into the child's routine of handling by the mother. At the end of 4 years, 75% of the 69 children who remained in the program demonstrated a normal gait. It was also observed that there were fewer mentally retarded children in the group than would be expected. Kong's impression was that early normal motor experience had given these children a chance to develop their normal potential.

Because of this study, and others by Denhoff and Holden (1954) and Jones, Barrett, Olonoff, and Anderson (1969), as well as much work by Bobath (1967) and Nancy Finnie (1975), the concept of neuro-developmental treatment and early intervention has received much support from professionals and the United Cerebral Palsy Association. The basic tenet of this approach seems to be that physical competence is the most important factor relating to later success, including the development of normal speech. Normal speech is dependent on the successful acquisition of feeding and prespeech skills, and the evaluation of these skills can, and must, be done early in life.

Prespeech Evaluation.   The advent of normal speech has, in addition to the cognitive and linguistic prerequisites, four sensorimotor prerequisites:

1. head control with stability of the neck and shoulder girdle, because stability provides for later mobility of the oral structure
2. a coordinated pattern of respiration and phonation, which is related to development of abdominal muscles
3. a variety of feeding experiences with foods of different textures, temperatures, and tastes, in order to provide normal development of feeding patterns
4. babbling practice

When evaluating oral motor function, it is necessary to note the presence or absence of these sensorimotor prerequisites. In addition, oral motor function must be assessed in relation to whole body movements, and in a variety of body positions. For example, a child may find sitting to be such an effort that there can be no control over the oral mechanism, whereas the same child, placed in a different position, will have more control. At this point, it is important to mention again the concept of a neuro-developmental treatment *team*. The speech pathologist can receive invaluable assistance from physical and occupational therapists in the evaluation and treatment of speech-related areas, such as head control and breathing.

The Pre-Speech Assessment Scale (Morris, 1975b) assists the speech pathologist on the team to evaluate systematically the areas of prespeech behavior in which cerebral-palsied children deviate from normal. The scale examines areas such as postural tone and movement, response to sensory stimuli, and the prespeech behaviors of (a) feeding, (b) biting and chewing, (c) sucking, (d) swallowing, (e) respiration and phonation, and (f) sound play.

In the Pre-Speech Assessment Scale, Morris suggests that the following observations be made regarding postural tone and movement patterns:

1.   Observe the general postural tone in terms of hypertonicity (excessive muscle tone) or hypotonicity (insufficient muscle tone), normalcy or fluctuation of tone. These observations should be made when the child is at rest, in various positions, and when the child tries to communicate or talk to someone. Typical patterns of tone and movement should be noted.
2.   Head and trunk control should be evaluated in terms of symmetry, positions that enhance control, and responses of head and trunk when the child rolls, sits, or talks.
3.   Responses to sensory stimulation should also be assessed. Auditory, visual, vestibular, and tactile modes should be questioned. The tactile mode is of special interest around the mouth. The clinician needs to know what responses the child has to sensory stimulation around the mouth, since many children are hypersensitive and must have a therapeutic approach to feeding and speech that incorporates a series of graded stimuli.

The prespeech skills section of the Pre-Speech Assessment Scale examines 12 components of prespeech behavior:

1.   The clinician and team should note the influence of abnormal body tone and movements on the speech mechanism. Are there certain tensions and movement patterns in the jaw, lips, tongue, etc. that are related to the gross movement abnormalities?
2.   Structural deviations and deformities of the speech mechanism, as well as of other parts of the body, should be noted.
3.   Facial expressions are very much a part of communication. Some cerebral-palsied children do not possess a repertoire of facial expressions because of poor muscle tone. The clinician needs to watch for variety and symmetry in facial expression and, especially, to see if the face is used communicatively.
4.   General feeding behavior is often abnormal in cerebral-palsied children. They do not suck well from the beginning, are slow, and do not tolerate new foods. Normal sucking activities, as well as normally coordinated actions of the tongue, lips, and mandible in chewing and swallowing prepare the child for the more precise oral movements necessary for articulation. Here again, the cerebral-palsied child is doubly penalized. The child was born with abnormal enervation and control to use the oral structure, and, because it cannot be used maximally, the child cannot profit from the developmental experiences that it provides. Therefore, the clinician needs to observe

length of time, and amount and types of foods needed by the child. Positioning and behavioral problems related to mealtime are also of interest.

5. Sucking behavior should be observed in terms of jaw, lip, and tongue involvement and control. What is sucking like when taking pureed foods from a spoon? Does a tongue thrust or bite reflex interfere with these activities?

6. Swallowing is reflex behavior in the normal infant. In the cerebral-palsied infant, it is often marked with coughing, choking, and leakage from the corners of the mouth. Some foods are easier to swallow than others. Drooling sometimes accompanies fine motor and speech activities because a voluntary swallow has not yet been accomplished.

7. The acts of biting and chewing are composed of a number of subskills and sometimes interfered with by reflexes, such as the bite reflex and a jaw thrust. The observer needs to see what kinds of food the child will chew or bite, and if there are overflow movements into the body while biting and chewing. Are the tongue, lips, and jaw active and efficient in chewing?

8. The clinician should observe what kinds of imitative control over the oral mechanism the child can demonstrate. Is there imitative behavior of basic oral movements such as puckering lips and protruding the tongue? In addition, the child needs to have some imitative responses for vowels, consonants, and syllables.

9. Two manners of breathing are recognized. Vegetative breathing, or silent involuntary breathing, is characterized by an almost even inspiratory and expiratory cycle through the nose. Breathing rates of children under 2 are also usually quite variable and may range from 20 to 40 breaths per minute. As the child matures, the rate decreases. In contrast to vegetative breathing is speech breathing, which is characterized by a quick inspiratory phase and a long expiratory phase, accomplished through the mouth. Productive speech breathing should be stabilized at the rate of about 20 breaths per minute. Breathing difficulties are reported to be seen in 40 to 80% of children with cerebral palsy. The problems include shallow breathing; incoordination of the thorax and abdomen, which produces simultaneous inspiratory and expiratory movements, or "oppositional breathing"; and a high rate of breaths per minute (over 30) (Crickmay, 1966). An additional difficulty may be the delay in changing from the state of vegetative breathing to the state of speech breathing. Some children cannot make the change at all. Morris (1975b) suggests that while looking at the child's breathing one should keep in mind tone of the musculature, depth and regularity of breathing, rib-flaring effects of other body movements, and use of the nose or mouth for breathing.

10. Control over breathing is essential to control over phonation, although there are abnormalities of phonation that may be present in spite of adequate breathing patterns. There may be poor control over the opening and closing of the vocal folds and/or velopharyngeal

port. There may be weakness and/or incoordination in the intrinsic and/or extrinsic muscles of the larynx. Among the things the clinician wants to note about the child's phonation patterns are the ease and variability of phonation. Are respiration and phonation well coordinated, or is there a voice quality problem of hoarseness or harshness? Does the child have appropriate stress patterns and does he or she use these as phonation patterns to communicate?

11.   In addition to assessing articulation in the usual way, the clinician on a neuro-developmental treatment team must also look for earlier articulatory gestures. Babbling and the variability, spontaneity, and speed of the articulators should be noted.

12.   Assessment for augmentative communication skills is also a necessity. Are the child's cognitive and linguistic abilities now more advanced than his speaking abilities? Can he use his eyes to indicate direction, or can he fingerpoint?

The prespeech assessment scale is a vital component in assessing the communication disorders of cerebral-palsied children. It should be used by a speech pathologist who is knowledgeable about normal oral motor development, because sometimes even subtle deficits in three or four areas of prespeech development can combine to produce a very complex clinical picture.

For several reasons, the evaluation of isolated articulation patterns can be done only after the clinician has evaluated the prespeech behaviors. One reason is that the isolated articulation evaluation should be done in terms of how prespeech behaviors have affected articulation. Secondly, due to the age at which the prespeech evaluation is done, an actual articulation evaluation is not appropriate until later. However, when the speech pathologist facilitates and stimulates normal bodily movements and prespeech behaviors, neuro-developmental theory postulates that articulation will begin more normally because other interfering variables have been eliminated and new patterns have been taught upon which articulation patterns can be based.

When a traditional articulation evaluation can be done, the methods suggested in chapter 4 are applicable. However, phonation, respiration, and resonation must also be assessed in the context of articulation, as suggested in the dysarthria section of this chapter.

Remediation

Prespeech Therapy.   Speech pathologists who are interested in serving the cerebral-palsied population must be prepared to be members of a team that will begin to deal with these children in infancy. The speech pathologist does not have to wait until speech fails to develop; the role is expanded to one of a pre–speech-language therapist. Therapies can be initiated in infancy, so that early interactions with the mother are productive for language learning and speech development. Early intervention by the speech pathologist can prevent, or lessen, the effects of poor head control, abnormal patterns of respiration and phonation, and feeding difficulties.

Neuro-developmental treatment (Bobath & Bobath, 1972) stresses that therapeutic physical handling by all professionals (as well as parents) will inhibit the abnormal and primitive reflexes, while providing stimulation for the development of more normal postural adjustments and coordinated movements. For example, a spastic child will experience extensor spasticity in the legs when he is carried. However, this pattern can be broken, and more normal patterns stimulated, if the mother will open the child's legs and carry him on her hip. This type of action also stimulates head control and balance reactions in the trunk. In other ways of physical handling, the child's breathing and oral activities can be stimulated into more normal patterns while the abnormal movements are extinguished.

In the pre–speech-and-language treatment of the cerebral-palsied infant, the speech pathologist has three priorities: (a) parent education, (b) communication and language stimulation, and (c) facilitation of prespeech skills.

Parent education is an integral part of treatment. The parent must be taught how to do all the things the therapist does. Early language stimulation is natural to most parents; the parents of cerebral-palsied children, however, are under special stresses, and they will need special help. One of the best ways to begin is to have them observe the therapist's interactions with the child.

Because cerebral-palsied children do not have normally integrated sensory systems, early initiation of graded sensory stimulation may be needed to facilitate development toward normal sensory experiences, which are important for language development. The therapist should verbalize the principle being demonstrated after the parents have observed it in action. Then the parent should be asked to practice the principle while being observed. Suggestions for placing the child so that he or she can obtain abundant visual stimulation are also helpful to language development. Facilitation of body positions should be of prime concern so that the child will be free of abnormal postures when directing attention to verbal and visual material.

The third priority in prespeech therapy is facilitation of prespeech skills. This includes work on the four sensorimotor prerequisites, which are head control, coordinated respiration and phonation, normal development of feeding skills, and babbling practice. The speech pathologist must consult with the physical therapist in order to learn how to facilitate the development of normal head control. For example, if there is an excess of movement, the speech pathologist must discuss with the physical therapist methods for stabilizing the trunk and extremities. The effectiveness of the entire prespeech program will often depend on the speech pathologist's ability to deal with abnormalities of postural tone, movement patterns, and reflex activities. Consequently, it is necessary for the clinician to maintain a good working relationship with the physical and occupational therapists.

Coordinated respiration and phonation, again, depend on the functioning of other larger muscles, particularly some abdominal muscles. Examples of some of the problems that the speech pathologist addresses are (a) lack of coordinated voicing and breathing and (b) inadequate duration of phonation to sustain babbling. Lack of coordinated voicing and breathing can be remediated by stimulating laughing or crying, and then using light vibration on the sternum during exhalation. This vibration then becomes associated with phonation on exhalation and can be used to initiate voice as control progresses. Increasing the duration of phonation can be aided by placing the child in a position that is conducive to phonation and babbling. This might be on the stomach (prone) or on the side. Another maneuver might be to use slow physical movement, such as lap jiggling or light rapid vibration of the therapist's hands over the chest and shoulders during exhalation.

A variety of feeding experiences are structured to assure normal development, as well as to inhibit abnormal reflexes and improve coordination of the jaw, lips, tongue, and soft palate in sucking, swallowing, biting, and chewing. Morris (1975d) presents the following principles:

1. Carefully analyze the task. For example, in chewing, there must be control of the jaw, lateral movement of the tongue, and inhibition from sucking and inward pressure of the cheeks. In what aspects is the child unable to succeed?
2. Observe what is happening in the rest of the body and use the positions that will facilitate or elicit the desired oral movements.
3. Because many cerebral-palsied children are hypersensitive to facial or oral stimulation, controlled stimulation must be used in the oral-facial area to reduce hypersensitivity, and build more normal oral sensory perception.
4. All types of food and liquids should be used. However, careful attention must be paid to grading of stimulation and variations of taste, texture, and temperature.
5. The mother should be an active participant in therapy. When she is skilled and confident, she can begin to incorporate the new routines in the home.
6. Successful experience of more normal feeding patterns will produce oral movements that can be modified for use in babbling and speech.

Because of the large amount of very specific information on therapeutic feeding, only the principles have been mentioned. More information on specific techniques can be found in Morris (1975d), Connor, Williamson, and Siepp (1978), and Finnie (1975).

The fourth sensorimotor prespeech skill is babbling practice. The child should be placed in a position that has been found to stimulate vocal play. Some techniques that have been used are facilitation of a sustained sound by using vibration, or by actually manipulating the jaw and lips to produce a variety of sounds. A wider variety of sound play may be stimulated by encouraging the child to voice while chewing. The therapist should praise jargon behaviors and set up little conversations by responding to jargoning with such statements as, "Oh, tell me more about that," or "Oh, that is very interesting." Imitating the child's babbling may also be helpful.

The therapeutic principles that have been discussed are taken from the philosophy of neuro-developmental treatment and are intended to apply to the very young child. However, some speech pathologists will be involved with cerebral-palsied children who are older and/or who have not had the benefit of early treatment. In addition to the articulatory remediation practices utilized with functional disorders, the following treatment strategies are applicable to these children.

Speech therapy for the older child without a language problem follows procedures similar to those discussed earlier in the treatment of dysarthria. However, there are modifications due to the nature of cerebral palsy as a developmental disorder.

A basic part of treatment is facilitating the desired movements while inhibiting the abnormal reflex patterns. Before the speech pathologist can address the problems of respiration, phonation, and articulation, the child must be able to assume and maintain some reflex-inhibiting postures that the physical therapist recommends. Articulation develops in the normal child when primitive reflexes have disappeared and coordination of respiration and phonation are established. A cerebral-palsied child who has been in a neuro-developmental treatment center since infancy will have experienced much therapy for inhibiting abnormal reflexes and stimulating normal movements before articulation develops. When this therapy is successful, articulation should begin and develop fairly normally. If there are errors, they can be treated in the same manner as articulation errors in a non–cerebral-palsied child would be treated (Newton, 1977). However, if the cerebral-palsied child is severely involved or has not had the advantage of neuro-developmental treatment, special procedures must be applied. Some children may still need therapeutic feeding and desensitization of the oral area before articulation therapy can be initiated.

The goals of articulation therapy are to increase the speed, range, and accuracy of the tongue, lips, and jaw movements. The goals are pursued in concert with the maintenance of body and head tones as well as respiration, phonation, and resonation normalcy (Myzak, 1980). Myzak divides therapy for articulation into three processes: (a) differentiation, or ability to move articulators in isolation from other body parts, (b) praxis, or the ability to make specific movements, and (c) diadochokinesia, or speeding up the movements.

In the differentiation phase, the child is stabilized and then asked to move his or her tongue or lips. If the child cannot do it, the clinician assists in this endeavor, but also should investigate why the child cannot make these movements. Is the difficulty related to body positioning, inability to perform some oral movement in feeding, or inability to inhibit abnormal reflex patterns? If these kinds of questions are not asked, treatment may be focusing on a symptom and not the cause. The sequence includes being able to independently move the mandible from the head, the tongue from the mandible, and the lips from the mandible. The final movements are when the child is able to move the mandible, lips, and tongue independently of the head and each other, as in normally articulated speech.

After independent movement is established, specific articulatory movements are introduced, such as lingua-alveolar, linguavelar, and linguadental. Movements should be carried out in conjunction with appropriate audio-visual stimulation by the clinician.

Speeding up the movements can be done by serial production of voiced and voiceless, or nasal and non-nasal sounds. Using phonemes that he or she can produce, the child can practice two-, three-, and four-syllable sets to increase speed. An example might be /na–ta/, /na–da/, /na–na/, /na–ka, /na–ga/. Three- and four-syllable combinations can be used and eventually two-word combinations can be introduced.

Although prognosis for a cerebral-palsied child is almost impossible to ascertain early in the treatment, it is a fact that all children will develop some kind of communicative skills, be it speech or not. Morris (1975a) suggests that all children be introduced to the use of augmentative communication early in their development. This addition is helpful in learning communicative acts, relieves the stress under which some children must communicate, and is a further enhancement of language learning. If the child cannot ultimately learn to use speech, he or she will be able to use augmentative communication systems more effectively, and without the feeling of failure in communicating.

Conclusion

There really is no specific articulation therapy program for the cerebral-palsied child. This child needs to begin at a much more basic level and needs to have articulation interrelated with all the other processes of bodily development and speech.

Neuro-developmental treatment is a philosophy of treatment that is based on early intervention. The basic tenets of this approach are to inhibit abnormal and primitive reflexes while stimulating the development of normal postural adjustments and the acquisition of coordinated movements. NDT appears to offer a new perspective on an old and yet-unsolved problem.

CLEFT PALATE

Cleft palate is a problem quite different from apraxia and dysarthria, but one that can have considerable effect upon speech. Speech problems result from inadequate structures, poor muscle function, compensatory strategies, and/or functional causes.

Treating the problems of cleft palate involves closing the actual defect as well as improving function of the structures for speech. Recently, many exciting medical/surgical and technological advancements have occurred that reduce or eliminate the devastating effects of cleft palate that once existed. However, the role of speech pathology in the management of cleft palate remains an important one.

Definition

Cleft palate is a structural anomaly that can affect the tissues, muscles, and bony processes of lip, alveolar process, hard palate, soft palate, and uvula. A cleft of these structures occurs during embyronic development, when there is a failure of structures to unite. Non-union most typically occurs between the median and lateral frontonasal processes that normally form the primary palate, including the lip, alveolar process, and incisive foramen; or at the midline between the palatal plates that form the secondary palate, including the hard and soft palates (Morley, 1970) (see Figure 10.1). This development takes place during the first trimester of pregnancy.

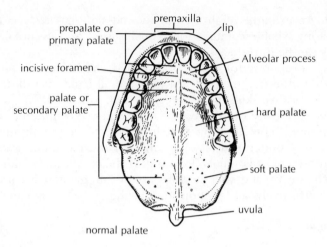

FIGURE 10.1
Normal palate.

Clefts of the lip and palate together affect boys more frequently than girls (2:1), while cleft palate only affects girls more frequently (2:1) (Koepp-Baker, 1971).

Although numerous classification systems exist, in an attempt to establish common terminology and an acceptable conceptual framework, a classification system was established by the American Cleft Palate Association (Harkins, Berlin, Harding, Longacre, & Snodgrass, 1962). It is based on embryological development and defines structures involved, location, size of cleft, and type of distortions present. The system includes submucous clefts, i.e., clefts that affect the underlying muscle and bony structures but leave the membrane covering intact, as well as palatal shortness, a frequently neglected problem in classification systems. This classification system is found in Table 10.2.

Etiology

Numerous causal factors have been associated with cleft palate, although no single explanatory factor has emerged (Koepp-Baker, 1971). Possible environmental causes cited by Morley (1970) include trauma, malnutrition, drugs, rubella, and viral disease during the first trimester of pregnancy. Interference from other embryonic structures such as the hands, feet, cord, or tongue which prevent the structures from uniting have also been cited as possible causes.

Genetic transmission is suggested by observation of a familial tendency, although the mode of transmission is not known (Longacre, 1970; Woolf, Woolf, & Broadbent, 1963). According to current literature, there may be a genetic predisposition which, when coupled with certain environmental factors, can result in a cleft (Koepp-Baker, 1971; McWilliams, 1982).

Speech Characteristics

Typical speech characteristics associated with cleft palate fall into the areas of resonation, articulation, and phonation. A brief summary of all three

TABLE 10.2
American Cleft Palate Association Classification System

Clefts of Pre-Palate*	*Cleft of Pre-Palate*
Cleft Lip	Any combination of foregoing types
Unilateral	Pre-palate protrusion
Right, Left	Pre-palate rotation
Extent in thirds (⅓, ⅔, ³⁄₃)	Pre-palate arrest (median cleft)
Bilateral	
Right, Left	*Clefts of Palate***
Extent in thirds	Clefts of soft palate
Median	Extent
Extent in thirds	Posteroanterior in thirds
Prolabium	Width (maximum in mm)
Small, medium, large	Palatal shortness
Cogenital Scar	None, slight, moderate, marked
Right, Left, Median	Submucous cleft
Extent in thirds	Extent in thirds
	Cleft hard palate
Cleft of Alveolar Process	Extent
Unilateral	Posteroanterior in thirds
Right, Left	Width (maximum in mm)
Extent in thirds	Vomer attachment
Bilateral	Right, Left, Absent
Right, Left	Submucous cleft
Extent in thirds	Extent in thirds
Median	Cleft of soft and hard palate
Extent in thirds	
Submucous	*Clefts of Pre-Palate and Palate*
Right, Left, Median	Any combination of clefts described under
	Clefts of Pre-Palate and Clefts of Palate

*Pre-palate or primary palate includes the lip, alveolus, and triangular area of the palate just behind the alveolus but anterior to the incisive foramen.
**Palate or secondary palate refers to the remaining portion of the palate lying posterior to the incisive foramen, i.e., hard palate and soft palate.
Source: "Classification of Cleft Lip and Palate" by A. J. Berlin. In *Cleft Lip and Palate: Surgical, Dental and Speech Aspects,* W. C. Grabb, S. W. Rosenstein, & K. Bzoch (Eds.), 1971, Boston: Little Brown & Co. Copyright 1971 by Little Brown & Co. Reprinted by permission.

areas is included because all three have an impact on overall intelligibility; they also have an interactive effect upon each other.

Resonation.   The most typical resonance characteristic associated with cleft palate is hypernasality. This results from inability of the velum to close off the nasal cavity in order to maintain a balance between oral and nasal resonance. Too much air is allowed to enter the nasal cavity. The cause may be structural, as in a short palate, submucous cleft, or an opening in the palate; or it may be functional, as in a repaired cleft with poor or uncoordinated velar mobility or poor tongue positioning. The phonemes most frequently affected are vowels. A symptom of hypernasality is nasal emission, which is a sound that results from air flow going through the nasal cavity. It is perceived as an audible nasal escape of air, especially on plosive, affricative and fricative phonemes.

Much less frequently found are problems of hyponasality and cul-de-sac resonation. Hyponasality is most often caused by an obstruction, or a pharyngeal flap (a type of surgical repair) that provides too much occlusion. Cul-de-sac resonance is a combination of hypernasality and hyponasality. This type of resonance could result from a blockage in the nasal passages.

Articulation.   Articulation may be affected in several different ways. The specific phonemic errors may vary according to cause as discussed in the following sections.

Decreased Intra-oral Pressure.   Hypernasality results in a decrease in intra-oral pressure and hence affects articulation. Stops (/p, b, t, d, k, g/), fricatives (/s, z, ʃ, ʒ/), and affricatives (/tʃ, dʒ/) are all affected since these phonemes require intra-oral pressure for accurate production.

When intra-oral pressure is limited, several effects might be anticipated. The consonant produced might be weak or distorted. If intra-oral air flow is increased, nasal emission results. Although the patient is often capable of normal articulatory placement, he or she may develop compensatory patterns in an attempt to prevent nasal emission. The two most common compensatory substitutions are glottal stops and pharyngeal fricatives. A glottal stop is an attempt to implode air before the oral cavity, especially on stop consonants, by creating a valve at the level of the glottis. Similarly, pharyngeal fricatives result from attempts to shift the valve to the pharynx to compensate for inadequate intra-oral breath pressure on fricatives and affricates. What the speaker is doing in both cases is attempting to close off the vocal tract at a point prior to where the air escapes through the nose.

Dental and Occlusal Abnormalities.   Although the specific effects of dental and occlusal anomalies remain unclear, both may interfere with normal articulation. Any deviations that produce a Class III malocclusion, or open bite, may have an effect on consonant production, especially the sibilant sounds (Starr, 1979). Any other dental abnormality that restricts tongue movement may likewise affect articulation. When there is a disproportionate relationship between the mandible (lower jaw) and maxilla (upper dental arch), bilabials, the fricatives /f/ and /v/, and lingual-alveolar consonants may also be affected. These kinds of problems may result in the development of compensatory movements and/or phoneme distortions or approximations. According to Starr (1979), the conditions most likely to result in an articulation problem are open bite, missing central incisors, or any anomaly affecting the relationship between the tongue and the lower incisors. However, although articulation problems may result from these problems, many individuals are able to compensate for dental and occlusal problems and have normal speech.

Hearing Loss.   Cleft-palate children have a higher incidence of conductive hearing loss than the normal population (McWilliams, 1982).

The prevalence of fluctuating hearing loss during the language-learning period has been commonly cited as a potential cause of articulation problems. The research to support this, however, has been poorly controlled (Ventry,

1980). This remains a viable possibility but needs further documentation to establish a cause/effect relationship.

Other Causes.   Finally, one must consider the possibility of functional articulation problems in the cleft-palate population. These are problems that are not caused by the organic deficit of cleft palate, and which the normal population is subject to as well.

Phonation.   Although problems of phonation are sometimes overlooked (Edwards, 1980), such problems as decreased loudness, which is used as a means of decreasing nasal resonance, often occur. This results in a weak and breathy voice. Individuals who have difficulty maintaining loudness levels may increase efforts to speak louder. This additional effort may produce hoarseness (Ross & Johnson, 1972). Vocal abuse, especially frequent glottal stops, may also contribute to phonatory problems, as seen by the increased incidence of vocal nodules in the cleft-palate population.

Associated Problems.   There are numerous other problems associated with cleft palate. The most frequently cited problems include hearing loss (Bluestone, 1978; Yules, 1970; Bennett, 1972; Walton, 1973; Chaudhuri & Bowen-Jones, 1978), impaired intelligence (Lencione, 1980; Ruess, 1965; Phillips & Harrison, 1969; Estes & Morris, 1973), psychological problems (Watson, 1964; Ruess, 1965; Wirls & Plotkin, 1971; Clifford, 1979), emotional problems of patient and family, medical complications, and feeding problems.

Assessment

The cleft-palate child can have numerous interrelated problems. Dealing with the deformity alone may require the skills of an oral surgeon, plastic surgeon, orthodontist and prosthodontist. When associated problems are present, additional specialists may be needed, such as a speech pathologist, audiologist, otologist, psychologist, cardiologist, radiologist, etc. Because of the numerous professionals who might be required, assessment and treatment are best carried out within the structural framework of a cleft-palate team, where an exchange of information and coordinated planning can occur. As with other types of articulation disorders, the assessment includes oral-facial examination and evaluation of function of nonspeech and speech tasks.

Oral-Facial Examination.   In performing the examination of the oral structures described in chapter 4, there are considerations specific to cleft palate. At this point, the reader might want to review the oral-facial examination procedures in chapter 4. In regard to cleft palate, the examiner should especially note the following:

Lips.   It has been found that the lips do not contribute significantly to articulation problems found in cleft-palate speech, although gross deviations of the lips might affect production of bilabial phonemes. The examiner should look for evidence of a cleft, location of the cleft, evidence of surgical repair, general appearance and symmetry of lips, tightness or mobility of the lips, and diadochokinetic rate of movement.

Occlusion and Dentition.   Although dental abnormalities can have an effect on articulation (especially the sibilant and fricative sounds), occlusion abnormalities have a greater effect. The examiner should observe the general condition of the teeth (healthy vs. carious), number of teeth, alignment of teeth, and occlusion pattern. When examining the occlusion pattern, one should particularly watch for anterior crossbite or Class III (open bite) malocclusion.

Alveolus.   Alveolar lingual phonemes such as /t, d, n, l/ are most notably related to the condition of the alveolus. Observations include: evidence of a cleft, location of the cleft, evidence of surgical repair, and use of an orthopedic appliance.

Palate.   Defects of the velum have a primary effect on resonance patterns. Articulation is also affected by the inability to implode adequate air pressure and by the consequent development of compensatory movements. As discussed in chapter 4, the velopharyngeal sphincter cannot be viewed via intraoral inspection. However, a certain amount of information can be obtained by observation of the visible structures. The hard palate should be examined for height and shape of the palatal arch, size and location of fistulas, evidence of a repair, and evidence of a submucous cleft.

The soft palate should be examined for height and shape of the arch, especially during phonation; extent and location of the cleft, if still unrepaired; evidence of submucous cleft, such as velar dimple or transparent appearance of membrane covering; bifid uvula; and length and mobility of velum. In most cases, the soft palate will have been repaired, since this is usually done early.

Pharynx.   The examiner should look for evidence of posterior and lateral pharyngeal wall movement. Other observations should include evidence of an abnormally deep pharyngeal area, previous surgical repair such as pharyngeal flap, and possible upper airway obstructions. Abnormalities should be noted but, since the velopharyngeal valve cannot be fully observed, normal appearance does not necessarily mean normal function.

Tonsils.   The examiner should observe whether tonsils are present or absent, and if present, size of the tonsils.

Tongue.   The positioning of the tongue in the mouth may have an influence on resonance. Observations of the tongue should include size of the tongue, ability to perform gross motor movements described in chapter 4, and position of the tongue at rest.

Speech Evaluation.   In the speech evaluation the following areas are especially important.

Resonance.   Both objective and subjective measures of resonance should be obtained. Objective measures include airflow studies, direct observation via nasopharyngoscopy, and X-ray studies such as videofluoroscopy and cineradiography. These measures can be employed to evaluate the balance between oral and nasal resonance and to determine the factors creating the resonance problem.

Additional testing for resonance is done in conjunction with articulation testing. Vowels, as well as the consonants described previously, are especially affected by hypernasality. Having the patient produce vowels and CV combinations with the nares occluded and unoccluded is a method of testing for hypernasality. The hypernasality will diminish when the nares are occluded. Hypernasality should also be evaluated at the single-word and sentence level. Some individuals are able to achieve proper balance for limited segments but cannot maintain it in ongoing speech.

Evidence of nasal emission, nasal snort, facial grimacing, nasal flaring, and compensatory productions such as glottal stops and pharyngeal fricatives should be noted.

Articulation.   The articulation evaluation is performed not only to determine specific deviant phonemes but, more importantly, to determine error patterns or deviations in the phonological system. The patient is routinely administered an articulation test. Tests that are frequently used include the McDonald Deep Test, (McDonald, 1964), Iowa Pressure Test (Morris, Spriestersbach, & Darley, 1961), C-PAC (Secord, 1981), or Bzoch Error Pattern Diagnostic Articulation Test (described in Bzoch, 1971). Typical substitutions, distortions, and omissions are noted as in any articulation evaluation. However, the examiner is particularly interested in types of errors and compensatory production.

Edwards (1980) points to a number of phonological differences that have been observed in the literature. Most of these are similar to those observed in children with functional articulation problems. Some cleft-palate children have been found to demonstrate final consonant omission, deletion of unstressed syllables, and cluster reduction. They also have difficulty in making binary contrasts such as oral vs. nasal, stop vs. continuant, and voice vs. voiceless.

In cleft palate speech, the resonance problem may be difficult to separate from the articulation problem. One of the most common problems when inadequate intra-oral air pressure is present is a weakness of consonants, despite normal placement. The examiner should attempt to determine the influence of resonance problems on articulation problems.

There are individuals who can produce isolated phonemes or even individual words due to the fact that the speech mechanism is able to function more efficiently at a slower rate. Therefore, analyzing spontaneous speech is as important as doing formal articulation testing. In addition, since cleft-palate children are subject to the typical delays of other children, the examiner should determine which problems are related to the cleft palate and which problems are due to other causes.

Phonation.   Breathiness is frequently found in cleft-palate individuals as they attempt to reduce pressure and use a soft attack. The examiner should look for signs of vocal abuse such as hard glottal attacks, abnormal head and neck postures, and excessive tension (Edwards, 1980). Hoarseness may be present if vocal nodules have developed. If phonatory problems are present, evaluation of the voice problem is indicated following typical voice evaluation procedures.

Other Evaluation Considerations.   All cleft-palate children should be suspected of having potential for language delay and hearing loss. Hearing testing and screening for both receptive and expressive language problems should be included in every evaluation.

Prognosis and Remediation

As mentioned at the beginning of this section, the prognosis for normal speech and language is quite good. Bzoch (1979) states that with appropriate intervention, 95% of cleft-palate children can achieve normal speech and language development.

The remainder of this section will focus on speech remediation. However, the earliest concerns for the cleft-palate child relate to surgical and/or prosthetic management. Cleft of the lip is generally repaired during the first few months of life. Repair of the alveolus may be done at the same time or may be delayed. In severe defects, orthodontic intervention may precede surgery to bring structures into better alignment for surgery. There has been some controversy over the timing of the surgical repair of the palate. Whether direct speech therapy is necessary depends upon the timing and success of these procedures.

For many children, no direct therapy will be needed. This is particularly true in early surgical repairs, i.e., when surgery occurs before speech development, assuming that a successful closure has been achieved. The rationale is that with an early structural correction, no faulty production patterns have yet developed, and speech will progress normally. While functional problems are still possible, they are less likely.

When surgery occurs after speech development, the need for speech therapy is more frequent. Despite a successful surgical result, the functional component often remains. Previous speech patterns are maintained, so even though immediate change in resonance may be noted, compensatory articulation patterns remain.

However, regardless of the timing of surgery, all cleft-palate children should be considered at risk for speech and language problems. Therefore, the most effective approach is of a preventative nature in order to minimize the risk of speech problems. This approach differs significantly from that for functional problems in that with functional problems, it is assumed that speech will develop normally, and so intervention does not occur until after symptoms begin to appear. For cleft-palate children, early speech and language stimulation is important. Philips (1979) feels that a stimulation program should begin as early as 18–24 months. Stimulation should be geared toward vocabulary, syntax, and phonological development.

When problems of resonance, articulation, and phonation occur, direct intervention is needed. Let us consider each of these areas.

Resonance.   Therapy will not improve resonance defects that are the result of an inadequate structure. When structures are deficient, surgical and/or prosthetic intervention should precede speech therapy. In unclear cases, a trial period of therapy can be attempted. If no improvement has occurred within 3 months, the child should be referred for re-evaluation to determine the need for secondary surgery or prosthetic alternatives.

Muscle-training techniques have been used by some to increase velopharyngeal function. According to Cole (1979), there are three approaches to muscle training for resonance problems: (a) indirect, as in articulation therapy; (b) semidirect, as in blowing and sucking exercises; and (c) direct, as in direct muscle stimulation designed to bring involuntary and reflexive muscle action under voluntary control. These approaches have had varying degrees of success.

Articulation therapy designed to improve resonance problems has not proven to be an effective approach for improving velopharyngeal closure. Sucking, and especially blowing exercises, have been used to redirect airflow into the oral cavity as well as to increase velopharyngeal closure. The efficacy of blowing techniques has been questioned on the basis that the closure pattern for blowing is different from that for speech (Edwards, 1980). The success of direct muscle-training techniques has been variable, and patient selection must be done carefully. Additional research into this area is needed to determine its value (Cole, 1979). Various biofeedback techniques have been used to offer visual and auditory feedback to develop kinesthetic and auditory awareness for reduced nasality. Therapy should also focus on eliminating extraneous movements such as facial grimacing, when such behaviors exist.

Articulation.   Riski and Millard (1979) suggest that articulation therapy should precede therapy for resonance disorders. The rationale for this is that often with improved articulatory postures, hypernasality will decrease as well, thereby saving unnecessary efforts in that area later on.

Many articulation defects relating to cleft palate are difficult to separate from resonance problems. However, the relationship between the two should be determined before establishing therapy goals. Although improved articulatory postures may decrease hypernasality, if there is a significant impairment of structure and/or function that causes hypernasality, articulatory postures will be unable to compensate totally. In planning therapy goals one must consider whether surgery or prosthodontia should precede extensive articulation therapy in order to achieve success.

Typical articulation and phonological procedures applicable to other types of articulation disorders are appropriate for therapy with cleft-palate individuals. Articulatory placement is important and should receive early emphasis. Auditory, visual, tactile, and kinesthetic cues can all be used to develop normal production. If structural distortions are present that obviate normal production, compensatory productions can be taught so that production may at least be improved.

Phonation.   Since there is a high incidence of vocal nodules due to abusive vocal behaviors, potentially abusive behaviors such as yelling and screaming should be identified and eliminated. Since many of the vocally abusive behaviors are associated with abnormal compensatory articulation productions and difficulty achieving intra-oral pressure, phonation therapy may sometimes be used simultaneously with resonance and articulation therapy. At other times, specific voice therapy techniques such as those used for decreasing breathiness or reduction of tension in the laryngeal area may be employed.

Conclusion

The outlook for the cleft-palate child today is very positive. Current diagnostic procedures are sophisticated enough to allow more specific definition of most parameters of the problem, thus making it possible for more effective treatment procedures to be undertaken. Surgical procedures have been refined to the point that, when these are combined with preventative speech therapy measures, many children can be expected to develop normal speech. Prognosis for children who do have residual speech problems is also good in light of advancements in secondary surgical procedures, available prosthodontic devices, and speech therapy. In order to accomplish the goal of normal speech development, the efforts of a coordinated team of professionals are essential.

REFERENCES

Bennett, M. (1972). The older cleft palate patient. *Laryngoscope, 82,* 1217–1225.

Bluestone, C. C. (1978). Prevalence of pathogenesis of ear disease and hearing loss. In M. Graham (Ed.), *Cleft palate, middle ear disease and hearing loss.* Springfield, IL: Charles C. Thomas Publisher.

Bobath, B. (1967). The very early treatment of cerebral palsy. *Developmental Medicine and Child Neurology, 9,* 373–390.

Bobath, K., & Bobath, B. (1972). Cerebral palsy. Part I: Diagnosis and assessment of cerebral palsy. Part II: The neurodevelopmental approach to treatment. In P. H. Pearson & C. E. Williams (Eds.), *Physical therapy services in the developmental disabilities.* Springfield, IL: Charles C. Thomas.

Boone, D. R. (1972). *Cerebral palsy.* Indianapolis, IN: The Bobbs-Merrill Co., Inc.

Bzoch, K. R. (1971). Introduction to section C: Measurement of parameters of cleft palate speech. In W. C. Grabb, S. W. Rosenstein, & K. Bzoch (Eds.), *Cleft lip and palate: Surgical, dental and speech aspects.* Boston: Little Brown & Co.

Bzoch, K. R. (1979). Rationale methods and techniques of cleft palate speech therapy. In K. R. Bzoch (Ed.), *Communication disorders related to cleft lip and palate.* Boston: Little, Brown, and Co.

Chappell, G. E. (1973). Childhood verbal apraxia and its treatment. *Journal of Speech and Hearing Disorders, 38,* 362–369.

Chaudhuri, P., & Bowen-Jones, E. (1978). An otorhinological study of children with cleft palate. *Journal of Laryngology and Otology, 92,* 29–40.

Clifford, E. (1979). Psychological aspects of cleft lip and palate. In K. R. Bzoch (Ed.), *Communicative disorders related to cleft lip and palate* (2nd ed.). Boston: Little, Brown, and Co.

Cole, R. M. (1979). Direct muscle training for the improvement of velopharyngeal activity. In K. R. Bzoch (Ed.), *Communicative disorders related to cleft lip and palate* (2nd ed.). Boston: Little, Brown and Co.

Connor, F. P., Williamson, G. G., & Siepp, J. M. (1978). *Program guide for infants and toddlers with neuromotor and other developmental disabilities.* New York: Teachers College Press, Columbia University.

Crothers, B., & Paine, R. S. (1959). *The natural history of cerebral palsy.* Cambridge, MA: Harvard University Press.

Cruickshank, W. (1976). The problem and its scope. In W. Cruickshank (Ed.), *Cerebral palsy: A developmental disability.* Syracuse, NY: Syracuse University Press.

Darley, F., Aronson, A., & Brown, J. (1975). *Motor speech disorders.* Philadelphia: W. B. Saunders.

Denhoff, E. (1976). Medical aspects. In W. Cruickshank (Ed.), *Cerebral palsy: A developmental disability.* Syracuse: Syracuse University Press.

Denhoff, E., & Holden, R. (1954). Family influence on successful school adjustment of cerebral palsied children. *Journal of International Council of Exceptional Children, 21,* 5–7.

Dworkin, J. P. (1984). Specific characteristics and treatments of the dysarthrias. In H. Winitz (Ed.), *Treating articulation disorders: For clinicians by clinicians.* Baltimore: University Park Press.

Edwards, M. (1980). Speech and language disability. In M. Edwards & A. C. H. Watson (Eds.), *Advances in the management of cleft palate.* New York: Churchill Livingston.

Estes, R. E., & Morris, H. L. (1973). Relationships among intelligence, speech proficiency, and hearing sensitivity in children with cleft palate. *Cleft Palate Journal, 7,* 763.

Finnie, N. R. (1975). *Handling the young cerebral palsied child at home.* New York: E. P. Dutton.

Geschwind, N. (1975). Apraxias: Neuromechanisms of disorders of learned movement. *American Science, 63,* 188–205.

Hanson, W. R., & Metter, E. J. (1980). DAF as instrumental treatment for dysarthria in progressive supranuclear palsy: A case report. *Journal of Speech and Hearing Disorders, 45,* 268–276.

Harkins, C. S., Berlin, A., Harding, R., Longacre, J., & Snodgrass, R. (1962). A classification of cleft lip and palate. *Plastic Reconstructive Surgery, 29,* 31.

Haynes, S. M. (1978). Developmental apraxia of speech. In D. Johns (Ed.), *Clinical management of neurogenic communicative disorders.* Boston: Little, Brown and Co.

Jones, M., Barrett, M., Olonoff, C., & Anderson, E. (1969). Two experiments in training handicapped children in nursery school. In P. Wolff & R. MacKeith (Eds.), *Planning for better living.* London: Heinemann.

Kimura, D. (1976). The neural basis of language qua gesture. In H. Whitaker & H. A. Whitaker (Eds.), *Studies in neurolinguistics* (Vol. 2). New York: Academic Press.

Koepp-Baker, H. (1971). Orofacial clefts: Their forms and effects. In L. E. Travis (Ed.), *Handbook of speech pathology and audiology.* Englewood Cliffs, NJ: Prentice-Hall.

Kong, E. (1966). Very early treatment of cerebral palsy. *Developmental Medicine and Child Neurology, 8,* 198–202.

LaPointe, L. L. (1982). Neurogenic disorders of speech. In G. H. Shames & E. H. Wiig (Eds.), *Human communication disorders.* Columbus: Charles E. Merrill Publishing Co.

Lapointe, L., & Wertz, R. (1974). Oral movement abilities and articulatory characteristics of brain injured adults. *Perceptual and Motor Skills, 39,* 39–46.

Lencione, R. M. (1980). Associated conditions. In M. Edwards & A. C. H. Watson (Eds.), *Advances in the management of cleft palate.* New York: Churchill Livingston.

Logemann, J. A. (1984). Management of acquired articulation disorders in adults. In H. Winitz (Ed.), *Treating articulation disorders: For clinicians by clinicians.* Baltimore: University Park Press.

Longacre, J. J. (1970). *Cleft palate deformation..* Springfield, IL: Charles C. Thomas.

Martin, A. D. (1974). Some objections to the term "apraxia of speech." *Journal of Speech and Hearing Disorders, 39,* 53–64.

McDonald, E. (1964). *A deep test of articulation.* Pittsburgh: Stanwix House.

McWilliams, B. J. (1982). The cleft palate. In G. S. Shames & E. Wiig (Eds.), *Human communication disorders.* Columbus, OH: Charles E. Merrill Publishing Co.

Minear, W. L. (1956). A classification of cerebral palsy. *Pediatrics, 18,* 841–852.

Morley, M. E. (1970). *Cleft palate and speech* (7th ed.). London: Churchill Livingston.

Morris, H. L., Spriestersbach, D. C., & Darley, F. L. (1961). An articulation test for assessing competency of velopharyngeal closure. *Journal of Speech and Hearing Research, 4,* 48–55.

Morris, S. E. (1975a). A neurodevelopmental approach to communication boards. In S. E. Morris (Ed.), *Pre-speech and language programming for the young child with cerebral palsy.* Wauwatosa, WI: Curative Rehabilitation Center.

Morris, S. E. (1975b). Pre-speech assessment. In S. E. Morris (Ed.), *Pre-speech and language programming for the young child with cerebral palsy.* Wauwatosa, WI: Curative Rehabilitation Center.

Morris, S. E. (1975c). Treatment principles: Respiration and phonation problems. In S. E. Morris (Ed.), *Pre-speech and language programming for the young child with cerebral palsy.* Wauwatosa, WI: Curative Rehabilitation Center.

Morris, S. E. (1975d). (Ed.) Program guidelines for children with feeding problems. In *Pre-speech and language programming for the young child with cerebral palsy.* Wauwatosa, WI: Curative Rehabilitation Center.

Myzak, E. D. (1980). *Neurospeech therapy for the cerebral palsied.* New York: Teachers College Press, Columbia University.

Netsell, R., & Cleeland, C. S. (1973). Modification of lip hypertonia in dysarthria using EMG feedback. *Journal of Speech and Hearing Disorders, 38,* 131.

Newton, M. (1977). *Cerebral palsy: Speech, hearing and language problems.* Lincoln, NE: Cliffs Notes.

Nober, E. H. (1976). Auditory processing. In W. Cruickshank (Ed.), *Cerebral palsy: A developmental disability.* Syracuse, NY: Syracuse University Press.

Pearlstone, A. D. (1969). Ocular defects in cerebral palsy. *Eye, Ear, Nose, Throat Monthly, 48,* 36–48.

Perlstein, M. A., Gibbs, E. L., & Gibbs, F. A. (1947). The electroencephalogram in infantile cerebral palsy. *Proceedings of Research in Nervous and Mental Disease, 2,* 377–384.

Peterson, H. A., & Marquardt, T. P. (1981). *Appraisal and diagnosis of speech and language disorders.* Englewood Cliffs, NJ: Prentice-Hall, Inc.

Philips, J. (1979). Stimulating syntactic and phonological development in infants with cleft palate. In K. R. Bzoch (Ed.), *Communicative disorders related to cleft lip and palate* (2nd ed.). Boston: Little, Brown, and Co.

Phillips, B., & Harrison, R. (1969). Language skills in pre-school cleft palate children. *Cleft Palate Journal, 6,* 108–119.

Ringel, R. L., House, A. S., Burk, K. W., & Dolinsky, J. P. (1970). Some relations between orosensory discrimination and articulatory aspects of speech production. *Journal of Speech and Hearing Disorders, 35,* 3–11.

Riski, J. E., & Millard, R. T. (1979). The processes of speech: Evaluation and treatment. In H. Cooper, R. Harding, W. Krogman, M. Mazaheri, & R. Millard (Eds.), *Cleft palate and lip: A team approach to clinical management and rehabilitation of the patient.* Philadelphia: W. B. Saunders Co.

Rosenbek, J. C., Hensen, R., Baughman, C., & Lemme, M. (1974). Treatment of developmental apraxia of speech: A case study. *Language, Speech and Hearing Services in Schools, 5,* 13–21.

Rosenbek, J. C., & LaPointe, L. L. (1979). The dysarthrias: Description, diagnosis and treatment. In D. F. Johns (Ed.), *Clinical management of neurogenic communicative disorders.* Boston: Little, Brown, and Co.

Rosenbek, J. C., & LaPointe, L. L. (1981). Aging communication processes and disorders. In D. Beasley & G. A. Davis (Eds.), *Aging communication processes and disorders.* New York: Grune and Stratton.

Rosenbek, J. C., Lemme, M., Ahern, M., Harris, E., & Wertz, R. T. (1973). A treatment for apraxia of speech in adults. *Journal of Speech and Hearing Disorders, 38*, 462–472.

Rosenbek, J. C., & Wertz, R. T. (1972). A review of 50 cases of developmental apraxia of speech. *Language, Speech and Hearing Services in the Schools, 3*, 23–30.

Rosenbek, J. C., Wertz, R. T., & Darley, F. L. (1973). Oral sensation and perception in apraxia of speech and aphasia. *Journal of Speech and Hearing Research, 16*, 22–36.

Ross, R. B., & Johnson, M. C. (1972). *Cleft lip and palate.* Baltimore: Williams and Wilkins.

Ruess, A. (1965). A comparative study of cleft palate children and their siblings. *Journal of Clinical Psychology, 21*, 354–360.

Secord, W. (1981). *C-PAC: Clinical probes of articulation consistency.* Columbus, OH: Charles Merrill Publishing Co.

Skelly, M., Schinsky, L., Smith, R., & Fust, R. (1974). American Indian Sign (Amerind) as a facilitator of verbalization for the oral-verbal apraxic. *Journal of Speech and Hearing Disorders, 39*, 445–456.

Sparks, R., Helm, N., & Albert, M. (1974). Aphasia rehabilitation resulting from melodic intonation therapy. *Cortex, 10*, 303–313.

Sparks, R., Holland, A. (1976). Method: Melodic intonation therapy for aphasia. *Journal of Speech and Hearing Disorders, 41*, 287–297.

Starr, C. (1979). Dental and occlusal hazards to normal speech production. In K. R. Bzoch (Ed.), *Communicative disorders related to cleft lip and palate.* Boston: Little, Brown and Co.

Trost, J., & Canter, G. (1974). Apraxia of speech in patients with Broca's aphasia. *Brain and Language, 1*, 63–80.

Ventry, I. M. (1980). Effects of conductive hearing loss: Fact or fiction. *Journal of Speech and Hearing Disorders, 45*, 143–156.

Vignolo, L. A. (1964). Evaluation of aphasia and language rehabilitation: A retrospective exploratory study. *Cortex, 1*, 344–459.

Walton, W. K. (1973). Audiometrically "normal" conductive hearing losses among the cleft palate. *Cleft Palate Journal, 10*, 99–103.

Watson, C. G. (1964). Personality adjustment in boys with cleft lips and palates. *Cleft Palate Journal, 1*, 130.

Wepman, J. M. (1958). The relationship between self-correction and recovery from aphasia. *Journal of Speech and Hearing Disorders, 25*, 302–308.

Wertz, R. T. (1978). Neuropathologies of speech and language. In D. Johns (Ed.), *Clinical management of neurogenic communication disorders.* Boston: Little, Brown, and Co.

Williams, R., Ingham, R., & Rosenthal, J. (1981). A further analysis for developmental apraxia of speech in children with defective articulation. *Journal of Speech and Hearing Research, 24*, 496–505.

Wirls, C. J., & Plotkin, R. R. (1971). A comparison of children with cleft palate and their siblings on projective test personality factors. *Cleft Palate Journal, 8*, 399.

Woolf, C. M., Woolf, R. M., & Broadbent, T. R. (1963). *American Journal of Genetics, 15*, 209.

Yorkston, K. M., & Beukelman, D. R. (1981a). *Assessment of intelligibility of dysarthric speech.* Tigard, OR: C. C. Publications.

Yorkston, K. M., & Beukelman, D. R. (1981b). Ataxic dysarthria: Treatment sequences based on intelligibility and prosodic considerations. *Journal of Speech and Hearing Disorders, 46*, 398–404.

Yoss, K. A., & Darley, F. L. (1974a). Developmental apraxia of speech in children with defective articulation. *Journal of Speech and Hearing Research, 17*, 399–416.

Yoss, K. A., & Darley, F. L. (1974b). Therapy in developmental apraxia of speech. *Language, Speech and Hearing Services in Schools, 5*, 23–31.

Yules, R. B. (1970). Hearing in cleft palate patients. *Arch. Otolaryngol., 91*, 319–323.

PART III

Specific Articulation Treatment Programs

In this section, four authors present the specific therapy methods or programs that they have developed. All of the programs are based on the general principles outlined earlier in Part II.

In chapter 11, Bradley describes a multiple-phoneme method that combines the multiphonemic emphasis of the linguistic model with the systematic application of behavioral principles.

Chapter 12 describes the paired-stimuli approach of Weston and Irwin, which uses the principle of generalization as the basis for a behavioral therapy design.

In the method of meaningful contrasts (chapter 13), Cooper advocates using minimal pairs, as described in the linguistic approach, for helping the child see the value of correct articulation, as emphasized in communication-centered therapy.

Blache's method (chapter 14) incorporates the minimal-pair strategy with distinctive-feature theory.

11

A Systematic Multiple-Phoneme Approach to Articulation Treatment

In recent years, the assessment and management of individuals with articulatory disorders has been influenced by theoretical work on distinctive features and phonological processes (see chapters 3 and 7). These developments have changed many aspects of articulatory therapy and support the idea of dealing with more than one phoneme at a time during therapy sessions (McReynolds & Engmann, 1975; Costello & Onstine, 1976; Singh, 1975; Weiner, 1978; Mowrer, 1978; Shriberg & Kwiatkowski, 1980; Ingram, 1981). Nevertheless, the need for a systematic approach to planning and monitoring therapy remains. There is also need for a clinically feasible means of assessing phoneme production in conversation. This is even a requirement of law in some states in order to establish the need for speech therapy within a public school system. The multiple-phoneme approach is a program that incorporates the following features: (a) simultaneous teaching of multiple phonemes, (b) systematic application of behavioral principles, and (c) analysis of phoneme production in conversational speech.

The method was first described by McCabe and Bradley (1973) as an intensive therapy program for individuals with six or more consonant error

Doris P. Bradley, Ph.D., is a professor of speech and hearing sciences and chairperson of the Department of Speech and Hearing Sciences at the University of Southern Mississippi, Hattiesburg, Mississippi.

phonemes in their articulatory patterns. Since then, various authors (Holtzapple & Marshall, 1977; Seaton & Bradley, 1978; Schissel & Doty, 1979) have reported its application with different populations and in several settings.

The purpose of this chapter is to explain the multiple-phoneme approach in detail so that students may use it effectively.

RATIONALE

The multiple-phoneme approach to articulation therapy was developed at the University of North Carolina in 1969 with support from grants (GRS RR 05333 USPHS and NIDR DE 42642 01). Its purpose at that time was to document and increase the efficiency of articulation therapy provided to children who had multiple phoneme errors with etiology of cleft palate and other children who had multiple errors and different etiologies. The development of this method included extensive documentation of articulatory skills prior to therapy and reassessment of articulatory skills after specified amounts of therapy. The success of the procedure has led to its continued use and adoption by others.

Since 1973, a number of authors have established the efficiency of teaching more than one phoneme at a time (Blache, Parsons, & Humphreys, 1981; Hodson & Paden, 1982) when working with children who have multiple errors (see chapter 7).

The multiple-phoneme approach maintains the traditional steps of therapy but uses them in some different ways (McCabe & Bradley, 1975). It stresses sound production skills at each level without any emphasis on auditory discrimination until after accurate production is well established, since there is evidence that production training also trains discrimination. During the establishment phase, all auditory monitoring is the responsibility of the speech pathologist. After accurate production of phonemes is achieved at the word level, the speaker begins to monitor the accuracy of phonemes. Many speech pathologists have questioned this part of the approach until they have tried it. Then, they have often agreed that undertaking auditory discrimination following the achievement of accurate sound production is beneficial and timesaving.

In keeping with behavioral methods, each step of the program is clearly outlined and sequenced so that increasingly complex behaviors are taught after it has been demonstrated that simpler behaviors have been mastered. Criteria for mastery are provided at each step. Several record-keeping forms are used to make tracking the client's performance in each session easy.

One of the measures used in pre- and post-therapy assessment is whole-word accuracy (WWA) in conversational speech. WWA is illustrated in Figure 11.1. It consists of a sample of a child's tape-recorded conversation typed in standard English form consisting of approximately 150 words. The examiner plays the tape recording and marks on the transcript each word spoken in error. A WWA score is derived simply by calculating the percentage of words spoken correctly. Bradley, Allen, and Clifford (1973) verified the consistency of WWA by testing a group of children during three different conversations. The reported consistency was within 8% across topics and time. More recently,

TABLE 11.1

Comparative Norms of Arizona Articulation Proficiency Scale and Whole Word Accuracy for Normally Speaking Children

Age	Mean		Standard Deviation		Median		Mode	
	AAPS	WWA	AAPS	WWA	AAPS	WWA	AAPS	WWA
3.0	86.3	68.53	5.5	10.28	85.5	70.5	90	73
3.6	90.93	76.4	5.79	10.72	92.17	75.25	94	72
4.0	90.93	80.0	5.73	10.32	91.83	82.5	96	74
4.6	93.57	83.77	3.58	3.46	93.5	83.0	92	83
5.0	95.13	87.97	3.6	6.04	95.5	90.7	97	91
5.6	96.5	88.6	3.18	7.75	97.3	90.0	100	96
6.0	96.4	91.87	3.27	4.9	97.25	92.83	100	96
7.0	98.57	95.4	1.4	1.1	98.87	95.72	100	96

Note.   These data are from "Conversational Speech Sampling in the Assessment of Articulation Proficiency" by L. S. Schmitt, B. H. Howard, and J. F. Schmitt, 1983, *Language Speech & Hearing Services in Schools, 14*, pp. 210–214.

Schmidt, Howard, and Schmidt (1983) reported data from assessments of 3- to 7-year-old children developing speech and language normally. The authors compared scores on the Arizona Articulation Proficiency Scale (Fudula, 1963) and WWA norms from conversational samples. These norms are shown in Table 11.1.

WWA can be used effectively to supplement information obtained from single-word articulation tests. The same conversational samples can be used to determine the distinctive features and/or the phonological processes present in the speaker's speech pattern. Figure 11.1 provides an example of a conversational sample that has been scored. The marked words were produced with at least one phoneme in error.

METHOD

The multiple-phoneme approach is divided into three phases: (I) establishment, (II) transfer, and (III) maintenance. In each phase, there are steps that lead to the goal for that phase. Each step has specific stimuli, response description, reinforcement schedule, and criterion level.

Phase I

Establishment, Phase I, has the goal that the speaker should produce each consonant phoneme of English in response to a grapheme or phonetic symbol representing it.

Step 1.   Accurate sound production is achieved through Step 1 of Phase I and is facilitated by the use of the sound production sheet (SPS), which appears as Figure 11.2. Consonants are arranged according to place of articulation going across the page. The SPS provides a recording system for each stimulus modality used to achieve accurate production of each phoneme in isolation.

NAME: SHANNON
DATE: 3-3-77
B.D.:   3-17-72
C.A.:   4-11

MAMA AND DADDY AND BOB AND SUSAN WAS GOING ON A PICNIC. AND BOB
WAS HAPPY ON WHEN HE WAS EATING HIS CEREAL. AND THAT WAS WHEN MAMA
AND BOB AND SUSAN AND DADDY WENT FOR A PICNIC. SO MAMA GOT IT READY
AND SUSAN PUT A APPLE AND BANANAS. AND MAMA MADE A JELLY AND PEANUT
BUTTER SANDWICH AND EGGS SANDWICH. AND DADDY MADE A BIG-WHAT WAS
THAT THING AGAIN—THERMOS OF LEMONADE. AND BOB PUT A STUFF OUT IN
A CAR. AND THEY WERE ON A WAY TO A PICNIC. SO THEY PUT DOWN THEM
BLANKET AND PUT THE BASKET ON THEM BLANKET. SO BOB SAID—WHY DON'T
WE PLAY THROW? SO DADDY THROW IT TO ONE TO A OTHER. SOMETIME HE PLAY
LAUGHING ON THEM AND DON'T THROW IT. SO A LITTLE LATER DADDY SAID—
DO YOU WANT TO GO A BOAT RIDE? AND BOB CRIED YES AND SUSAN CRIED YES.
SO DAD AND SUSAN AND BOB WENT ON A BOAT FOR A RIDE.

Total Words: 168
Total Accurate: 110
% Accurate: 65%

FIGURE 11.1
Conversational whole word accuracy.

Because phonemes cannot be produced in true isolation, a neutral vowel is used in a CV syllable at this step. Each response is recorded. For example, if the client is attempting to produce /k/, the section of the SPS would look like this:

    K
    A-1 2 3 4 5
    B-1 2 3 4 5
    C-1 2 3 4 5

The speech pathologist shows the client the grapheme for /k/, which may be an upper- or lower-case letter, and asks "Do you know what sound this letter makes?" If the client indicates yes, the speech pathologist asks the client to

Name:_____

Date: _____

Age: _____

Time: _____

Code:
A = Visual stim.
B = Aud-Visual
C = Aud-Visual Phonetic Placement
Correct = /
Incorrect = −

p	b	m
A - 1 2 3 4 5	A - 1 2 3 4 5	A - 1 2 3 4 5
B - 1 2 3 4 5	B - 1 2 3 4 5	B - 1 2 3 4 5
C - 1 2 3 4 5	C - 1 2 3 4 5	C - 1 2 3 4 5

w	t	d
A - 1 2 3 4 5	A - 1 2 3 4 5	A - 1 2 3 4 5
B - 1 2 3 4 5	B - 1 2 3 4 5	B - 1 2 3 4 5
C - 1 2 3 4 5	C - 1 2 3 4 5	C - 1 2 3 4 5

n	l	k
A - 1 2 3 4 5	A - 1 2 3 4 5	A - 1 2 3 4 5
B - 1 2 3 4 5	B - 1 2 3 4 5	B - 1 2 3 4 5
C - 1 2 3 4 5	C - 1 2 3 4 5	C - 1 2 3 4 5

g	f	v
A - 1 2 3 4 5	A - 1 2 3 4 5	A - 1 2 3 4 5
B - 1 2 3 4 5	B - 1 2 3 4 5	B - 1 2 3 4 5
C - 1 2 3 4 5	C - 1 2 3 4 5	C - 1 2 3 4 5

s	z	th[1]
A - 1 2 3 4 5	A - 1 2 3 4 5	A - 1 2 3 4 5
B - 1 2 3 4 5	B - 1 2 3 4 5	B - 1 2 3 4 5
C - 1 2 3 4 5	C - 1 2 3 4 5	C - 1 2 3 4 5

th[2]	ch	j
A - 1 2 3 4 5	A - 1 2 3 4 5	A - 1 2 3 4 5
B - 1 2 3 4 5	B - 1 2 3 4 5	B - 1 2 3 4 5
C - 1 2 3 4 5	C - 1 2 3 4 5	C - 1 2 3 4 5

y	sh	zh
A - 1 2 3 4 5	A - 1 2 3 4 5	A - 1 2 3 4 5
B - 1 2 3 4 5	B - 1 2 3 4 5	B - 1 2 3 4 5
C - 1 2 3 4 5	C - 1 2 3 4 5	C - 1 2 3 4 5

h	r	ng
A - 1 2 3 4 5	A - 1 2 3 4 5	A - 1 2 3 4 5
B - 1 2 3 4 5	B - 1 2 3 4 5	B - 1 2 3 4 5
C - 1 2 3 4 5	C - 1 2 3 4 5	C - 1 2 3 4 5

Total Reponses	Total Correct	% Correct
A_____	A_____	A_____
B_____	B_____	B_____
C_____	C_____	C_____

FIGURE 11.2
Multiple-phoneme articulation therapy sound production sheet. (*Source:* Reprinted with permission from C. Denham, R.B. McCabe, and D.P. Bradley (1980), *Multiple Articulation Approach.* Tempe, Arizona: Ideas, Inc., page 9)

319

attempt production of /k/ in isolation and records the accuracy of five successive attempts in the A modality using a / for accurate and − for error.

If the client indicates a lack of knowledge of the sound the symbol /k/ represents, the speech pathologist says "I'll help you" and moves to Level C, which provides the most clues to promote an accurate production.

In this stimulus modality, verbal directions for producing /k/ are provided, along with tactile stimulation or any other technique that will achieve accurate production of the /k/. Assistance is repeated prior to each response until the client can produce at least four accurate /k/ sounds in five successive trials. Since this procedure is followed for all sounds on the SPS, only five trials are provided for each sound in any session. If a speaker fails to show progress in three sessions, it may be wise to branch to intensive isolation work as shown on the branch index, which is discussed later.

Criterion for movement from one stimulus modality to the next on the SPS is five consecutive accurate productions for one session or four of five for two consecutive sessions. When criterion is reached at Level C, which utilizes auditory, visual, and phonetic-placement stimuli, the shift is made to auditory and visual stimuli only at Level B. Only one auditory-visual stimulus (simultaneous presentation of letter and sound) is modeled for the client, who is then asked to produce five responses. When criterion is reached at Level B, the shift is made to Level A, where only the written (visual) stimulus is provided. When working with children under 5 years of age, one may omit the Level A stimuli and move on to other parts of the therapy because 5-year-old children are not expected to have established symbol/sound associations.

Throughout this phase, reinforcement for correct responses is provided by marking correct and incorrect responses on the SPS. Token or social reinforcement may be provided if appropriate to the client's needs.

Speakers for whom the multiple-phoneme approach is considered appropriate usually have six or more phonemes that are not produced accurately on single-word articulation tests or in conversational speech. The SPS is used during the first therapy session with the procedures just described. It is carried out with all consonants—both those produced accurately and those produced inaccurately in conversational speech. Usually, the speaker will reach criterion on all phonemes not considered error phonemes during the first or second session. Including non-error phonemes helps provide initial success. The phonemes not found to be in error on articulation testing or in whole-word accuracy analysis are not worked with in subsequent steps of therapy. Experience has shown that 20 to 25 minutes are required to go through all the sounds on the SPS if phonetic placement is necessary for several sounds. After the first two to three therapy sessions, no more than 15 minutes is usually spent on the SPS.

Step 2.   This step of Phase I is a holding procedure. This is sometimes necessary if many phonemes reach criterion on the sound production sheet at one time but cannot be advanced into the next step of therapy for several sessions. *Holding* requires the client to give one accurate response in Modality A during every therapy session until that phoneme is advanced to the next level of therapy. This is sufficient to maintain the symbol-to-sound association and keep the phoneme in accurate production.

Phase II

Phase II, transfer, has the ultimate goal of using all the error phonemes accurately in conversational speech. It includes five conventional steps of therapy. The difference between this procedure and traditional therapeutic methods is that five or more phonemes are worked on during each therapy session and each phoneme may be at a different step. Specific considerations important at each step are discussed next. The plan for each session is recorded on the articulation data sheet, which appears as Figure 11.3.

Step 1: Syllable.   This step is used only if the client fails a word probe. If the client is successful in producing the target phoneme in 6 of 10 monosyllabic words, the syllable step is not necessary, and work proceeds at the word level until 90% accuracy is achieved. It is reasonable to include in the probe five words with the target phoneme at the beginning and five with it at the end. Selection of words based on frequency of occurrence has been suggested by Denham, McCabe, and Bradley (1979). Another good word probe is the Mc-Donald deep test (McDonald, 1964). If the deep test is used, an accuracy level of 60% should be achieved before eliminating the syllable step.

In syllable practice, the consonant target phoneme is produced in conjunction with a variety of vowels. Syllable practice should include a high front vowel such as /i/, a low front vowel such as /æ/, a neutral vowel like /ʌ/, a high back vowel such as /u/, and a low back vowel like /ɑ/. It is helpful to use line drawings of tongue positions appropriate to each vowel along with the standard spelling of the vowel. The consonant target phoneme is practiced in both initial and final positions of syllables. The clinician may provide one auditory-visual model or one visual stimulus and then the client should produce five syllables. The ratio of stimulus models to the number of syllable productions should be recorded in the comments section of the articulation data sheet if it is necessary to use a ratio other than 1:5. In a typical 1-to-2-minute syllable task, 25 or more responses should be obtained.

Criterion for Step 1, syllable practice, is 80% accuracy in two consecutive sessions or 90% accuracy in one session.

Step 2: Words.   At the word step, the objective is accurate production of the target phoneme in specific words. Appropriate selection of words is critical because the words will be used later in sentences, and it is also important to select a variety of words: verbs, nouns, modifiers, and prepositions. Denham et al. (1979) suggested a core vocabulary based on frequency of occurrence of words. The clinician should also be sure that the words contain a variety of vowels. Clinicians usually make the mistake of choosing too many words for practice at this level. If the client masters 25 to 30 words, that is sufficient to provide a base for producing phrases and sentences.

Criterion for moving from the word step is production of the target phoneme at 90% accuracy level for one session or 80% accuracy for two sessions. Phonemes in the practice words, other than the target phoneme, may still be in error at this level. Sometimes a client will show 100% accuracy for words beginning with the target phoneme and 10% accuracy for words ending

Patient: _____ Establishment: _____
Clinician: _____ Transfer: _____
Date: _____ Maintenance: _____

Date	Session	Activity	Iso.	Syl.	Words	Sent.	Read	Conv.	Time	Total Error	Total Correct	% Correct	Comments

FIGURE 11.3

Multiple-phoneme articulation therapy articulation data sheet. (*Source:* Reprinted with permission from C. Denham, R.B. McCabe, and D.P. Bradley (1980), *Multiple Articulation Approach.* Tempe, Arizona: Ideas, Inc., page 10) with that phoneme. In such situations, the clinician should move on to the sentence level with initial-position words while continuing practice at the word level with final-position words.

Step 3: Phrase/Sentence.   The objective at the phrase/sentence step is accurate word production. This means that the response unit is the word instead of the phoneme, and all sounds in the word should be produced accurately. Control of vocabulary may be needed to make accurate word production possible. This is also the step in which the client begins to monitor productions of phonemes and words. It is helpful to incorporate the words practiced in step 2 in the phrase/sentence-level productions along with new words needed to complete the sentence. Clients who are nonreaders can use rebus symbols (Woodcock, Clark, & Oakes, 1979) to aid in sentence productions. Bliss symbols (McDonald, 1980) are useful in the same way. Another approach, used by Denham et al. (1979), is to provide pictures that assist children in remembering sentences.

At first, some children will find it difficult to formulate phrases and sentences. They may be assisted by having them repeat phrases or sentences after the clinician. When possible, reading may also be used. Variety in the types of sentences is also important because it facilitates natural stress and rhythm. The use of imperative, declarative, and interrogative sentence types is essential as a foundation for conversations at later stages of therapy.

In the phrase/sentence step, errors associated with coarticulation may become evident. In these instances, the client will use target phonemes accurately in one sentence and not in another due to the influence of preceding and following phonemes that vary from sentence to sentence. A complete analysis of the phonetic environments in which accurate production occurs may not be necessary if the clinician notes errors and retains exactly the same phonetic environments for additional practice phrases. It is extremely important to provide additional trials for error words at this step of therapy. Practice may be done on the error word and the word which preceded or followed it, or the clinician may choose to use a phonological process analysis of conversational speech to identify assimilation processes (see chapters 4 and 7). The clinician should vary stress, rhythm, timing, and accent patterns in the auditory models provided to assist the client in achieving normalcy of utterance as well as accuracy of word productions in the context in which the error phoneme occurred.

Criterion for leaving the phrase/sentence step is 80% accuracy for two consecutive sessions or 90% for one session. In some instances, when calculating accuracy, the clinician must use only the words containing the target phoneme instead of all words in the sentences because the client who formulates sentences may use many words containing phonemes not yet at this level of therapy. This variation should be noted on the articulation data sheet.

Step 4: Reading/Story.   The reading step requires several special considerations. Because some clients with articulatory errors are poor readers, material selected for use in speech therapy should be at a comfortable reading level rather than at an instructional level. This enables the client to attend to the accurate production of target phonemes without the distraction of word-recognition struggles. Some clients are nonreaders and need a substitute activity. Comic books, picture books, and sequence cards provide this. The objective at this level is accurate production of target phonemes in connected speech in utterances of four to six word units. Therefore, any technique that encourages the client to speak long strings of words is useful. Repeating a story read or told by the clinician is also acceptable. Culatta, Page, and Ellis (1983) described a procedure for use of story retelling as a screening tool that is equally useful in therapy. Sometimes this is more efficient than taking the time necessary for a child to formulate a story or struggle with reading aloud.

Storytelling may be facilitated by helping the speaker understand the elements of a story. According to Rumelhart (1975), a story has a setting and an episode. The episode consists of an event and a reaction. The event may be a change of state, an action that people carry out, or a series of events. The reaction may be an internal response, such as emotion or desire, or it may be overt, such as an action or an attempt. Through questions and comments that follow this structure, the clinician is able to assist the speaker in creating a meaningful story.

At the reading/story step, accurate production of the target phonemes in words is expected. Whole-word accuracy of every word spoken is the criterion base. Sometimes it is necessary to tape-record responses so that phrases containing errors can be identified and used for additional practice. As at the phrase/sentence level, specific assimilation processes may be identified through analysis of the recording using systems for phonological analysis described in chapter 4.

Criterion at the reading/story step is 80% for two consecutive sessions or 90% for one session. This is whole-word accuracy for all words spoken.

Figure 11.4 is an example of an articulation data sheet that contains the plan for session number 11 on a child who has several sounds at different steps of the program. It is typical for a client at this stage of therapy.

Step 5: Conversation.   The objective of this step is accurate production of all phonemes used in conversational speech. Sometimes in the early sessions, a conversation may be held in which the clinician only monitors one or two phonemes that have moved to that level. In such cases, only those words containing the target phonemes are counted as responses. Sometimes the clinician finds it necessary to monitor 10 or 12 phonemes simultaneously in conversation. In order to accomplish this difficult task, sounds are grouped according to a process or a place of articulation. The clinician then listens for that group for a designated time period of 3 to 5 minutes. After recording responses, attention is turned to another group of sounds. When most phonemes are being monitored at the conversational step, every spoken word is counted as a response. The procedure for determining percentage of accuracy becomes the same as the whole-word accuracy measure of conversational speech.

At the conversational level, it is critical that error words be noted in the context in which they occur so that these phrases or sentences may be used as practice material. Such phrases may be entered on the articulation data sheet as "trouble" phrases. At the conversational level, no single-word practice is needed,

Patient Shannon

Clinician KPS

Date 1/24/77

Transfer x

Maintenance

Step

Date	Session	Activity	Iso.	Syl.	Words	Sent.	Read.	Conv.	Time	Tot. Resp.	Tot. Error	Tot. Corr.	% Corr.	Comments
1/24/77	11	SPS							5					
		/k/			x				3	50	10	40	80	
		/f/				x			3	40	0	40	100	move to read
		/t/					x		5	60	10	50	83	
		/s/		x					3	50	0	50	100	move to words
		/pbm/							10	40	2	38	95	
		/g/			x				5	40	10	30	75	
		/r/	ii*						10	50	40	10	20	

*intensive isolation

FIGURE 11.4
Multiple-phoneme articulation approach articulation data sheet.

since it is usually the phonetic environment of the sound that is causing an error production. Use of the tape recorder enables the client and clinician to recheck some of the errors. It is more time-efficient if the clinician writes the phrase and stops after short segments of 2 or 3 minutes to practice the phrases in which errors occurred.

Conversations should be more than questions and answers. The clinician should use comments to extend the discussion or introduce a related topic. The client should be encouraged to ask questions, clarify meanings, describe events, state cause-and-effect relationships, and identify emotions and desires, as well as stating facts. Techniques for developing conversational skills of speakers are not well described in the literature, but recent material on pragmatics contains information that is helpful (Lucas, 1980; Culatta & Horn, 1982; Gallagher & Prutting, 1983).

Criterion for completion of the conversational step is 80% accuracy on all words spoken during the entire session for two consecutive sessions or 90% for one entire session. The criterion suggested in this program is higher than the 75% suggested by Diedrich and Bangert (1980). However, since data are not available to validate the use of 75% with this approach, the criterion previously used has been retained. In view of the whole-word accuracy norms presented by Schmidt, Howard, and Schmidt (1983), some adjustments should be made for age level. For example, 3-year-old children should be held only to a criterion of 69% whole-word accuracy, the level found in children thought to be developing speech normally. Any speaker 6 years or older should reach the 90% accuracy level.

Phase III

Phase III is maintenance, and its purpose is to maintain at least 90% whole-word accuracy in various speaking situations without support from therapy sessions or other external monitoring. It is typical for a speaker to lose about 5% accuracy within 3 months after the termination of therapy. Thereafter, the accuracy level is maintained or moves to around the 95% accuracy level. Most adults have about 97% accuracy in articulatory skills during conversational speech (Faircloth, 1977).

Maintenance can be conducted by return clinic visits, clinician visits to classrooms, telephone conversations, or reports from others who associate with the client. Accuracy should be monitored in various speaking situations during the maintenance phase. The length of time for maintenance used with this approach is 3 months. Since data are not available for other time spans, there is no basis for determining if other intervals would be adequate.

VALUE

The most important advantage of the multiple-phoneme approach is the speed with which intelligibility of speech is improved. In 6 to 8 weeks of daily therapy, consisting of one hour per day, most speakers with multiple articulatory errors can be understood. Whole-word accuracy should increase from a starting point of 10% to 60% or greater.

NAME: SHANNON

B.D.:   3-17-72

C.A.:   5 yrs.

| | W.W.A. | |
Date	Percentage	Arizona
9-2-75	12%	40.5
10-6-75	19%	39.5
10-10-75	29%	56.0
12-1-76	30%	56.0
1-17-77	30%	N.A.*
1-24-77	39%	N.A.
1-31-77	35%	N.A.
2-7-77	40%	N.A.
2-14-77	40%	N.A.
2-21-77	66%	N.A.
2-28-77	72%	N.A.
3-7-77	83%	N.A.
One week home.		
3-21-77	91%	N.A.
3-24-77	91%	90.0

*Not available.

FIGURE 11.5

Data on progress of a child whose treatment was relatively inconsistent until an intensive multiple-phoneme approach was instituted covering the last 2 months.

Figure 11.5 presents data on a child with whom this approach was used. He was evaluated in September of 1975 and showed 12% whole-word accuracy in conversational speech. The following month, he was seen for one week of therapy, which consisted of one-hour individual sessions each day. His whole-word accuracy increased to 29%, and a home program of therapy was initiated. A year later, in December of 1976, little change had occurred and it was decided to provide a 2-month period of intensive therapy. At the end of 2 months, his whole-word accuracy was 91%. When he started to school, the teacher reported no evidence of a speech problem.

At the present time, no research has come to the attention of the author that would allow comparison of results achieved with this approach and with other articulation therapy.

The multiple-phoneme approach was developed during the years when behavioral or operant programs were fashionable. The current emphasis on the pragmatics of communication does not make it any less desirable to use efficient, effective procedures to change articulatory skills. Neither does current information on phonological process development negate the need for attention to specific phonemes in a structured therapy situation for some speakers. Other approaches to articulation may be more efficient than the multiple-phoneme approach, and research is needed to determine this.

The multiple-phoneme approach is applicable in a number of situations. It is most often used for individual therapy sessions because speakers with severe problems are usually scheduled individually. However, Kasica (1978) described its use in group therapy. It can also be used with clients of various ages. The age range of clients in the report by McCabe and Bradley (1975) was 5 to 14 years. Holtzapple and Marshall (1977) used it with adult aphasic clients. The only age limitations relate to selecting an appropriate criterion for conversational speech accuracy and to the need for modification of the reading level with nonreaders.

LIMITATIONS

Since the multiple-phoneme approach is not a definitive program, some users have indicated that too many decisions are left to the clinician. This might be considered an advantage because it allows the clinician to incorporate other techniques at appropriate steps of the therapy. For example, if a client fails to meet criterion at the word level during several sessions, it is possible to branch to the paired-stimuli technique (see chapter 12) until criterion is reached (Weston & Irwin, 1971). If sessions are too short to cover all error phonemes, the "wedge" approach suggested by Sommers and Kane (1974) might be used to select two or three phonemes to use with this approach. In a similar manner, a distinctive-feature analysis (see chapter 14) might suggest which sounds should be selected.

For readers who desire more structure, a progression model developed by McCabe and Bradley (1973) is offered in Appendix 11.1. This model suggests the type of stimulus, indicates the target response, states criterion, provides a reinforcement schedule, and indicates points in therapy when branching may be necessary. A branch index appears as Appendix 11.2, which suggests changes in one or more of the variables controlled in establishing the steps of this procedure. Appendix 11.3 contains the key to the symbols used in the progression model and the branch index.

When using the branch for open stimuli, the clinician should use all known techniques to develop the accurate response.

The multiple-phoneme articulation data record which appears as Appendix 11.4 provides a quick way to summarize the information from the data sheets. This facilitates report writing and allows the clinician to report precise information regarding the time required to change error phonemes to correct use in conversational speech.

SUMMARY

The multiple-phoneme approach to articulation therapy is organized to provide therapy on all error phonemes during each session of therapy. Each phoneme may be at a different step of therapy. In a 30-minute session, time allocations should be made for each phoneme and each therapy step. This ensures some activity on each phoneme. The sound productions at Step 1 of Phase I are recorded on the sound production sheet. As soon as a phoneme is moved to Phase II, Step 1, the accuracy of responses is recorded on the articulation data sheet. When phonemes are accurate in conversation, the time required for their correction is recorded on the multiple-phoneme articulation data record.

The traditional steps of therapy are used with behavioral criterion and reinforcement schedules. Criterion for moving from each step to the next is provided. Accuracy of all sounds in conversational speech at the 95% level is measured by whole-word accuracy and is the criterion for dismissal from therapy.

Effectiveness of the program is determined through follow-up evaluations 3 months after dismissal from therapy.

The principal advantages of the approach are its comprehensiveness (working on all errors rather than one at a time) and the speed of acquisition of intelligible speech.

Appendix 11.1

SUGGESTED PROGRESSION MODEL, MULTIPLE PHONEME ARTICULATION

Phase	Step	Stimulus	Target Response	Criterion	Reinforcement Schedule	Branch
I. Establishment	1-SPS	V,V-A, V-A-PP	ph	4/5-2	1:1	ii
	2-H	V	ph	100%	1:1	I, 1-SPS V-A
II. Transfer	1-WP	A	ph	60%	None	+ = II,3 − = II,2
	2-S	V-O	ph	90%-2	1:2	ii
	3-W	V-O	ph	95-100%-1 90%-2	1:3	II,2
	4a-phr/st	V-A	ph	"	1:3	II,3
	4b-phr/st	V-A	ww	"	1:3	II,3
	4c-phr/st	V-O	ph	"	1:3	II,3
	4d-phr/st	V-O	ww	"	1:5	II,3,ww
	5a-R	V	ph	"	1:4	11,4a
	5b-R	V	ww	"	1:10	II,4b
	5c-TW	V	ww	"	1:1	II,5a
	6a-C	A	ph	"	1:10	II,5a
	6b-C	A	ww	"	1:15	II,5b
	6c-TW	A	ww	"	1:1	II,6a
III. Maintenance	I-IC-C	A	ww	90% EX	Var. Int.	II,6b
	2-OC-C	Env.	ww	-	-	-

Appendix 11.2

BRANCH INDEX, MULTIPLE PHONEME ARTICULATION

Branch	Step	Stimulus	Target Response	Criterion	Reinforcement Schedule
1	I,ii	0	ph	95%-2	1:1
2	I,1	V-A	ph	4/5-2	1:1
3	−II,2	V-O	ph	90%-2	1:2
	+II,3	V-O	ph	90%-2	1:3
4	I,ii	O	ph	95%-1	1:1
5	II,2	V-O	ph	″	1:1
6	II,3	V-O	ph	″	1:1
7	II,3	V-O	ph	″	1:1
8	II,3	V-O	ph	″	1:1
9	II,3ww	V-O	ww	″	1:1
10	II,4a	V-A	ph	″	1:1
11	II,4b	V-A	ww	″	1:1
12	II,5a	V-A	ph	″	1:1
13	II,5a	V	ph	″	1:1
14	II,5b	V	ww	″	1:1
15	II,6a	A	ph	″	1:1
16	II,6b	A	ww	″	1:1

Appendix 11.3

KEY TO SYMBOLS, MULTIPLE PHONEME ARTICULATION

Symbols:

ii	Intensive isolation
V	Visual stimulation
A	Auditory
V-A	Visual-Auditory stimulation
V-A-PP	Visual-Auditory-Phonetic Placement stimulation
O	Open (any type of stimulation needed)
S	Syllable
W	Word
phr	Phrase
st	Sentence
R	Reading
C	Conversation
IC	In clinic
OC	Out of Clinic
ph	Phoneme
ww	Whole word
WP	Word probe
H	Hold
EX	Exit

Criterion:
1. SPS—three days, one response at B and four/five at A, move to Step 2. (Continue on SPS for visual recognition.) Three days with less than three/five at C, move to ii.
2. General:
    1. Below 70% two consecutive days, branch to previous step.
    2. 70–90% two consecutive days, re-program at same step.
    3. 90–95% two consecutive days, move to next step.
    4. 95% and above, one day, move to next step.

Appendix 11.4

MULTIPLE PHONEME ARTICULATION DATA RECORD

Name_____   Year_____

Phoneme	Isolation		Syllable		Word		Phrase/Sent.		Reading		Conversation	
	Date Init.	Date Comp.	Date Init.	Date Comp.	Date Init.	Date Comp.	Date Init.	Date Comp.	Date Init.	Date Comp.	Date Init.	Date Comp.

TEST DATA: (Articulation Test Scores and whole word accuracy)

Source: Reprinted with permission from C. Denham, R.B. McCabe and D.P. Bradley (1980), *Multiple Articulation Approach*. Tempe, Arizona: Ideas, Inc., page 11.

REFERENCES

Blache, S. E., Parsons, C. L., & Humphreys, J. M. (1981). A minimal-word-pair model for teaching the linguistic significance of distinctive features. *Journal of Speech and Hearing Disorders, 46* (3), 291–295.

Bradley, D. P., Allen, G. D., & Clifford V. V. (1973). Reliability of assessment of articulation skills in conversational speech. *Division of Council on Communication Disorders Bulletin, 11,* 28–31.

Costello, J., & Onstine, J. M. (1976). The modification of multiple articulation errors based on distinctive feature theory. *Journal of Speech and Hearing Disorders, 41,* 199–215.

Culatta, B., Page, J. L., & Ellis, J. (1983). Story retelling as a communicative performance screening tool. *Language Speech & Hearing Services in Schools, 14* (2), 66–74.

Culatta, B., & Horn, D. (1982). A program for achieving generalization of grammatical rules to spontaneous discourse. *Journal of Speech and Hearing Disorders, 27* (2).

Denham, C. D., McCabe, R. B., & Bradley, D. P. (1979). *Multiple phoneme articulation approach.* Tempe, AZ: Ideas.

Diedrich, W. D., & Bangert, J. (1980). *Articulation learning.* Houston: College-Hill Press.

Faircloth, M. A. (1977, November). *Conversational speech analysis.* Short course presented at the meeting of the American Speech and Hearing Association, Chicago.

Fudula, J. B. (1963). *Arizona articulation proficiency scale, revised.* Los Angeles: Western Psychological Services.

Gallagher, T. M., & Prutting, C. A. (Eds.) (1983). *Pragmatic assessment and intervention issues in language.* San Diego: College-Hill Press.

Hodson, B., & Paden, E. (1982). *Targeting intelligible speech: A phonological approach to remediation.* San Diego: College-Hill Press.

Holtzapple, P., & Marshall, N. (1977). Application of multiple phonemic articulation therapy with apraxic patients. In R. Brookshire (Ed.), *Clinical Aphasiology Conference Proceedings.* Minneapolis: BRK Publishers.

Ingram, D. (1981). *Procedures for the phonological analysis of children's language.* Baltimore: University Park Press.

Kasica, A. (1978). *Multiple phoneme approach to articulation therapy in group setting.* Unpublished manuscript, University of Kentucky, Department of Special Education, Lexington.

Lucas, E. V. (1980). *Semantic and pragmatic language disorders.* Rockville, MD: Aspen Systems Corporation.

McCabe, R. B., & Bradley, D. P. (1973). *The systematic multiphonemic approach to articulation therapy.* Short course presented at American Speech and Hearing Association South Eastern Regional Conference, Atlanta.

McCabe, R. B., & Bradley, D. P. (1975). Systematic multiple phonemic approach to articulation therapy. *Acta Symbolica, 6,* 2–18.

McDonald, E. (1964). *A deep test of articulation.* Pittsburgh: Stanwix House, Inc.

McDonald, E. (1980). *Teaching and using Bliss symbols.* Toronto: Bliss Symbolics Institute.

McReynolds, L. V., & Engmann, D. L. (1975). *Distinctive feature analysis of misarticulations.* Baltimore: University Park Press.

Mowrer, D. W. (1978). Phonological processes and articulation therapy. In L. J. Bradford & R. T. Wertz (Eds.), *Communication disorders: An audio journal for continuing education.* New York: Grune and Stratton, Inc.

Rumelhart, D. E. (1975). Notes on a schema for stories. In D. G. Bobrow & A. Collins (Eds.), *Representation and understanding.* New York: Academic Press, Inc.

Schissel, R. J., & Doty, M. H. (1979). Application of the systematic multiple phonemic approach to articulation therapy: A case study. *Language Speech & Hearing Services in Schools, 3*, 178–184.

Schmidt, L. S., Howard, B. H., & Schmidt, J. F. (1983). Conversational speech sampling in the assessment of articulation proficiency. *Language Speech & Hearing Services in Schools, 14*(4), 210–214.

Seaton, K. P., & Bradley, D. P. (1978, November). *Application of multiple phonemic approach to articulation therapy.* Mini-seminar presented at the meeting of the American Speech and Hearing Association, San Francisco.

Shriberg, L. D., & Kwiatkowski, J. (1980). *Natural process analysis.* New York: John Wiley and Sons.

Singh, S. (1975). *Distinctive features: Theory and validation.* Baltimore: University Park Press.

Sommers, R. K., & Kane, A. R. (1974). Nature and remediation of functional articulation disorders. In S. Dickson (Ed.), *Communication disorders: Remedial principles and practices.* Glenview: Scott, Foresman, and Co.

Weiner, F. (1978). *Phonological process analysis.* Baltimore: University Park Press.

Weston, A., & Irwin, J. (1971). The use of paired-stimuli in the modification of articulation. *Perceptual Motor Skills, 32*, 947–957.

Woodcock, R. W., Clark, R., & Oakes, D. (1979). *Peabody rebus reading program.* Circle Pines, MN: American Guidance Service.

12 Paired-Stimuli Treatment

RATIONALE

The rationale for the paired-stimuli technique is based on several considerations. These will be discussed briefly before the details of the method are presented.

When one reviews the research in the area of articulation, certain inconsistencies become apparent. For example, the admitting of a client for articulation therapy is generally done on the basis of a sound-in-word articulation test, whereas the criterion for dismissal from therapy is frequently the intelligibility of conversational speech (Irwin & Weston, 1971; Irwin, 1975; Sommers, Leiss, Delp, Gerber, Fundrella, Smith, Revucky, Ellis, & Haley, 1967; Weston & Leonard, 1976). The measurement of the effectiveness of articulation therapy is equally equivocal. Variables that must be considered include frequency and intensity of therapy, consistency of errors, types and patterns of errors, and stimulability performance (Sommers et al., 1967). Until paired-stimuli research was developed, controlled experiments that planned for these variables were not available.

Alan J. Weston, Ph.D., is a professor in the Department of Speech Pathology and Audiology at the University of Wisconsin-Milwaukee. John V. Irwin, Ph.D., is a professor emeritus at Memphis State University, Memphis, Tennessee, and currently resides in Lexington, Kentucky.

Many investigators (Irwin, Huskey, Knight, & Oltman, 1974; Poole, 1934; Roe & Milisen, 1942; Templin, 1957) have shown that, at least until fourth grade, children's articulation improves as they grow older. On the basis of these studies, the speech-language clinician might conclude that to save time one should devote time to those older children who would not improve without therapy. Sayler's (1949) study showed that only a slight or inconsistent improvement in articulation occurred among students between the 4th and 12th grades. The opposing argument, that therapy should begin as early as possible, is based on learning theory and studies in child development (Weston & Leonard, 1976; Winitz, 1969). This argument suggests that children may be learning defective articulatory skills in the sense that they are practicing them daily. The longer they use an articulatory pattern, the more difficult it will be to change it. It may be hypothesized that some children are not growing out of their immature articulation; they are growing into it through the repetition of a faulty pattern that has achieved communication, hence reinforcement. To date, there is no method for determining the strength of articulatory learning at different ages. It is only through prognostic testing that identification of those children who do not show promise of developing their articulation without therapy becomes possible.

Traditionally, articulatory therapy has centered on two major methods: the phonetic-placement method and the auditory or ear-training method (see chapter 5). Research in acoustic phonetics has tended to place the phonetic-placement method in doubt (Ladefoged, 1962). Peterson and Barney (1952) and Fairbanks and Grubb (1961) demonstrated that a given acoustic result can be achieved by a variety of positionings in different individuals. Therefore, what may be optimum articulator placement for one child may not necessarily achieve satisfactory results with another. Another criticism of the phonetic-placement approach has been the overawareness of the mechanics of sound production on the part of the child, which creates an artificial and unnatural attitude about speech, and thus may have an inhibiting effect. The primary objection is that it gives a child little help in judging his own speech.

The auditory or ear-training method (Van Riper, 1963) is still used by the majority of speech-language pathologists working with articulatory disorders today. The presumption is that hearing is the primary basis for acquisition of articulation in childhood. This concept and its related procedures are explained in chapter 5. More recent views on auditory considerations are presented in chapter 9.

The major emphasis of the traditional approach on sound discrimination training (ear training) is supported by several studies (Cohen & Diehl, 1963; Sherman & Gerth, 1967; Travis & Rasmus, 1931) showing that children with poor discrimination scores have less-than-adequate articulation. However, some studies (Hall, 1938; Hansen, 1944; Prins, 1963) show little or no relationship. Furthermore, how do we account for the large percentage of children with auditory perceptual disturbances who demonstrate poor auditory discrimination yet have adequate articulatory skills?

With reference to the paired-stimuli technique, two studies deserve special discussion. McLean (1970) proposed a therapeutic procedure of teaching phonemes in a variety of contexts; this procedure is known as *stimulus shift generalization*. Using echoic stimulation, McLean taught the child to produce the target phoneme correctly. Using 5 subjects who consistently misarticulated phonemes that they could produce under stimulation, he began his therapeutic procedure. A correctly articulated stimulus word was paired with pictures of words wherein the phoneme was consistently misarticulated. The next steps involved successive pairing of pictures with printed words and of printed words with words in context. In all cases, correct responses were reinforced, and the preceding condition was phased out. In short, this program was designed to transfer the correctly articulated response from the control of an auditory stimulus to pictures, printed words, and then into complete spoken sentences, using reinforcement until the subjects achieved stable levels of correct responding.

Leonard and Webb (1971) studied the effects of an automated therapy program involving several phonemes. Essentially, the program consisted of reinforcing the child's correct imitation of tape-recorded material by playing his correct response back to him immediately thereafter. Before and after treatment, a 30-word list was administered in which each of the words contained the target phoneme at least one time. Results indicated improvement as measured on the pre- and posttest scores.

Operant conditioning, with its focus on symptoms, has often been unattractive to the conventionally trained speech-language pathologist. However, because of its demonstrated effectiveness in modifying behavior both within and without the realm of communication, speech-language pathologists have found it difficult to ignore the concept (Weston & Irwin, 1971). Behavioral principles are discussed in greater detail in chapter 6.

The major question raised regarding the use of behavior modification principles in changing articulatory behavior is whether the child will be able to use the learned sound in his everyday conversational speech. Generally, in the past it was thought that specific attention to promoting the newly acquired phoneme was needed in order to ensure correct usage. However, past therapeutic techniques have been exceedingly time-consuming, and carry-over procedures have had inconsistent results (Engle, Brandriet, Erikson, Gronhound, & Gunderson, 1966; Sommers et al., 1967). The measurement of carry-over has also been a problem. The effectiveness of an articulatory modification program is determined by two principles: the rate of acquisition of the target phoneme in training materials and the effect of the program on the use of the corrected phoneme in the child's normal environment.

In many therapeutic approaches, writers have indicated that the client may be given an additional model in the form of his own correct production using key words (words in which the usually defective sound is made correctly under certain conditions) (Ainsworth, 1948; Van Riper, 1963; Van Riper & Irwin, 1958). However, although Van Riper (1963) described the function of the key word and its possible impact on articulatory acquisition, he did not recommend the key word as a replacement for strong stimulation by the clinician. He and others suggested it only as an additional model. Irwin and Wong (1983) demonstrated that the probability of finding or teaching a key word—based on the availability of consonants—should be typically high even by age 3 or 4. The paired-stimuli technique (Weston, 1969) is based on the premise that the client can transfer correct production in a key word to correct production in other training words without the traditional stimulation and practice in imitating the clinician. In this program acquisition is rapid, and success has been achieved with a wide range of functional articulatory problems. Carry-over has been good, and the technique has been used successfully by student clinicians with but a modicum of training.

Obviously, effective treatment programs for the modification of articulatory behaviors have existed for many years. However, despite satisfactory outcomes, it has frequently been difficult to assess the extent to which a given outcome is attributable to clearly identified variables within the treatment program itself. The carefully structured sequences of specific training procedures that characterize programmed instruction make possible the identification of each particular element of treatment whose influence can be studied and thus assessed. In recent years, the use of programmed instruction in speech and language pathology has become well established (Griffith, Irwin, & Weston, 1980). Gerber (1977) wrote that "numerous pre-constructed programs are available that apply principles of programming to the modification of articulation in an attempt to increase the effectiveness and efficiency of the process of remediation" (p. 29). She stated also that "the procedures in these programs represent, in most cases, a radical departure from previous practices that were all too often unduly protracted and not demonstrably effectual" (Gerber, 1977, p. 29).

Griffith et al. (1980) cited criteria for an effective articulatory intervention program. According to these writers, effective articulatory modification programs have the following characteristics: They (a) are applicable to a wide variety of phonological deviations, (b) are adaptable to a broad range of subjects with reference to age and levels of ability, (c) are limited only by behavioral baselines and not etiology, (d) specify entry and exit criteria clearly, (e) require no special equipment, (f) are consistent in structure and form, (g) are amenable to use by paraprofessionals, (h) provide intrinsic motivation to keep the client progressing in the learning task, (i) bring about a rapid achievement of goals, (j) ensure generalization and maintenance of newly learned behavior, and (k) create no negative side effects. From our study and experience, the paired-stimuli technique meets these criteria.

METHOD

The paired-stimuli technique for the modification of articulatory errors was developed by Weston (1969) and influenced by McLean's (1970) work. The basic assumption underlying the technique is that a target phoneme produced in a socially acceptable way can be generalized from selected phonetic contexts to a variety of phonetic contexts through a program of behavior modification (Weston & Irwin, 1971). In many of the other therapeutic approaches discussed in this text, the importance of the clinician's model for the client has been stressed. These approaches have generally not recommended the use of the client's own correct production as a general substitute for the clinician's model (Weston & Rampp, 1973).

Essentially, the paired-stimuli procedure (Weston & Irwin, 1971) involves identification of target phonemes, key words, and training words. Target sounds and potential key words may be identified by such devices as the Triota Screening Battery (Irwin, 1972), the Templin-Darley Tests of Articulation (Templin & Darley, 1969) or the Screening Deep Test of Articulation (McDonald, 1968). A *key word* is defined as one in which the subject produces the target sound in a socially acceptable manner at least 9 out of 10 times. The word must have the target sound in it only once, in either the initial or final position. If a key word cannot be found in the vocabulary of the child, current procedure is to teach one or more key words. Key-word teaching techniques are developed later in the chapter.

A *training word* is one in which the target sound appears only once, in either the initial or final position, and in which the target sound is misarticulated in at least two of three attempts to say the word. A minimum of 10 training words must be found for both the initial and final word positions. If, however, training is needed in only one position, then training words would be selected with the target sound in that position.

After all training words for a particular sound have been located, the procedure consists of the subject's naming alternately the key word and each of the training words for the target sound in a particular position. During the pairing procedure, the child is given a tangible reinforcer for every socially acceptable production of the target sound, whether it is in the key word or in the training word. This occurs irrespective of the subject's articulation of the other sounds in the words.

Throughout the procedure, probes are used. Probes are designed to measure the extent to which a subject produces a target sound acceptably in a conversational speech sample under conditions of no reinforcement. Criterion is defined as the socially acceptable production of at least 80% of the target sounds in conversation with a minimum of 15 to 20 occurrences. The purpose of evaluating the untrained words is to determine whether any generalization to them occurs as a result of training on the selected training words.

The paired-stimuli approach, then, is based on the assumption that a target sound produced in a word in a socially acceptable manner can be generalized from a selected phonetic environment to a variety of other word contexts. This is accomplished through a behavior modification program that emphasizes building procedures. During the initial pairing procedure, a contin- uous reinforcement schedule is applied to all socially acceptable productions of the target sound. The criterion for terminating training on a sound in a given position is the socially acceptable production of the target sound in at least 8 out of 10 training words over two successive probes. A step-by-step summary of the G-F paired-stimuli procedures is presented in Figure 12.1.

FIGURE 12.1

G-F paired stimuli procedures. (*Source:* From *Paired Stimuli Kit* by J. V. Irwin and A. J. Weston, 1971/1975, Milwaukee: Fox Point Press. Copyright 1971/1975 by Fox Point Press. Reprinted by permission.)

PAIRED-STIMULI G-f PROTOCOL

STEP I

OPERATION	RESPONSE REQUIRED FOR REINFORCEMENT	REINFORCEMENT	CRITERION	THEN
I-A	I-A	I-A	I-A	
Teach Key Word #1.* See Appendix for assigned Key Words for each phoneme and Key Word teaching procedures.	Correct production of the target phoneme within the context of the assigned Key Word.	One token for each correct response.	A successful stability test is required for criterion and is defined as the correct productions of the target phoneme in at least 9 out of 10 productions of the Key Word under conditions of no reinforcement. Administration of the stability test is described in the Key Word teaching procedures. See Appendix.	If successful, go to I-B. If unsuccessful, continue in I-A.
I-B	I-B	I-B	I-B	
Pair Key Word #1 with its ten Training Words. Two words are elicited each containing the target phoneme in the same position of words, e.g., (for phoneme /s/ with "this" as the Key Word) this-bus, this-house, etc. Go clockwise, start with Training Word #1. The pairing of the Key Word with each of the 10 Training Words is defined as a training string.	Correct production of the target phoneme in either or both of the words elicited (Key Word and/or Training Word).	One token for each correct production of the target phoneme. The child may earn two tokens, one for the Key Word and one for the Training Word.	Correct production of the target phoneme in at least 8 of the 10 Training Words on two successive training strings.	Go to I-C.

*It is possible that children who begin the protocol with some correct productions of the target phoneme may already produce the assigned Key Word(s) correctly. If the child does have the correct production of the Key Word(s) in repertoire, those sub- step(s) dealing with the teaching of the Key Word(s) should be omitted, i.e., I-A, I-C, I-E, I-G. A test for stability should be administered to determine if the production of the target phoneme in the repertoire Key Word(s) is sufficiently stable to continue in the protocol.

OPERATION	RESPONSE REQUIRED FOR REINFORCEMENT	REINFORCEMENT	CRITERION	THEN
I-C	**I-C**	**I-C**	**I-C**	**THEN**
Teach Key Word #2 using the same teaching procedure as in I-A. See the Appendix for the assigned Key Word. The position of the target phoneme in Key Words is alternated. If the final position is taught in I-A, then the initial position is taught here and vice versa.	Correct production of the target phoneme within the context of the assigned Key Word. (Same as I-A).	One token for each correct response. (Same as I-A).	A successful stability test is required for criterion which is the correct production of the target phoneme in at least 9 out of 10 productions of the Key Word under conditions of no reinforcement. (Same as I-A).	If successful, go to I-D. If unsuccessful, continued in I-C.
I-D	**I-D**	**I-D**	**I-D**	**THEN**
Pair Key Word #2 with its 10 Training Words. Two words are elicited each containing the target phoneme in the same position of words, e.g., (for phoneme /s/ with "see" as the Key Word) see-sun, see-sock, etc. Go clockwise and start with Training Word #1. The pairing of the Key Word with each of the 10 Training Words is defined as a Training String.	Correct production of the target phoneme in either or both of the two words elicited (Key Word and/or Training Word). (Same as I-B).	One token for each correct production of the target phoneme. The child may earn two tokens, one for the Key Word and one for the Training Word. (Same as I-B).	Correct production of the target phoneme in at least 8 of the 10 Training Words on two successive training strings. (Same as I-B).	Go to I-E.

343

FIGURE 12.1 (*continued*)

STEP I (*continued*)

OPERATION	RESPONSE REQUIRED FOR REINFORCEMENT	REINFORCEMENT	CRITERION	THEN
I-E	I-E	I-E	I-E	I-E
Teach Key Word #3 using the same teaching procedure as in I-A and I-C. See Appendix for assigned Key Word.	Correct production of the target phoneme within the context of the assigned Key Word. (Same as I-A and I-C).	One token for each correct response. (Same as I-A and I-C).	A successful stability test is required. (Same as I-A and I-C).	If successful, go to I-F. If unsuccessful, continue in I-E.
I-F	I-F	I-F	I-F	I-F
Pair Key Word #3 with its ten Training Words, e.g., (for phoneme /s/ with "that's" as the Key Word) that's-moose, that's-cats, etc. In this sub-step, the two words should be elicited as a "unit" with only a brief pause between the two words. This is defined as a unit response. A training string is now defined as ten unit responses, each unit containing the Key Word and one of its Training Words.	Correct production of the target phoneme in both the Key Word and the Training Word. The two words must be said as a unit. The target phoneme must be produced correctly in both words for the unit to be a correct unit.	One token following each correct unit. The target phoneme must be produced correctly in both the Key Word and the Training Word for the token to be given. The value of the token is increased to two. The frequency of delivery of reinforcement begins to decrease at this point in the protocol while the value of the token increases.	8 out ot 10 correct *units* over two successive training strings.	Go to I-G.

OPERATION	RESPONSE REQUIRED FOR REINFORCEMENT	REINFORCEMENT	CRITERION	THEN
I-G	I-G	I-G	I-G	
Teach Key Word #4 using the same teaching procedures as in I-A, I-C, I-E. See Appendix for assigned Key Word.	Correct production of the target phoneme within the context of the assigned Key Word. (Same as I-A, I-C, and I-E).	One token for each correct response. The value of the token remains at two.	A successful stability test is required. (Same as I-A, I-C, and I-E).	If successful, go to I-H. If unsuccessful, continue in I-G.
I-H	I-H	I-H	I-H	THEN
Pair Key Word #4 with its ten Training Words, e.g., (for phoneme /s/ with "said" as the Key Word) said-skate, said-salad, etc. The Key Word and one Training Word are elicited as a unit.	Correct production of the target phoneme in both words when the Key Word and Training Word are said as a unit. (Same as I-F).	One token following two correct units in succession. The target phoneme must be produced correctly in 4 words — the Key Word twice and two different Training Words. *The two successful units must be successive.* The value of each token given is increased to four.	8 out of 10 correct units over two successive training strings. (Same as I-F).	Probe.* See Appendix for instructions.

*Probes are inserted in the protocol at various points to check on the generalization effects of the training to that point. It is recommended that Probes be given in Steps I and II at the clinician's discretion but preferably at the end of each step. Probes are mandatory in Step III and designated as such in the protocol. Although only two probes are designated in Step III, more frequent probing can be done in that step if the clinician desires.

FIGURE 12.1 (continued)

STEP II

	OPERATION	RESPONSE REQUIRED FOR REINFORCEMENT	REINFORCEMENT	CRITERION	THEN
	II-A	II-A	II-A	II-A	
	Use Key Word #1 and its ten Training Words. Point to a Training Word and ask the assigned question for the Key Word being used. See Appendix for assigned Key Word Question, e.g., (for phoneme /s/ with "this" as the Key Word) "What is this?" Go clockwise and start with Training Word #1. A training string is now defined as ten questions.	Child must answer the question with a prescribed part of a sentence and insert the correct production of the Training Word to which the clinician is pointing. For example, the clinician points to Training Word #1 (bus) and asks, "What is this?" The child responds, "This is a bus."*	One token following three correct sentences in succession. The target phoneme must be correct in both the Key Word and Training Word of the sentence to be considered correct. The target phoneme must be correct in 6 words — the Key Word three times and three different Training Words. *The three correct sentences must be successive.* The value of the token is increased to six.	8 out of 10 correct sentences over two successive training strings.	Go to II-B.

*Some children automatically expand the prescribed sentence, e.g. saying "I see some soup" instead of "I see soup." The clinician may accept either. If the sentence is expanded, however, usage of the target phoneme other than in the Key Word and Training Word should be disregarded.

346

STEP II (continued)

OPERATION	RESPONSE REQUIRED FOR REINFORCEMENT	REINFORCEMENT	CRITERION	THEN
II-B	II-B	II-B	II-B	
Use Key Word #2 and its ten Training Words. *Two questions are alternated,* one using Key Word #2 and one using Key Word #3. See Appendix for the assigned questions for the appropriate Key Words, e.g., (for phoneme /s/ with Key Word #2 "see" and Key Word #3 "That's") "What do you see?" and "That's what?" The clinician points to Training Word #1 and asks, "What do you see? The child responds. The clinician then points to Training Word #2 and asks, "That's what?" and the child responds. A training string is defined as ten questions. Go clockwise and start with Training Word #1.	The child must answer the question with a prescribed part of a sentence and insert the correct production of the Training Word to which the clinician is pointing, e.g. "I see (a) bus" or "That's grapes."	One token following three correct sentences in succession. The target phoneme must be correct in all six occurrences — two target phoneme words per sentence. The three correct sentences must be successive for the token to be given. The value of the token remains at six. (Same as III-A).	8 out of 10 correct sentences over two successive strings.	Go to II-C.

347

FIGURE 12.1 *(continued)*

STEP II *(continued)*

OPERATION	RESPONSE REQUIRED FOR REINFORCEMENT	REINFORCEMENT	CRITERION	THEN
II-C	II-C	II-C	II-C	
Use two Key Word sheets — Key Word #1 and its ten training Words and Key Word #4 and its ten Training Words. Place both before the child. *Four* questions are asked alternately. See Appendix, e.g., (for phoneme/s/) 1. What is this? 2. What do you see? 3. That's what? 4. What did you say that was?	The child must answer the question with a prescribed part of a sentence and insert the correct production of the Training Word to which the clinician is pointing, e.g., "This is (a) bus," "I see a box," "That's grapes," or "I said that was a sock."	One token following three correct sentences in succession. The value of the token is six. (Same as II-A and II-B)	8 out of 10 correct sentences over two successive training strings. (Same as II-A and II-B)	Probe.*
The clinician points to Training Word #1 and asks the first question. The child responds. The clinician then points to Training Word #11 and asks the second question. The child responds, etc. The order of presentation of the Training Words is not clockwise. The Training Words to be used are designated by Roman Numerals on the two picture sheets. Ten of the twenty Training Words before the child will be used and are scattered throughout the sheets in random order. A training string is still defined as ten questions (Training Words I-X).				

*Optional

348

STEP III

OPERATION	RESPONSE REQUIRED FOR REINFORCEMENT	REINFORCEMENT	CRITERION	THEN
III-A	III-A	III-A	III-A	
Engage the child in conversation. Score each word containing the target phoneme as right or wrong on the basis of his production of the phoneme. A score sheet should be used with a right and wrong column. The child must be permitted to see the score sheet and the scoring as it occurs. *Stop* the conversation when the child has correctly produced the target phoneme in any 4 words containing the target phoneme. All occurrences of the target phoneme within those 4 words must be correct. This is considered a successful segment. Give the child brief verbal feedback on each word correctly produced. OR *Stop* the conversation when the child incorrectly produces the target phoneme in any one word. This is considered an unsuccessful segment. Immediately give the child brief verbal feedback as to words produced correctly with the target phoneme prior to the incorrect production. Then the clinician should correctly produce the misarticulated word to give auditory and visual stimulation for correct production to the child. The child is required to repeat the word once immediately after the stimulation is given but correct production is not required of the child. This is intended to be a stimulation procedure and not a practice procedure.	A conversation which includes four words containing the target phoneme. Correct production is required of all occurences of the target phoneme in those four words.	No tangible reinforcement is given. Reinforcement is visual as the child is allowed to see the scoring of target phoneme words as they are produced. Reinforcement is also verbal in that feedback is given to the child regarding his productions of the target phoneme words.	One 4-word segment in which the target phoneme is produced correctly in all occurrences.	Go to III-B.

349

FIGURE 12.1 (continued)

STEP III (continued)

OPERATION	RESPONSE REQUIRED FOR REINFORCEMENT	REINFORCEMENT	CRITERION	THEN
III-B	III-B	III-B	III-B	
Follow the same format as in III-A but extend the segment to include seven words containing the target phoneme. *Stop* the child when he has correctly produced all occurrences of the target phoneme in 7 words. This is a successful segment. No verbal feedback is given on each word. The clinician states that all were correct. OR *Stop* the child when he has incorrectly produced the target phoneme in any one word. Do not give verbal feedback on correct productions but do give the stimulation procedure for the misarticulated word as described in III-A.	A conversation which includes seven words containing the target phoneme. All occurrences of the target phoneme must be correct in those seven target phoneme words.	No tangible reinforcement. Visual reinforcement is used as described in III-A and verbal feedback is used on error words as described in III-A.	One 7-word segment in which the target phoneme was produced correctly in all occurrences.	Probe.*

*Mandatory

STEP III (continued)

OPERATION	RESPONSE REQUIRED FOR REINFORCEMENT	REINFORCEMENT	CRITERION	THEN
III-C	**III-C**	**III-C**	**III-C**	
Use the same format as in III-A and III-B but extend the conversation to include 10 words containing the target phoneme. *Stop* the child when he has correctly produced the target phoneme in all 10 words. This is a successful segment. No verbal feedback is given except to say that all words were produced correctly. OR *Stop* the child when he incorrectly produces the target phoneme in any one word. Follow the same stimulation procedures as in III-B.	A conversation which includes 10 words containing the target phoneme. All occurrences of the target phoneme must be correct in those 10 target phoneme words.	No tangible reinforcement but visual and verbal is given as in III-B.	One 10-word segment in which the target phoneme was produced correctly in all occurrences.	Go to III-D.
III-D	**III-D**	**III-D**	**III-D**	**THEN**
Follow the same format, stopping procedures, and feedback procedures as in III-C but extend the conversation to include 13 words containing the target phoneme.	A conversation which includes 13 words containing the target phoneme. All occurrences of the target phoneme must be correct in those 13 target phoneme words.	Same as III-B and III-C.	One 13-word segment in which the target phoneme was produced correctly in all occurrences.	Probe.* If unsuccessful, repeat III-D.

*Mandatory

351

FIGURE 12.1 (*continued*)

APPENDIX I
KEY WORDS, QUESTION STIMULI, AND SENTENCE RESPONSES

Target Phoneme	Key Words	Questions for Step II	Sentence Responses for Step II
/s/	#1 see	What do you see?	I see (a/an) _____ .
	#2 this	What is this?	This is (a/an) _____ .
	#3 said	What did you say that was?	I said that that was (a/an) _____ .
	#4 that's	That's what?	That's (a/an) _____ .
/l/	#1 like	What do you like?	I like (a/an) _____ .
	#2 tell	What can you tell me about?	I can tell you about (a/an) _____ .
	#3 look	What do you look at?	I look at (a/an) _____ .
	#4 will	What will you say?	I will say _____ .
/tʃ/	#1 check	What do you check?	I check (a/an) _____ .
	#2 touch	What can you touch?	I can touch (a(an) _____ .
	#3 choose	What do you choose?	I choose (a/an) _____ .
	#4 reach	What can you reach?	I can reach (a/an) _____ .
/r/	#1 write	What do you write?	I write (a/an) _____ .
	#2 here	What is here?	Here is (a/an) _____ .
	#3 read	What can you read?	I can read _____ .
	#4 there	What is there?	There is (a/an) _____ .
/k/	#1 call	What do you call?	I call (a/an) _____ .
	#2 ask	What do you ask for?	I ask for (a/an) _____ .
	#3 keep	What do you want to keep?	I want to keep (a/an) _____ .
	#4 look	What do you look for?	I look for (a/an) _____ .

APPENDIX I
KEY WORDS, QUESTION STIMULI, AND SENTENCE RESPONSES

Target Phoneme	Key Words	Questions for Step II	Sentence Responses for Step II
/f/	#1 for	What are you looking for?	I'm looking for (a/an) _____ .
	#2 laugh	What do you laugh at?	I laugh at (a/an) _____ .
	#3 find	What do you find?	I find (a/an) _____ .
	#4 off	What did you take off?	I took off (a/an) _____ .
/ʃ/	#1 show	What can you show me?	I can show you (a/an) _____ .
	#2 fresh	What's fresh?	This is a fresh _____ .
	#3 should	What should you say?	I should say _____ .
	#4 mash	What do you mash?	I mash (a/an) _____ .
/g/	#1 got	What did you get?	I got (a/an) _____ .
	#2 big	What's big?	This is a big _____ .
	#3 give	What do you give?	I give (a/an) _____ .
	#4 beg	What do you beg for?	I beg for (a/an) _____ .
/dʒ/	#1 join	What do you join?	I join (a/an) _____ .
	#2 change	What do you change?	I change (a/an) _____ .
	#3 joke	What do you joke about?	I joke about (a/an) _____ .
	#4 huge	What's huge?	This is a huge _____ .
/d/	#1 do	What do you see?	I do see (a/an) _____ .
	#2 made	What did you make?	I made (a/an) _____ .
	#3 does	What does it look like?	It does look like (a/an) _____ .
	#4 had	What did you have?	I had (a/an) _____ .

FIGURE 12.1 *(continued)*

APPENDIX I
KEY WORDS, QUESTION STIMULI, AND SENTENCE RESPONSES

Target Phoneme	Key Words	Questions for Step II	Sentence Responses for Step II
/θ/	#1 t<u>h</u>ank	What do you t<u>h</u>ank?	I t<u>h</u>ank (a/an) ———— .
	#2 wit<u>h</u>	This is a picture wit<u>h</u> what?	This is a picture wit<u>h</u> ———— .
	#3 <u>th</u>ought	What did you <u>th</u>ink it was?	I <u>th</u>ought it was (a/an) ———— .
	#4 benea<u>th</u>	What is benea<u>th</u> my finger?	Benea<u>th</u> it is (a/an) ———— .
/v/	#1 <u>v</u>isit	What can you <u>v</u>isit?	I can <u>v</u>isit (a/an) ———— .
	#2 mo<u>v</u>e	What can you mo<u>v</u>e?	I can mo<u>v</u>e (a/an) ———— .
	#3 <u>v</u>iew	What do you <u>v</u>iew?	I <u>v</u>iew (a/an) ———— .
	#4 ha<u>v</u>e	What do you ha<u>v</u>e?	I ha<u>v</u>e (a/an) ———— .
/t/	#1 tal<u>k</u>	What do you tal<u>k</u> about?	I tal<u>k</u> about ———— .
	#2 tha<u>t</u>	What is tha<u>t</u>?	Tha<u>t</u> is (a/an) ———— .
	#3 <u>t</u>ake	What do you <u>t</u>ake?	I <u>t</u>ake (a/an) ———— .
	#4 i<u>t</u>	What is i<u>t</u>?	I<u>t</u> is (a/an) ———— .
/z/ final only	#1 u<u>s</u>e	What do you u<u>s</u>e?	I u<u>s</u>e (a/an) ———— .
	#2 i<u>s</u>	What is thi<u>s</u>?	This is (a/an) ———— .
	#3 the<u>s</u>e	What are the<u>s</u>e?	The<u>s</u>e are ———— .
	#4 wa<u>s</u>	What was thi<u>s</u>?	This was (a/an) ———— .

APPENDIX II

GUIDELINES FOR TEACHING A KEY WORD

Present a line drawing picture of the Key Word. Name the picture and ask the child to imitate your production of the word. Direct the child's attention to your production of the word by asking him to watch and listen carefully as you say it.

When the child repeats the word in a socially acceptable manner, give him a token. Indicate the reason for which the child was given the token. Exchange the tokens for back-up reinforcers at the end of the session.

Give the child a token only for a Key Word in which the target phoneme is produce acceptably. That is, if the child usually omits the target phoneme but then distorts it, no reinforcer should be given for this "more nearly acceptable" production.

If necessary, the target phoneme can be taken out of context so that you may present the child a verbal model of the sound in isolation. This should be done only a few times; then the sound should be put back into the word context. You may give the child verbal feedback about the acceptability of the target phoneme in isolation, but do not give the child a token for acceptable production of the target phoneme in isolation.

When the child has correctly produced the target phoneme in the word several times in succession, you may test it to see if it is stable enough to use in the protocol procedures. The stability test procedure is to ask the child to say the Key Word ten times. *Do not reinforce correct productions of the target phoneme in the Key Word during this test for stability.* Judge each production as correct or incorrect. If the child produces the target phoneme in the Key Word in a socially acceptable manner at least nine out of 10 times (or, at least 90% correct production), you may discontinue training on the word. The Key Word can now be used in the protocol procedure.

The target phoneme of a Key Word occasionally breaks down during the protocol procedures. If, in Step I, the Key Word is produced incorrectly three or more times in two successive training strings within any one sub-step, therapy should be discontinued immediately at that point and the Key Word retrained to stability criterion (9/10 correct productions of the target phoneme under conditions of no reinforcement). If the Key Word breaks down in the sentence procedures of Step II, therapy should be discontinued immediately at that point and the child prompted as to the nature of his errors. A Key Word breakdown in Step II is usually due to either the child not understanding the required task or his having difficulty in producing the Key Word in a sentence structure. Retraining of the word in isolation would not be beneficial at that point, but further explanation of the required task with emphasis on the correct production of a word already trained could be helpful.

FIGURE 12.1 *(continued)*

APPENDIX III
PROBE

A Probe is a sample of the child's conversational speech with the purpose of checking on the generalization effects of the training. The clinician engages the child in a conversation and records the words produced by the child containing the target phoneme. The clinician judges the production of the target phoneme as either correct or incorrect. The child should not be able to see the recording of words by the clinician. All occurrences of the target phoneme must be produced correctly for the word to be considered a correct target phoneme word.

A probe should be given at each point designated on the protocol, but additional probes can be given at the clinician's option. Additional probes should be given only after criterion has been reached on an OPERATION.

Possible Outcomes:

A. If the target phoneme is produced correctly on the first 15 successive occurrences, the probe is considered successful and therapy should be discontinued for that day and another probe administered on the next therapy day.

If the first 15 occurrences of the target phoneme are produced correctly on the second day, then therapy should be terminated on the target phoneme.

B. If the production of the target phoneme is incorrect on any occurrence of the first 15 required, either on the first or second day of probing, proceed to the next part of the protocol.

Thus, *terminal criterion* for the teaching of a phoneme is correct production of the target phoneme in 100% of 15 successive occurrences during two probes separated by at least one day.

FIGURE 12.1 ***(continued)***

STEP III SCORE SHEET

NAME: ____________________ CLIN. ____________ PHONEME: / / DATE: __________

		RIGHT	WRONG		RIGHT	WRONG
	1.			1.		
	2.			2.		
	3.			3.		
STEP III-A	4			4		
	5.			5.		
	6.			6.		
STEP III-B	7.			7.		
	8.			8.		
	9.			9.		
STEP III-C	10.			10.		
	11.			11.		
	12.			12.		
STEP III-D	13			13		

	1.			1.		
	2.			2.		
	3.			3.		
STEP III-A	4.			4		
	5.			5.		
	6.			6.		
STEP III-B	7.			7.		
	8.			8.		
	9.			9.		
STEP III-C	10.			10.		
	11.			11.		
	12.			12.		
STEP III-D	13.			13		

FIGURE 12.1 *(continued)*

PROBE SCORE SHEET

NAME: _____CLIN. _____ PHONEME: /   /   DATE: _____

	RIGHT	WRONG		RIGHT	WRONG
1.			1.		
2.			2.		
3.			3.		
4.			4.		
5.			5.		
6.			6.		
7.			7.		
8.			8.		
9.			9.		
10.			10.		
11.			11.		
12.			12.		
13.			13.		

1.			1.		
2.			2.		
3.			3.		
4.			4.		
5.			5.		
6.			6.		
7.			7.		
8.			8.		
9.			9.		
10.			10.		
11.			11.		
12.			12.		
13.			13.		

TRAINING STRING SCORE SHEET

NAME _____ CLIN. _____ PHONEME ___ / ___ / ___ DATE _____

TRAINING STRINGS

Step ___		Step ___		Step ___		Step ___		Step ___		Step ___		Step ___	
I	F	I	F	I	F	I	F	I	F	I	F	I	F
K	1	K	1	K	1	K	1	K	1	K	1	K	1
K	2	K	2	K	2	K	2	K	2	K	2	K	2
K	3	K	3	K	3	K	3	K	3	K	3	K	3
K	4	K	4	K	4	K	4	K	4	K	4	K	4
K	5	K	5	K	5	K	5	K	5	K	5	K	5
K	6	K	6	K	6	K	6	K	6	K	6	K	6
K	7	K	7	K	7	K	7	K	7	K	7	K	7
K	8	K	8	K	8	K	8	K	8	K	8	K	8
K	9	K	9	K	9	K	9	K	9	K	9	K	9
K	10	K	10	K	10	K	10	K	10	K	10	K	10

TRAINING STRINGS

Step ___		Step ___		Step ___		Step ___		Step ___		Step ___		Step ___	
I	F	I	F	I	F	I	F	I	F	I	F	I	F
K	1	K	1	K	1	K	1	K	1	K	1	K	1
K	2	K	2	K	2	K	2	K	2	K	2	K	2
K	3	K	3	K	3	K	3	K	3	K	3	K	3
K	4	K	4	K	4	K	4	K	4	K	4	K	4
K	5	K	5	K	5	K	5	K	5	K	5	K	5
K	6	K	6	K	6	K	6	K	6	K	6	K	6
K	7	K	7	K	7	K	7	K	7	K	7	K	7
K	8	K	8	K	8	K	8	K	8	K	8	K	8
K	9	K	9	K	9	K	9	K	9	K	9	K	9
K	10	K	10	K	10	K	10	K	10	K	10	K	10

TRAINING STRINGS

Step ___		Step ___		Step ___		Step ___		Step ___		Step ___		Step ___	
I	F	I	F	I	F	I	F	I	F	I	F	I	F
K	1	K	1	K	1	K	1	K	1	K	1	K	1
K	2	K	2	K	2	K	2	K	2	K	2	K	2
K	3	K	3	K	3	K	3	K	3	K	3	K	3
K	4	K	4	K	4	K	4	K	4	K	4	K	4
K	5	K	5	K	5	K	5	K	5	K	5	K	5
K	6	K	6	K	6	K	6	K	6	K	6	K	6
K	7	K	7	K	7	K	7	K	7	K	7	K	7
K	8	K	8	K	8	K	8	K	8	K	8	K	8
K	9	K	9	K	9	K	9	K	9	K	9	K	9
K	10	K	10	K	10	K	10	K	10	K	10	K	10

Error = Slash

PST - TS

FIGURE 12.1 *(continued)*

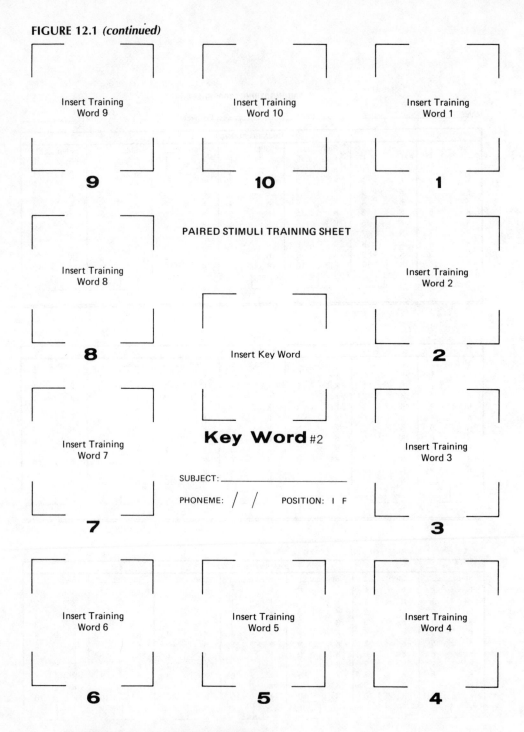

Insert Training Word 9

9

Insert Training Word 10

10

Insert Training Word 1

1

PAIRED STIMULI TRAINING SHEET

Insert Training Word 8

8

Insert Key Word

Insert Training Word 2

2

Insert Training Word 7

Key Word #2

Insert Training Word 3

SUBJECT: _____

PHONEME: / / POSITION: I F

7

3

Insert Training Word 6

6

Insert Training Word 5

5

Insert Training Word 4

4

ANALYSIS OF THE PROCEDURES

Following is a detailed analysis of the learning principles used in the paired-stimuli G-F protocol. It is designed to help the reader understand and evaluate all of the pertinent variables as they are used initially and as they change throughout the course of the program.

Major Operations in Step I

The paired-stimuli G-F protocol consists of three major steps, each having several substeps. Major steps and substeps are designated by number and letter; for example, Step I-B or Step II-D. In the first step, children who misarticulate the target phoneme in both the initial and final positions of training words are taught (if necessary) two final-position and two initial-position key words. The position of the target phoneme within each key word is alternated. The first final-position key word (such as *this*) is designated Key Word #1, the first initial-position key word (such as *see*) is Key Word #2, the second final-position key word (such as *that's*) is Key Word #3, and the second initial-position key word (such as *said*) is Key Word #4.

The major operations involved in Step I consist of the following:

1. Steps I-A, I-C, I-E and I-G involve teaching each key word under continuous reinforcement for correct responses, to a stability criterion of 90% correct production of the target phoneme within the key word (9 correct responses out of 10 consecutive trials), under conditions of no reinforcement. (Specific suggestions for key-word training are included as part of the protocol.) The purpose of key-word training is to establish the target phoneme in the key word as a discriminative stimulus. This goal is accomplished by providing the child reinforcement for each production of the key word in which the target phoneme is produced correctly, thus increasing the likelihood that the child will produce the target phoneme correctly in other words that contain the target phoneme.

2. Steps I-B and I-D pair Key Words #1 and #2 with the group of 10 training words associated with each of them. The names of each pictured key word and each pictured training word are produced alternately by the child. The pairing of the key word with each of its 10 training words is called a training string. Reinforcement is provided following the correct production of the target phoneme in the key word and in each training word. Criterion for these substeps is correct production of the target phoneme in at least 8 of the 10 training words on two successive contingent training strings. The learning strategy used in this activity is to shift the discriminative stimulus from the key word to each of the training words, which contain the target phoneme in the same position as in the key word, by reinforcing correct production of the target phoneme in untaught words (the training words). This shift of stimulus control from key word to training word is also facilitated by the temporal pairing of the names of the key word and each training word alternately.

3. In Step I-F, three changes occur involving (a) response definition, (b) reinforcement schedule, and (c) criterion. In previous pairing steps (I-B and I-D), a time lag was permitted between the child's naming of the key-word picture and his naming of a training-word picture, and he or she could earn a token for each word in a pairing

(or one or none, depending on the correctness of production of the target phoneme in either or both words). Thus, if the target phoneme was produced correctly in all occurrences of the key word and in each of the ten training words, a total of twenty tokens could be earned for that training string. In Step I-F, the response definition requires that the child produce each pairing rapidly, resulting in a two-word unit, such as *this-house*. In order to be reinforced for any pairing, the child must produce the target phoneme correctly in both the key word and its training word. Thus, a training string is now defined as 10 unit responses, each unit containing the key word and one of its training words. The reinforcement contingency is shifted, so that a token is given following each correct unit, and the value of each token is increased to 2. In this way, the total number of tokens available for errorless performance remains 20, but an error in any pairing means that two tokens are withheld rather than one. Criterion now becomes correct production of at least 8 out of 10 units over two successive training strings. The purpose of these shifts is to decrease the temporal gap between key-word and training-word pairings to approximate compound words or phrases. The shift in reinforcement contingency is designed to ensure the discrimination of target-phoneme accuracy as the behavior that controls the delivery of reinforcement. That is, if the child fails to receive a token following a unit, he has no external feedback as to whether the failure to earn a token represented a target-phoneme error in his production of the key word, the training word, or both. Therefore, in order to receive the token, he must be vigilant to produce the target phoneme correctly in both words of each unit.

4. Step I-H is identical to Step I-F in response definition and criterion, but the reinforcement contingency is shifted again. Here, two successive units must be produced correctly, and the value of each token is increased to 4. Operationally, this step represents primarily a leaning out of the reinforcement schedule, in that token delivery follows after two consecutive correct units. However, the increased value of each token maintains the token ratio established at the beginning of the program.

Major Operations in Step II

Step II represents an important departure from Step I in that the key words and training words learned earlier are systematically incorporated into sentence units in response to questions asked by the clinician. The major format is presented in II-A, where the clinician points to each training word associated with Key Word #1 and asks a question, such as "What is this?" where *this* is the key word. The child responds with a prescribed sentence in which the key word appears before the training word, e.g., "This is a house." Reinforcement is delivered after three consecutively correct sentences, with token value placed at 6. Step II was added to provide a transitional stage between pairs of words, which may have little or no linguistic significance for some children, and conversational speech. The prescribed sentences provide an opportunity for the child to perceive that the words learned in Step I can be used in meaningful linguistic units, with no demand made upon the child for spontaneous syntactic formulation.

1. Step II-B requires the child to respond to each of two questions asked alternately by the clinician, with the pictured training words associated with Key Word #2 as the stimuli. In this substep, two important changes occur, First, the child is required to listen carefully to the form of each question in order to give the appropriate sentence response. Thus, the child is asked to rely on cognitive processing more than he has in earlier steps. Second, every other sentence response places the key word and the required training word in a new relationship with one another. At this point in the training program, a final-position key word occurs in conjunction with an initial-position training word for the first time. For example, in response to the questions for Key Word #3, "What's that?" the child says, "That's soap," or "That's the sun." Prior to this substep, the pairing of key words and training words was always one where the position of the target phoneme in the key word was identical with the position of the target phoneme in the training word. Thus, the stimulus support provided by the constancy of target phoneme position has been faded out of the required responses.

2. Step II-C makes additional demands on the child's cognitive processing of the stimuli. Here, the four structured questions associated with each of the four key words are asked alternately, using the 20 training-word pictures associated with Key Words #1 and #4. Only 10 of these 20 pictures are used, and they are presented in random order, distributed across the two training-word picture sheets. The assumption is made that the child's having to process each of four questions and to retrieve the responses appropriate to the randomly presented pictures approximates the requirements of conversational speech. It is also assumed that these cognitive requirements are such that the child's ability to produce the target phoneme in the key word and in the training word for each sentence has become relatively automatic.

Major Operations in Step III

Having successfully moved the child toward closer approximation of the activities that occur in actual communicative interchanges via Step II, the clinician should use Step III to extend the child's ability to retain the trained response in conversational units under conditions of no tangible reinforcement. Certain feedback alterations are provided for in Step III, as follows:

1. In Step III-A, the child's spontaneous speech is monitored for the occurrence of correct productions of the target phoneme in four successive words. If a child misarticulates the target phoneme in a

target word prior to four successful consecutive occurrences, the clinician gives the child feedback on target words produced correctly and the word on which the error occurred. Visual feedback about correctness/incorrectness is also available to the child by his observing the clinician write the words under the appropriate column of the scoring sheet. The clinician models the correct production of the misarticulated target word and requires the child to say the word once before beginning the next trial. Thus, in this substep, the child receives visual and auditory feedback about correct productions and errors and is given a verbal model of his misarticulated target word.

2.   In Step III-B, stimulation continues to be given for any target word misarticulated within the first seven occurrences in the child's conversations, but reinforcement about correct production is withdrawn. This procedure of calling attention only to the first misarticulated target word in a prescribed sequence is followed for the remaining substeps of Step III. Thus in Step III, verbal feedback about correctness of production of the target phoneme in words is faded rapidly, leaving the child with only visual information about correctly produced words and with visual and verbal feedback about errors.

The responses required in the substeps of Step III are identical; the substeps vary only by requiring increasingly larger numbers of consecutively correct occurrences of target words, varying from 4 in Step III-A to 13 in Step III-D.

Despite the fact that Step III-D is the final training step of the program, its criterion—unlike that of certain other programs—is not identical with the terminal criterion for the training program. Terminal criterion requires 15 consecutive correctly produced target words over two different days, with no reinforcement provided for correct production of the target phoneme in the words. The tacit assumption underlying the terminal criterion is that the ability to produce 15 target words correctly in succession in conversational speech is highly correlated with the child's ability to produce the target phoneme correctly at a very high rate in all target words in conversation outside the clinical environment.

VALUE OF THE PROGRAM

Earlier, the criteria for effective articulatory intervention cited by Griffith et al. (1980) were reviewed. The paired-stimuli articulation program fares well on these criteria. It (a) can be used with a large variety of consonant sounds, (b) is usable with a wide range of subjects, (c) is independent of etiology as long as the specified baselines are achieved, (d) clearly specifies entry and exit criteria, (e) requires no specialized equipment, (f) provides a consistent program format, (g) enjoys a high potential for use by paraprofessionals, (h) has intrinsic motivational value, (i) brings about rapid achievement of goals, (j) yields good generalization, and (k) does not produce any negative side effects.

Until 1970, available data consisted of the original 13 subjects in the Weston (1969) study, 6 subjects in the unpublished Freilinger studies in 1970, and 13 subjects studied by Weston and Irwin in 1970—a total of 32 children all of whom satisfied criteria under carefully controlled conditions. However, in a major research project undertaken in 1970, Irwin, Weston, Griffith, and Muma studied 396 children representing 498 phonemes. Results of this unpublished study indicated that 480 (96%) of 498 phonemes were taught successfully, 15 (3%) were considered failures, and 3 (1%) were classified as other outcomes.

The total number of children available for analysis was 338. For this group, the average child was able to learn to articulate his error phoneme correctly in conversational speech in 82.59 minutes, with a range of 11 to 267 minutes, and standard deviation of 52.93 minutes.

Based on the results of this large study, Irwin, Weston, Griffith, and Muma studied 160 additional children in 1972. The subjects were divided into an experimental group (n = 80), who received paired-stimuli training, and a control group (n = 80). All children demonstrated an error percentage on /s/ in conversation of 87% or greater.

The effects of intervention on correct production of /s/ and the time required for completion of the intervention steps were studied. Because it was recognized that the reliability of live judgments of /s/ in free conversation had major implications for any clinical application of the paired-stimuli technique, the design included an observer at each test conversation and, for one half of the subjects, a conversational measurement on two separate days.

The data demonstrated that the experimental group's mean scores at each of the testing times were significantly higher than the scores for the control subjects at the same times (Griffith, Irwin, & Weston, 1980). The data from this investigation revealed that:

1. "Whether measured immediately after the intervention or one month subsequent to the termination of intervention, the experimental group showed a significantly higher percentage of correct /s/ responses in conversation than the control group" (Irwin & Weston, 1975, p. 23).
2. Scores immediately following intervention were significantly higher than pre-intervention scores. Conversational scores were slightly lower 1 month following intervention than at the time of termination of the program but continued to show a high rate of correct production of /s/ in conversational speech as compared with baseline data.
3. Mean intervention time for the experimental subjects was greatest for Step III of the program, and mean intervention time for the entire program was less than 2 hours.

These data suggest that the paired-stimuli articulation program is an effective and efficient means of teaching the /s/ to a high rate in conversational speech in a very brief period of treatment time.

LIMITATIONS

The data accumulated since 1969 continue to demonstrate the success of the paired-stimuli therapy procedure for children and adults with articulatory disorders of nonorganic origins. Some clinicians have reported success with the use of paired-stimuli therapy with clients with severe hearing impairments. At this time we know of no specific data as to the use of PST with clients who have organically based speech disorders. Therefore, clinicians using PST with clients with organically based disorders should note behavioral changes, quantify them, and share these results with others.

SUMMARY

The paired-stimuli technique is based on the assumption that production of an acceptable target sound in one word can be generalized to other words through programmed behavior modification. Specifically, through contextual testing or through instruction, a word is located in which the subject produces the target phoneme acceptably. This word is termed a *key word*. The subject produces this word alternately with 10 other words in which the target phoneme is produced in error. Words in which the target phoneme is incorrectly produced are termed *training words*. Reinforcement of socially acceptable responses is administered on a continuous schedule, whether the correct utterance occurs in the key word or in a training word. This continues until specified criteria are met. Procedures are described that bring the client from acquisition of the target phoneme in words to generalization in conversation.

This technique is supported by one of the most complete sets of data available on the modification of articulatory behavior. Of particular importance are the time studies that range from the acquisition of the original key word to the acquisition of acceptable conversational usage. Of course, more research needs to be done with respect to many factors, such as spontaneous acquisition and the prediction of conversational usage. The effects of etiological conditions need careful examination. The contributions of current phonological research—with its emphasis on distinctive features and processes—should be carefully considered. Contributions from such research may well influence subject selection, details of technique, and criteria. The individual clinician must, of course, evaluate the appropriateness of the paired-stimuli technique in the modification of articulatory behavior with each client. It is hoped that many clinicians will attempt replication of the procedure as part of their decision-making process.

REFERENCES

Ainsworth, S. (1948). *Speech correction methods.* Englewood Cliffs, NJ: Prentice-Hall.

Cohen, J. H., & Diehl, C. F. (1963). Relation of speech-sound discrimination ability to articulation-type speech defects. *Journal of Speech and Hearing Disorders, 28,* 187–190.

Engle, D., Brandriet, S., Erikson, K., Gronhound, K., & Gunderson, G. (1966). Carryover. *Journal of Speech and Hearing Disorders, 31,* 227–233.

Fairbanks, G., & Grubb, P. A. (1961). A psychophysical investigation of vowel formants. *Journal of Speech and Hearing Research, 4,* 203–219.

Gerber, A. (1977). Programming for articulation modification. *Journal of Speech and Hearing Disorders, 42,* 29–43.

Griffith, F. A., Irwin, J. V., & Weston, A. J. (1980). A historical overview and critical assessment of the paired-stimuli technique for the modification of articulatory disorders. In W. D. Wolfe & D. J. Goulding (Eds.), *Articulation and learning* (pp. 218–268). Springfield: Charles C. Thomas.

Hall, M. E. (1938). Auditory factors in functional articulatory speech defects. *Journal of Experimental Education, 7,* 110–132.

Hansen, B. F. (1944). The application of sound discrimination tests to functional articulatory defectives with normal hearing. *Journal of Speech and Hearing Disorders, 9,* 347–355.

Irwin, J. V. (1972). The triota: A computerized screening battery. *Acta Symbolica, 3,* 26–38.

Irwin, J. V. (1975). Normal articulatory function: Detection, diagnosis and management of abnormal articulatory function. In E. L. Eagles (Ed.), *The nervous system* (Vol. 3, pp. 515–523). New York: Raven Press.

Irwin, J., Huskey, R., Knight, N., & Oltman, S. (1974). A longitudinal study of the spontaneous remission of articulatory defects of 1665 school children in grades 1, 2, and 3. Part III: The study group. *Acta Symbolica, 5,* 9–17.

Irwin, J. V., & Weston, A. (1971). *A manual for the clinical utilization of the paired-stimuli technique articulation modification.* Memphis: National Educator Service.

Irwin, J. V., & Weston, A. J. (1975). The paired-stimuli monograph. *Acta Symbolica, 6,* 1–76.

Irwin, J. V., & Weston, A. J. (1981). *Paired stimuli therapy kit.* Covina, CA: Fox Point Publishing, Ltd.

Irwin, J., & Wong, S. (1983). Summary. In J. Irwin & S. Wong (Eds.), *Phonological development in children: 18 to 72 months.* Carbondale, IL: Southern Illinois University Press.

Ladefoged, P. (1962). *Elements of acoustic phonetics.* Chicago: University of Chicago Press.

Leonard, L., & Webb, C. (1971). An automated therapy program for articulation correction. *Journal of Speech and Hearing Research, 14,* 338–344.

McDonald, E. (1968). *A screening deep test of articulation.* Pittsburgh: Stanwix House.

McLean, J. (1970). Extending stimulus control of phoneme articulation by operant techniques. *ASHA Monograph, 14,* 24–47.

Peterson, G., & Barney, H. L. (1952). Control methods used in a central study of vowels. *Journal of the Acoustical Society of America, 42,* 175.

Poole, I. (1934). Genetic development of articulation of consonant sounds in speech. *Elementary English 11,* 159–161.

Prins, T. D. (1963). Relations among specific articulatory deviations and responses to a clinical measure of sound discrimination ability. *Journal of Speech and Hearing Disorders, 28,* 382–388.

Roe, V., & Milisen, R. (1942). The effect of maturation upon defective articulation in elementary grades. *Journal of Speech and Hearing Disorders, 7,* 37–45.

Sayler, H. K. (1949). The effect of maturation upon defective articulation in grades seven through twelve. *Journal of Speech and Hearing Disorders, 14,* 202–207.

Sherman, D., & Gerth, A. (1967). Speech sound discrimination and articulation skill. *Journal of Speech and Hearing Research, 10,* 277–280.

Sommers, R., Leiss, R., Delp, M., Gerber, A., Fundrella, D., Smith, R., Revucky, M., Ellis, D., & Haley, V. (1967). Factors related to the effectiveness of articulation therapy for kindergarten, first and second grade children. *Journal of Speech and Hearing Research, 10,* 428–437.

Templin, M. (1957). *Certain language skills in children.* Minneapolis: University of Minnesota Press.

Templin, M., & Darley, F. (1969). *Templin-Darley tests of articulation* (2nd ed.). Iowa City, IA: Bureau of Educational Research and Service, University of Iowa.

Travis, L. E., & Rasmus, B. (1931). The speech sound discrimination ability of cases with functional disorders of articulation. *Quarterly Journal of Speech, 17,* 217–226.

Van Riper, C. (1963). *Speech correction: Principles and methods* (4th ed.). Englewood Cliffs, NJ: Prentice Hall.

Van Riper, C., & Irwin, J. V. (1958). *Voice and articulation.* Englewood Cliffs, NJ: Prentice Hall.

Weston, A. J. (1969). *The use of paired-stimuli in the modification of articulation.* (Doctoral dissertation, University of Kansas, 1969). *Dissertation Abstracts International, 30B,* 5738.

Weston, A., & Irwin, J. V. (1971). The use of paired-stimuli in the modification of articulation. *Perceptual Motor Skills, 32,* 947–957.

Weston, A., & Leonard, L. (1976). *Articulation disorders: Methods of evaluation and therapy.* Lincoln: Cliff Notes, Inc.

Weston, A., & Rampp, D. (1973). Articulation intervention. In J. Wingo & G. Holloway (Eds.), *An appraisal of speech pathology and audiology: A symposium* (pp. 96–114). Springfield, IL: Charles C. Thomas.

Winitz, H. (1969). *Articulatory acquisition and behavior.* New York: Appleton-Century-Crofts.

13

The Method of Meaningful Minimal Contrasts

RATIONALE

Meaning, while obviously at the core of language learning, has sometimes been ignored as a variable in the treatment of functional articulation disorders. Traditional speech therapy tends to focus on formal aspects of language, such as establishing target phonemes in isolation, learning to apply rules for the manner and place of articulation or to use distinctive features, and, finally, attempting to join the discrete phonemes or features to the flow of speech. These procedures result from assumptions that phonemes and their phonetic expression are discrete, invariant signal units of phonology that children can perceive and produce as such.

What is overlooked in this approach is that speech reception and expression depend on a multidimensional complex where acoustic and neurological events overlap, where coarticulation or parallel processing is characteristic, and where redundancy of phonemes and allophonic variation is inherent. As a result, in traditional therapy, structure may become separated from meaning, form from content. The therapy may also fail to place the burden of speech modification where it belongs—on the children themselves. This chapter takes

Reuben Cooper is a professor emeritus of speech at Old Dominion University, Norfolk, Virginia.

the position that it is essential to restore the role of meaning in therapy. The evidence for this view will be presented in the ensuing brief survey of selected publications.

Phoneme Variance and Redundancy

It was well known to phoneticians such as Wise (1957), Kantner and West (1960), and numerous others that phonemes are modified within the vast number of phonetic environments in which they occur. For some of these conditions, regressive and progressive assimilation rules were devised. However, it remained for acoustic and psycholinguistic studies to add hard evidence concerning the variance of phonemes and the problems in phoneme detection and reception. The work of Peters (1963), Graham and House (1971), and Singh (1975) provides sufficient documentation that phonemic perception cannot be accounted for by auditory and articulatory principles alone. Singh states that the acoustic and articulatory parameters provide only a manifesting medium for the perceptual process, or, in other words, a basis for the evocation of meaning.

Liberman, Cooper, Shankweiler, and Studdert-Kennedy (1972) are more explicit. They point out that phoneme boundaries disappear in the flow of speech, that the speech signal typically does not contain segments corresponding to discrete phonemes, and that there is a marked lack of correspondence between sound and perceived phoneme. These are central facts of speech perception. Of unusual interest in this connection are Harris's experiments, quoted by Liberman, which showed that speech based on one building block for each vowel and consonant not only sounds unnatural but is mostly unintelligible. Liberman concluded that acoustic cues cannot be divided on the time axis into segments of phonemic size, nor can the sound stream be cut along the time dimension so as to recover segments that will be perceived as separate phonemes. Furthermore, he points out that the temporal, resolving power of the ear sets a relatively low limit on the rate at which discrete acoustic segments can be perceived so that the average rate of speech, from about 10 to 15 phonemes per second, could neither be perceived nor produced. From such data it is obvious that phoneme perception, per se, in the flow of speech must be dependent on more complex dimensions and most certainly must involve meaning.

At this point, the question of children's capabilities in perceiving phonemes naturally arises. Cutting and Pisoni (1978) described Liberman's attempt to answer this question when he examined the ability of nursery-school and kindergarten children to tap out the number of syllables and phonemes in common words. The findings were that the ability to segment by syllable was shown by half of the 4-year-olds, but none of them could segment by phoneme. Among the 6-year-olds, 90% could segment by syllable but only 70% by phoneme.

The Multilevel Complex Representing Phoneme Perception and Production

How does the listener, then, manage to decode the ever-changing complexity of the speech flow? Part of the answer lies in the fact, as Cutting and

Pisoni (1978) affirm, that the listener treats speech as a multidimensional display, the attributes of which occur more or less in parallel. The display necessarily involves the total set of communication behaviors that underlie the expression of meaning. These are auditory, phonetic, and phonological features; nonverbal, pragmatic, and contextual aspects. Nor is it possible to ignore the redundancy inherent in natural languages, which makes it possible to understand meaning more efficiently by reducing the need to decode and encode all of the segments.

The study of speech production, like that of its counterpart, speech perception, reveals a multidimensional complex that therapy programs may not ignore. For example, from the work of Daniloff (1968), Liberman et al. (1972), McClean (1973), Öhman (1973), Gay (1974), Cutting and Pisoni (1978), and Starkweather (1980), it is reasonable to conclude that the speech load is being divided among the articulators in the course of normal speech production. This distribution of output is referred to generally as *coarticulation* or *parallel processing*. For example, in producing the word *hello,* by the time /h/ is about to be produced, the mandible is already lowered, the tongue is moving up to the /ɛ/ position, and the tongue tip is approaching the alveolar ridge to perform the /l/ while the lips are beginning to round for the /ou/. It becomes clear that the features belonging to the successive phonemes overlap in time, and the speaker can produce the phonemes at a rate much faster than would be possible if each phoneme required a discrete movement. In this way, parallel processing makes conversational speech possible.

Speech-perception, phoneme-identification, and speech-production data as part of a multilevel complex should significantly alter therapeutic approaches to speech pathology and place the burden where it belongs—on meaning. I recall a mother, by way of illustration, teaching her 6-year-old boy to read the word *run,* which he read out loud as "walk." As she demanded, he repeated after her the discrete segments [r] . . . [ʌ] . . . [n]. Then she waited for the miracle as the boy gleefully uttered [wɔk]. Which is more meaningful to a child—his natural, deep [di mi mi] or an artificial, surface /gɪv mi mɪlk/?

Data on speech production predict that the learning of discrete phonemes and attempts to join them to connected speech so that the speech is meaningful are, in general, doomed to failure. It seems that if a child could learn to say the separate phonemes /k/ . . . /eɪ/ . . . /k/ and then put them together like three notes on a piano, saying /keɪk/ should be readily accomplished. However, such is not the reality. /keɪk/ is a big leap in meaning from /k/ . . . /eɪ/ . . . /k/. It must be emphasized again that phonemes are indivisible from the flow of speech and the meanings they evoke. Complex problems are generated by attempts to isolate them, establish them, and then join them to syllables and words and then to connected discourse. These problems consist, in part, of nonnatural attempts at a prescribed manner and/or place of articulation. Often a physiological preoccupation develops, along with a psychological loss of speech spontaneity and the risk of interference with the flow of speech. In addition, the newly learned discrete phonemes are often placed into bizarre positions. For example, in therapy a child who is taught the /ʃ/ and learns to say [dɪʃ] may also produce [hauʃ] for [haus] and [miʃ] for [mit]. One comes away with the feeling that the child is producing the sound to please the therapist and has not added it to the phonemic repertoire.

The Significance of Meaning

The data already presented suggest a multilevel complex in speech perception and production in which meaning must be considered a key factor. However, more direct evidence of the significance of meaning for speech-language pathology is also available. Grey and Stunden (1961) studied responses to auditory stimuli of high and low meaning, comparing children with so-called functional articulatory disturbances and those whose speech was judged to be free of speech problems. They concluded that meaning influences the ability of the individual to make phonetic discriminations. They also state: "It is apparent that evaluating only the patient's response to phonetic stimuli disregards the foundation upon which the phoneme rests, namely, the meaningful nature of the stimulus" (p. 341). Carroll (1961) claims that the child discovers the critical distinctions in his language by an unconscious trial and error process where his errors result from failure to recognize a critical distinction in sound, form, or meaning. Studying selected auditory perceptual factors and articulation ability, Mange (1960) examined the hypothesis that "one of the principal causative factors in certain functional articulatory defects is the presence of some auditory deficiency" (p. 67). It is interesting that the one factor he found that appeared significant was phonetic word-synthesis ability, defined as "meaningful interpretation of auditory stimuli under conditions of distortion" (p. 68).

In addition, studies not directly related to articulatory disorders but involving verbal learning suggest the importance of meaning. Underwood and Schulz (1960), in a series of well-designed experiments, sought answers to the question of how meaningfulness exerts its influence in rote learning in the adult. The pertinent conclusions warranted by the evidence were that (a) as meaning increases, the rate of learning increases, and (b) whether the verbal units are placed in serial lists or in paired-associate lists, learning and meaning are directly related. The findings of Parker and Noble (1960) and of Ruder, Hermann, and Schiefelbusch (1977) give further support to these conclusions.

Such evidence suggests a methodological approach to articulation therapy in which "meaning" is used as an important variable. *Meaning* is here defined operationally as the conditioning of a referent to an utterance so that the subject will reliably point to the referent with the utterance as a stimulus. In general, the method is based on the principle that in paired contrasts of defective and standard productions of words where the defective utterance already possesses a standard meaning or is conditioned to a new meaning, children will tend to alter the articulation of their defective utterances. This principle is based not only on studies in meaning (Osgood, Suci, & Tannenbaum, 1957; Staats, 1968; Cooper, 1970, 1971) but also on linguistic principles emphasized by Leopold (1961) and Carroll (1961).

The Need to Rely on Children

So far the rationale for the method of meaningful minimal contrasts has considered primarily the multilevel complex in which phoneme variance, phoneme perception, parallel processing, and meaning are important features. However, for a therapy to be effective, clients themselves must undertake to make the necessary changes in their speech behavior, and these changes must grow out of the clients' communicative and psychological needs. Traditional therapies sometimes move from the top down—from adult speech to the child's, often in violation of the child's dialect and communication needs. If the child is to succeed in therapy, the process must be reversed and come from the bottom up—from where the child is. Children, in other words, must undertake to make their own corrections at their own speed, motivation, and conceptual ability, as provided for in meaningful minimal contrast therapy. They must experience the pleasure of success in their own achievements.

Summary of Rationale

The rationale underlying the theory of meaningful minimal contrast therapy, then, arises out of the following facts:

1. phoneme variance and redundancy
2. the multilevel complex representing phoneme perception and production
3. the significance of meaning as a variable in the alteration of children's articulation errors, and
4. the need to rely on children to alter their articulation in a natural process arising from their own conceptual abilities, needs, and motivation.

The next section will elaborate the methodology of meaningful minimal contrast therapy. Further rationale for suggested procedures will be included in the discussion.

METHOD

The Development of Contrasts in Normal Children

It seems that language develops in children as they learn to differentiate between various human sounds because of the effects these sounds have on their existence. The logic of meaning in language requires the use of different sounds for different events. Therefore, if *mommy, daddy,* and *bye-bye* evoke different meaningful events, the child will naturally learn to use different sounds in the context of these events. The impetus, then, to word, phrase, or sentence differentiation lies in the child's communicative need to use different words or expressions for different events where these are perceived as different. Children will thus utter their words for "mother" and "father" in ways that both distinguish between these two noble creatures and approximate the articulation for the words used in their environment. At first, gross sound differentiations are made by children until gradually finer discriminations are demanded by the number of meaningful words and phrases in their vocabularies. These discriminations arise necessarily out of two kinds of pressure: the functional need for linguistic differentiation in meaningful contexts and the social need to conform to the communication requirements of particular dialects.

An example of the linguistic need is the minimal contrast found in the words *won/run.* The social need is the rejection of [wʌn] for [rʌn]. In this example, the linguistic and social needs converge. In the case of the substitution of [kæ-] or [tæ-] for [kæt], the social requirement prevails. (The hyphen symbol is used here to indicate the unknown features that may be present in a so-called substitution or distortion.) The linguistic relationship between [kæ-], [tæ-] and [kæt], therefore, may be said to be allophonic. Because no word or nonword stands in minimal contrast to [kæ-] or [tæ-], these forms function in communication within a particular context to elicit meaning. Furthermore, [kæ-] or [tæ-] do not exist as nonwords in the child's expressive repertoire, and the referent "cat" is precisely what is evoked by the utterance [tæ-] or [kæ-].

Similar allophonic conditions prevail with many other substitutions, omissions, or distortions used to describe children's functional articulation problems. Now, if a child's defective articulation of a target phoneme could be placed into meaningful contrast with its standard articulation, the child would be placed under a logical and linguistic compulsion to alter the articulation. In other words, the allophonic difference would be made phonemic by the creation of a conceptual need to differentiate between the defective utterance and the standard utterance. Then the child would alter the articulation of the defective utterance in the direction of the standard form, or at least, attempt such an alteration.

This can be brought about if

1. in a minimal-contrast pair, a meaning is available for a defective utterance; for example, the articulation of [tɑr] for [kɑr] or [wʌn] for [rʌn];
2. a meaning is established for a defective utterance to create a minimal-contrast pair; for example, to the child's word [tup] a temporary meaning is established to contrast with the meaning of the standard word [sup];
3. the child can make the target sound required in the standard utterance, or if no physical inability to do so is present;
4. in general, the child also notes as many other features of the multilevel complex as are normally available, such as visible, situational, and acoustic cues, all of which are related to meaning;
5. the child is confronted with the defective word and the standard word, which are now in meaningful contrast;
6. the child is asked to name each, one at a time, in a more or less normal conversational temporal sequence—first, the defective form, the articulation of which presents no problem, and then the standard form;
7. the child is assisted in differentiating the articulation of the standard form in any way that seems needed; and
8. whatever articulatory efforts the child makes to distinguish the events is accepted temporarily by the speech pathologist as a movement in the direction of a change to the standard form of the utterance.

In accordance with these principles, a bare outline follows of a suggested procedure whose rationale is defined by Mowrer (1958) as follows:

If a word is heard and is then shortly followed by the experience of some thing, this sequence of events, if repeated a few times, will reliably cause the word to come to *mean* the associated thing. Part of the total reaction elicited by the thing stimulus gets conditioned to the word stimulus, and in this way the latter, as one may say, acquires *meaning*. (p. 143)

Miller (1951), in his studies of the verbal behavior of children between the ages of 2 and 5, concluded that after learning to react verbally to one object, children learn verbal reactions to other objects more quickly. These principles are particularly applicable to the ability of children to generalize from the correct production of one paradigmatic contrast pair to those within the set. Once one minimal contrast is achieved, like [kæt] for [kæ-], other related articulations are readily made, such as [hæt]/[hæ-], [mæt]/[mæ-], [sæt]/[sæ-], and so on. With one contrast pair established as a paradigm, other substitutions or omissions will generalize to related contrasts, and the child will readily correct such errors. It is most effective to maintain grammatical uniformity for paradigmatic generalizations, that is, such as nouns with nouns, or verbs with verbs. Yet, where such contrasts are not available, grammatical forms may be mixed— nouns with verbs, verbs with adjectives, and so on. Such mixtures, requiring more ingenuity from the speech-language pathologist to develop meaningful contexts, can still be effective. Based on studies with children, McReynolds (1978) reports these observations, which have a bearing on this approach:

A child uses an incorrect form during several stages in acquisition but he will later spontaneously produce the correct form. . . . Children generalize a new sound or combination of sounds almost immediately after they produce it correctly in one context. . . . they begin to produce the sound correctly in the appropriate words and only in that set of words, with little overgeneralization. (p. 148)

While these findings apply to children with normal speech development, they also hold for children with functional articulation problems and accord well with the method of meaningful minimal contrasts.

Speech-language pathologists, in accordance with their philosophies, have adapted this theory to situations in which they work, and to the nature of the children. For example, Sommers and Kane (1974) describe its use in the framework of a Backus-and-Beasley (1951) type of structure that is based on interpersonal communication as the medium of therapy. Weiner (1981) used the method in a game situation to achieve final [t] articulation. He placed into contrast, for example, the words *bow* and *boat*. The stimuli were five pictures of *boat* and four pictures of *bow*. And the instructions were: "We are going to play a game. The object of the game is to get me to pick up all five pictures of the boat. Every time you say *boat*, I will pick one up. When I have all five, you may paste a star on your paper." All the games he played were variations of the above procedure. If the child said *bow*, the therapist picked up the *bow* picture. Then he would offer a helping instruction such as: "You keep saying bow. If you want me to pick up the *boat* picture, you must say the [t] sound at the end. Listen, *boat, boat, boat.* You try it. Okay. Let's begin again."

In the next chapter, Blache describes the use of minimal pairs in a distinctive feature approach to articulation therapy. Numerous other tactics are possible, including informal methods, all of which can be effective. The following procedures are suggested bearing these qualifications in mind.

Choosing the Word Pairs

As a first step in planning therapy, after case histories have been taken and after testing, speech analyses, and diagnoses have been accomplished, it is necessary to set up in advance the word contrasts to be used for each child or group of children. These should be arranged as paradigms for any set of misarticulations involving phoneme substitutions and omissions as these terms are generally used in speech pathology. The contrasts may be CV, CVC, or VC words or utterances, and, depending on the conditions, words or defective utterances that are bisyllabic or that contain blends. The criteria for the selection of the paradigms should include the ease with which articulation changes could be made as well as the overall effect of the particular changes in improving the child's communication.

Therapy Using Simulated Word/Real Word Pairs

When a series of simulated word/real word sets are to be used, the following procedures are effective. If, for example, the first problem to be dealt with is a so-called substitution of [t/s] in initial position because these consonants are among the most frequent in English, the paradigmatic contrast pair could be any of these pairs: for *soap*, [toup/soup]; for *soup*, [tup/sup]; for *salt*, [tɔlt/sɔlt]. Articulation errors not directly related to the phoneme contrasts are temporarily ignored.

The program may start with one pair of contrasts for which a nonsense object or picture that is novel to the child is to be temporarily associated with the defective word, and a real object or picture is associated with the real word for contrast. In the example given above, the unknown or nonsense object or picture is to be associated with the word [toup]. I have with success used small abstract sculptures readily available from our Art Department, devised nonsense pictures, and selected pictures of unusual objects from *Scientific American*. Children can also create their own nonsense forms, either drawn with crayons or made out of wire or clay, and this activity provides extra dimensions to the therapy sessions. The speech pathologist may say: "You know what you made? You made a [toup]!" or "Let's call what you made a [toup]" or some such formulation. Of course, one must avoid asking the child to name the object or drawing unless it was agreed upon to make a [toup] or the name was part of the game.

Establishing Meaning for the Contrast Pair

The therapist should explain: "We are going to play a game. I will show you some pictures (or things) and you tell me what they are." Correct responses are reinforced by the clinician. The type of reinforcement used is optional. Social reinforcers are appropriate as are other more precision-oriented systems such as those discussed in chapter 6. The nature of reinforcements used is not crucial to the program. It is assumed that the clinician will motivate the child in an effective manner.

The therapist continues: "This is the *soap*." He points to the appropriate picture or object. "Now show me the *soap*." The child is rewarded in accordance with the rules of the game as they are set up. The therapist then points to the contrast picture and says: "This is the *toap*. Show me the *toap*." The child is rewarded. The therapist then asks the child to point to the appropriate picture or objects in response to the contrast words, randomly presented, until the child identifies each without error and with assurance. In this step and the one following, the child is not asked to speak the nonword or the standard word.

The next step requires that the therapist and child play with the functions of each of the words, fabricating functions for the nonwords so that a greater significance than just the name of the object is temporarily established for the contrast word. Where objects are used, tactile associations are available. For example, with the word *soap*, the therapist may say: "What is this for?" or "What do we do with this?" (Points to the *soap*.) Then, "What is this for?" (Points to the *toap*.) When the uses of the contrast words are well established and the child understands their functions by responding to the above questions or similar ones without error, either in speech or gestures or both, the final step is begun. With retarded children, the procedure takes longer, but can be effective. Rather than following a mere formal routine, the therapist and the child should actually play the objects in accordance with their alleged functions. The greater the number of associations established, the greater will be the compulsion of the child to differentiate the articulation of the contrast words.

Learning to Produce the Defective Word

When the new meaning is clearly established for the defective utterance, the therapist says to the child, starting with the nonword first: "This is the *toap*. Show me the *toap*. What is *toap* for?" After the child answers, the therapist says (pointing to the *toap*): "What is this?" The child will have no difficulty in saying the initial consonant in [toup]. He or she is rewarded for the response. The therapist then points to the other picture and says: "This is the *soap*. Show me the *soap*. What is *soap* for? This is *soap*. What is this?" If the child responds by saying [toup], then he or she is referred back to the contrast picture or object. Then again, the therapist points to the soap and says: "This is *soap*. What is this?" The child will make an effort to change his or her articulation—any effort is encouraged. Should a child, in attempting to alter [toup] to [soup], emit [stoup], this change should be accepted, the child rewarded, and the play stopped or switched to *st* words. At the next session, new contrasts may be used, such as [stoup/soup]. Sometimes when children are confronted with forced choices, they may feel "stuck" and refuse to continue the game. This too, of course, is progress. The play should change, and the session end with speech successes.

At this stage is it appropriate to help the child to say the word correctly. Any device such as stimulation, phonetic placement, prompting, or simple encouragement may be used to obtain a correct production. The child can also be shown how different sounds can be used at the beginning of a word. Using sounds the child can say, the clinician might ask the child to say words that rhyme with the target word *soap*, such as *mope, cope, dope, hope, lope, "nope,"* and *rope*. The object is to get the word spoken correctly, and at this stage any reasonable technique may be used.

Therapy Using Real Word Pairs

Where both contrast words are real words, the method of meaningful minimal contrasts is much simplified. For example, if the pair for a t/k substitution is *tar/car*, no temporary meanings need be established, nor will there be a need to learn, in general, the difference in meaning, although such assumptions may not be automatically made. The basic approach of reinforcing the meanings of these words and building up experiences and pragmatic applications of them will still be applicable. The procedure outlined for simulated words may be used in these instances. Again, such opportunity as exists to assist the children in making the necessary contrasts is taken advantage of. For example, in the fronting problem in real words where the children make the effort to distinguish the words [kɑr]/[tɑr], they can be made to produce [kɑə] instead of [tɑə] by taking a tongue depressor and holding the tip and the adjacent section of the blade of the tongue down so that [kɑə] emerges. This same technique can be used for words without final alveolars in contrasts such as *key/tea, cake/take,* or *kick/tick*. After these contrasts are established, the /k/ phoneme can readily be generalized to other initial /k/ words in the child's vocabulary. (See *One-Syllable Words* collected by Henry Moser (1969) for a comprehensive source for selection of contrasts in one-syllable words.) Generalizations will be more effectively accomplished where minimal pairs are in the same grammatical categories, such as nouns with nouns, or verbs with verbs. Yet where such contrasts are not available, mixed grammatical forms may be tried, as previously suggested.

Once one pair of contrasts is established and generalized to related articulation, the child is ready for the second paradigmatic pair, which will be completed more rapidly. The remaining pairs can go at a faster pace.

Carry-over

Having produced standard speech forms by their own efforts, the children are now ready for carry-over procedures. These should arise out of real or play situations in which normal conversation prevails so that the meanings of the correct articulations take on pragmatic significance. The more situations in which the children use their now-standard forms, the greater will be the permanence of the therapy. Obvious activities for *soap* include washing hands, washing dolls, cleaning, making up TV ads for soap, and so on. For establishing more securely the generalizations from the model form, such as *soup, salt, seat,* etc., a series of brief play or real activities can be developed. Children can create their own practice books using pictures, words, and drawings. Counseling of parents should encourage home use of the new forms; teachers can assist in classroom practice.

The advantages of the method of meaningful minimal contrasts as well as contraindications for its use are discussed in the following sections.

VALUE

The method of meaningful minimal contrasts has the potential for reducing the time required to achieve correction because it avoids the phonological complexities of establishing phonemes in isolation and then joining them to words. Furthermore, the paradigmatic technique fosters generalization to other contrasts in the series. For example, if k/t initial contrast is used, after [kɑr] for [tɑr] is established, [ki] for [ti] and [kʌp] for [tʌp] are readily produced. For contrasts created by temporary artificial meanings, as with [bæf] in contrast to [bæθ], other final [θ] words are soon corrected, such as [tiθ], [mɑʊθ], [tuθ], and [sɑʊθ]. When the responsibility of a forced choice is placed on the clients themselves, they are the ones who alter their speech and who therefore experience delight in their own achievements. Speech spontaneity is preserved by the avoidance of drills and preoccupation with the physiological aspects of manner and place of articulation or of distinctive features. The method is also flexible enough to apply to groups as well as individual children. It is variable and adaptable to the needs of different children.

Some of these values have been reported in a study by Weiner (1981). Although he worked with only 2 subjects, he reported that "the meaningful minimal contrast method . . . was effective in reducing the frequency of phonological processes. Furthermore, there was generalization of the treatment effect to words not included in the training task." Weiner reports also that both of his subjects were able to "change their productive systems without specific articulatory instructions. . . . In addition, there was no need for specific auditory discrimination training or production practice at an isolated sound or syllable level before attempting the sound in words." The method was considered efficient "in the sense that the frequency of phonological processes in two children decreased rather dramatically in a relatively short period of time. The employment of minimal-contrast also resulted in decreases in the frequency of several sound errors . . ." (p. 102).

The meaningful minimal contrast technique may also contribute to the permanence of the corrections the children make because they are similar to the alterations children make in their speech naturally in their efforts to distinguish between speech events which occur in similar contexts.

LIMITATIONS

No clients should be placed in a position where they cannot achieve the goals of therapy even when the structure of the sessions appears to be optimum. In the therapy described, the speech-language pathologist should be certain that the child possesses no physical inability to produce the required phonemes. In any case, if frustration appears, the procedure should be quickly altered, postponed, or rescheduled.

With older children or adults, minimal contrasts using real words is without doubt the best approach, although even older children, 6 to 10, may be willing to play a make-believe meaning game, especially with computer-generated pictures. In general, however, with older children the temporary fabrication of meanings may not be indicated where pragmatic contrasts could be equally effective. For example, the therapist may stress that there are two ways to say a particular word and the differences could be role-played.

Another limitation that might be considered relates to atypical placements that yield normal or near-normal acoustic results. In these cases the problem is the visual impact on the listener and not the sound of the utterance. For example, some speakers dentalize the alveolar consonants, such as [t, d, n, l], and sometimes there is a marked tongue protrusion even though the sound is adequate acoustically. The linguadental fricatives [ð, θ] are also subject to visible placement distortions. In such instances, where the acoustic differences between normal production and the abnormal are difficult to detect, the meaningful minimal contrasts may not be applicable. Situations of this type would require the development of a system of visible contrasts. Also, there are some phonetic or acoustic deviances that do not lend themselves readily to this approach. For example, a lisp characterized by excessive sibilance is not easily managed. However, contrasts can still be used by the method of "two ways of saying something," or modified by imitation or phonetic placement.

In a sense, many language-delayed children may be included in the functional articulation therapy. The chief difference in modifying their articulation would be the need for patience, solid building up of meaningful contrasts, increasing the quantity of their communication, and adhering closely to their functional needs. Whether the method is applicable to all language-impaired people is a matter of diagnosis, prognosis, and experimentation.

It is tempting to consider the value of minimal-contrast techniques for other than functional articulation problems. With hearing-impaired children the method would have to be modified to include visible and tactile contrasts related to meaningful differences. This could prove to be an additional method in assisting such children. Applications to dyspraxias and dysarthrias may also prove useful in certain instances, but in general, the method is contraindicated without adjunct therapies because of the need to provide remediation for motor function as described in chapter 10.

The contrast method between deviant and standard syntactic or morphological forms may also be useful for language problems. Meanings would be developed for the incorrect forms, which would be placed into contrast with standard forms within the client's dialect.

These speculations may be worth inquiry. On the whole, the method of meaningful minimal contrasts may not be applicable to communication-handicapped children where physical problems interfere significantly with speech function or where speech inhibition is a basic condition. But where speech requires modification for social or linguistic reasons in functional articulation problems, the method appears to be effective.

SUMMARY

In brief, then, it is well established that natural languages have accumulated differentiation of enough signals or phonemes to constitute a code. The language of children, with which this chapter has been concerned, appears to evolve in a similar fashion. The first words require few differentiating sounds, but with the growth of language, greater demands are made for distinguishing one utterance from another. Since the utterances of children in communication are associated with meaning, even so-called linguistically inadequate word approximations are tied to meaningful associations. As a result of this fact, children are not prompted, in general, to change articulations that are functioning for them. If, therefore, children's defective utterances, preferably where one target phoneme is singled out, could be placed into meaningful contrast with the standard articulation of such utterances, the children would be placed under a logical and linguistic need to alter their articulations. In other words, if a need were created to differentiate between the defective and the standard utterances, then the children would alter the articulations of the defective utterances in the direction of the standard forms, or, in any case, attempt such alterations. This therapeutic method, referred to as the method of meaningful minimal contrasts, has been found to be clinically effective.

REFERENCES

Backus, O., & Beasley, J. (1951). *Speech therapy with children.* Cambridge: The Riverside Press.

Carroll, J. B. (1961). Language development in children. In S. Saporta (Ed.), *Psycholinguistics* (pp. 331–345). New York: Holt Rinehart and Winston.

Cooper, R. (1970). Semiology and speech, Part I. *Journal of the Speech and Hearing Association of Virginia, 12,* 6–10.

Cooper, R. (1971). Semiology and speech, Part II. *Journal of the Speech and Hearing Association of Virginia, 13,* 6–10.

Cutting, J. E., & Pisoni, D. B. (1978). An information-processing approach to speech perception.In J. F. Kavanaugh & W. Strange (Eds.), *Speech and language in the laboratory, school, and clinic* (pp. 38–64). Cambridge: MIT Press.

Daniloff, R. G., & Moll, K. I. (1968). Coarticulation of lip rounding. *Journal of Speech and Hearing Research, 11,* 707–721.

Gay, T. (1974). Some electromyographic measures of coarticulation in VCV utterances. Haskins Laboratories Status Report on Speech Research (SR-44, 137–145). New Haven, CT: Haskins Laboratories.

Graham, L., & House, A. (1971). Phonological opposition in children: A perceptual study. *Journal of the Acoustical Society of America, 49,* 559–566.

Grey, H. A., & Stunden, A. A. (1961). A preliminary study of the effect of meaning as a variable in the auditory discrimination ability of speech handicapped and normal grade school children. *ASHA, 3,* 10.

Kantner, C. E., & West, R. (1960). *Phonetics* (Rev. ed.) New York: Harper and Brothers.

Leopold, W. F. (1961). Patterning in children's language. In S. Saporta (Ed.), *Psycholinguistics.* New York: Holt, Rinehart and Winston.

Liberman, A. M., Cooper, F. S., Shankweiler, D. P., & Studdert-Kennedy, M. (1972). The perception of the speech code. In E. E. David, Jr. & P. B. Denes (Eds.), *Human communication: A unified view* (pp. 13–44). New York: McGraw Hill Book Co.

Mange, C. V. (1960). Relationships between selected auditory perceptual factors and articulation ability. *Journal of Speech and Hearing Research, 3*(1), 67–74.

McClean, M. (1973). Forward coarticulation of velar movements at marked junctural boundaries. *Journal of Speech and Hearing Research, 16,* 286–296.

McReynolds, V. (1978). Behavioral and linguistic considerations in children's speech production. In J. F. Kavanagh and W. Strange (Eds.), *Speech and language in the laboratory, school, and clinic* (pp. 127–164). Cambridge: M.I.T. Press.

Miller, G. A. (1951). *Language and communication.* New York: McGraw-Hill Book Company, Inc.

Moser, H. M. (1969). *One-syllable words.* Columbus: Charles E. Merrill Publishing Co.

Mowrer, O. H. (1958). Hearing and speaking: an analysis of language learning. *Journal of Speech and Hearing Disorders, 23*(2), 143–152.

Öhman, S. E. G. (1973). Coarticulation in VCV utterances: Spectrographic measurements. *Journal of the Acoustical Society of America, 54,* 1235–1247.

Osgood, C. E., Suci, G. J., & Tannenbaum, P. H. (1957). *The measurement of meaning.* Urbana: University of Illinois Press.

Parker, G. V. C., & Noble, C. E. (1960). Effects of experimentally-produced meaningfulness on paired-associate learning. *American Psychologist, 15,* 451.

Peters, R. W. (1963). Dimensions of perception for consonants. *Journal of the Acoustical Society of America, 35,* 1985–1989.

Ruder, K. F., Hermann, P., & Schiefelbusch, R. L. (1977). Effects of verbal imitation and comprehension training on verbal production. *Journal of Psycholinguistic Research, 6*(1), 59–72.

Singh, S. (1975). Distinctive features: A measure of consonant perception. In S. Singh (Ed.), *Measurement procedures in speech, hearing and language* (pp. 93–153). Baltimore: University Park Press.

Sommers, R. K., & Kane, A. R. (1974). The nature and remediation of functional articulation disorders. In S. Dickson (Ed.), *Communication disorders, remedial principles and practices* (pp. 104–193). Glenview, IL.: Scott, Foresman and Co.

Staats, A. W. (1968). *Learning, language, and cognition.* New York: Holt, Rinehart and Winston, Inc.

Starkweather, C. W. (1980). Speech fluency in normal children. In N. J. Lass (Ed.), *Speech and language: Advances in basic research and practice* (pp. 143–200). New York: Academic Press, Inc.

Underwood, B. J., & Schultz, R. W. (1960). *Meaningfulness and verbal learning.* New York: J. R. Lippincott Co.

Weiner, F. F. (1981). Treatment of phonological disability using the method of meaningful minimal contrast: Two case studies. *Journal of Speech and Hearing Disorders, 46,* 97–103.

Wise, C. M. (1957). *Applied phonetics.* Englewood Cliffs, NJ: Prentice Hall, Inc.

14

A Distinctive-Feature Approach to Articulation Therapy

Since the publication in 1952 of *Preliminaries to Speech Analysis: The Distinctive Features and Their Correlates* by Roman Jakobson, Gunnar Fant, and Morris Halle, momentum has been generated to discover the true nature of the entities called *phonemes*. While Jakobson, Fant, and Halle's book is very technical and difficult to apply clinically, it was preceded by a more pertinent book called *Child Language, Aphasia and Phonological Universals* (Jakobson, 1941/1968). This work contained an explanation of the manner in which children acquire speech sounds—in a step-by-step fashion. In *The Acquisition of Distinctive Features* (Blache, 1978), the distinctive-feature theory of these texts was applied to the establishment of a clinical method to correct speech sound errors. This chapter is devoted to a presentation of the manner in which distinctive-feature principles may be used to correct deviant articulation.

This discussion presumes no prior knowledge of distinctive-feature theory. It is organized in such a way that basic concepts are introduced first. This is followed by a discussion of the application of these basic principles in the clinical setting. A variety of ways in which the basic teaching format may be modified so that it may be integrated into existing remedial approaches are

Stephen E. Blache, Ph.D., is an associate professor of communication disorders and sciences at Southern Illinois University, Carbondale, Illinois.

discussed. Finally, the strengths and limitations of the approach are commented upon.

While the term *theory* may be disconcerting to some, it should be remembered that a theory is nothing more than speculation in the process of becoming scientific law. Today the scientific community is fairly certain of those sound properties that are used in human communication. Computers are being programmed to produce and recognize human speech. While arguments do develop concerning some aspects of the communication process, enough information is readily available to outline the basic elements of speech sound acquisition. From this perspective, it is possible to infer a remedial program.

RATIONALE

Basic Concepts

The term *distinctive feature*, as described in chapter 7, is a by-product of the idea that a speech sound or phoneme is a complex unit. Each speech sound has component parts, i.e., manner features, place features, voicing features, etc. At the same time, these component parts have a linguistic function: They are *used to make words different*. A speaker must have enough articulatory control to stabilize his or her sound gestures so that they result in an acoustic end product that is recognizable to other listeners in the culture (Jakobson, 1932/1962).

The terms *distinctive* and *feature* should be given equal weight. In this discussion, *feature* implies the physical postures used to generate the utterance and the subsequent acoustic properties. *Distinctive* indicates the psycholinguistic use of these properties, i.e., making words different. It implies a speaker and a listener from the same language, exchanging ideas using a motor-acoustic code. In all, the transmission of an idea involves a code that is physiologically generated, acoustically transmitted, psychologically perceived, and culturally standardized.

The Training Unit

Formally, a phoneme is *a set of concurrent motor-acoustic properties that are used to differentiate words in a given language*. While the set of properties constitutes the phoneme's structure, the use of the properties to distinguish utterances constitutes its function. The distinctive-feature approach places a great deal of emphasis on the importance of isolating a single sound property as a training goal rather than training phonemes as a whole. Because the phoneme is so complex, it is considered easier to work with the component parts, one at a time, rather than confuse the child with several different challenges at the same time. This strategy also permits the therapist to concentrate on one goal at a time.

In many traditional articulation approaches, the child has been expected to produce an ideal sound as an all-or-nothing task. Irrespective of the subtle shifts in place or manner of articulation, the therapist reinforces the child on the basis of standard articulatory ideals. The current approach, however, uses a form of progressive approximation, in which the child is reinforced for articulatory changes that represent significant shifts toward the target phoneme. By concentrating on the features, rather than the sound, the therapist is able to concentrate on one phonemic property at a time. Because of the nature of the sound system, a significant shift in a distinctive-feature property signals a sound that is different from the original utterance. The therapist is expected to assess whether or not the new sound represents phonemic progress.

The Phonemic System

The sound properties or features that separate the consonantal phonemes of American English are illustrated in Figure 14.1. Each of the lines represents a distinctive feature and a possible training goal. To organize the consonantal phonemes, the child must control six distinctive features: velopharyngeal movement (*nasality*), laryngeal vibration (*voicing*), labial/lingual production (*front*), front/back lingual production (*back*), the duration of the utterance (*continuation*), and turbulent dental friction (*stridency*). While these concepts may seem simple, the manner in which the properties may be combined to produce 19 different phonemic units results in a complex learning task. The physiological requirements of the system are substantial. Also, the acoustic signals that result from the feature combinations represent difficult learning goals. The average child takes between 4 and 6 years to gain mastery over such a system.

Using the Phonemic Model

The phonemic model in Figure 14.1 may be used in several ways. For example, it can be used to analyze the nature of sound substitution errors. If a child substitutes an [m] for an [n] sound, the child is confusing the lips with the tongue. The model can also be used to assess the severity of the substitution. A child who substitutes an [m] for [b] has a milder problem than a child who substitutes [m] for [ʃ]. The former child has forgotten to close the velum, the latter has additional problems with laryngeal inhibition, dental approximation, prolonging the signal, and two place-of-articulation errors. If one counts the lines from intersection to intersection that separate the two different substitutions, it will be noted that the former substitution involves one line; the latter, six lines. This model is called a *city-block* model. It represents the type and number of distinctive features that separate any 2 of the 19 phonemes.

In clinical practice, this model is used to assess the appropriateness of new speech sound approximations. For instance, if one is trying to teach the child the importance of the front/back lingual contrast due to a [t] for [k] substitution, the following might happen. Once the child abandons production of the [t] in attempting to produce [k], the child sometimes opts for [tʃ]. It can be noted on the model that to get from [t] to [k], the child must generate *back place*. The [tʃ] represents back place plus *continuation*. The child, then, has produced the correct feature, back tongue position, plus an extra one. As was noted earlier, the child would be reinforced at this stage, and then would be taught the significance of not prolonging the back lingual utterance. We have found that children who are not reinforced for creative, though imperfect, utterances tend to stop experimenting with sound properties.

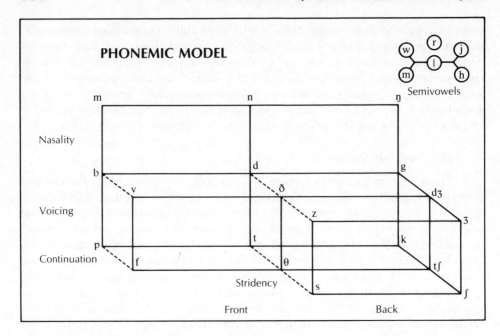

FIGURE 14.1
Configuration used to display the distinctive features that separate the consonants of American English. Each line on the city-block model represents one of
the six distinctive features. (*Source:* "Minimal Word-Pairs and Distinctive Feature Training" by S. E. Blache, in *Phonological Intervention: Concepts and
Procedures* (p. 67), M. Crary (Ed.), 1982, San Diego: College-Hill Press, Inc.
Copyright 1982 by College-Hill Press. Reprinted by permission.)

Stimulating Creative Phonemic Behavior

The main vehicle for stimulating new sound properties is the *minimal word-
pair*. We define a *minimal word-pair* as any two phonetically equivalent words that
only differ by a *single sound property*. Therapy consists of teaching the motor-
acoustic characteristics and the linguistic importance of each of these sound-pair
contrasts.

To develop word-pairs, as described in chapter 12, the therapist must
have two words with an equal number of segments. The words may be of any
length, but they both must have the same number of phonemes. In addition to
this requirement, in all but one position, the words must contain the same
sounds in the same order. The contrast may be in any position in the words, but
all other segments must be identical. Here are some examples:

[pi/bi]	*pea/bee*	2 segments, prevocalic contrast
[pɪt/bɪt]	*pit/bit*	3 segments, prevocalic contrast
[slæp/slæb]	*slap/slab*	4 segments, postvocalic contrast
[nɪpəl/nɪbəl]	*nipple/nibble*	5 segments, intervocalic contrast

As noted above, it is possible to have two matching words that are not
minimal distinctive-feature contrasts. While *pea* and *me* have an equal number

of segments and the contrast is prevocalic, the sound-pair involves two features, nasality and voicing. If a sound contrast such as this is used during discrimination testing, it will not be possible to determine which feature is being used. The child may use one or both features to perceive the difference between the pronunciation of the two words; hence, the therapist will not be sure if the child is detecting the target feature. Because of this ambiguity, it is suggested that all minimal word-pairs used in this method be restricted to single distinctive-feature contrasts.

The Semantic Referent

Once the two words have the proper phonetic balance, it is important to make sure that the child understands the ideas behind the words. Strategies for establishing meaning were discussed in chapter 13. If the child does not have the concept to be labeled, it is extremely difficult for the child to associate the motor-acoustic utterance with meaning. Although it is possible to teach the child the lexical concept in question and then do phonemic training, it is often much easier to choose other words from the child's lexicon to obtain the desired feature contrast.

METHOD

The minimal word-pairs teaching approach is organized into four basic steps (see Figure 14.2—B. *Presentation Phase*). The therapist first determines whether the child knows the concept to be used, i.e., the words to be transmitted (Step 1). In Step 2, the therapist checks to see if the child can perceive the difference in pronunciation that separates the two words. In Step 3, the therapist stimulates the child to experiment with new utterances and shapes the behavior. Finally, the therapist integrates the acquired feature into longer and longer verbal utterances and different social situations (Step 4). Because of the importance of each of these steps, they will be discussed in detail.

Step 1: Discussion of Words

Once a minimal word-pair contrast has been chosen to teach a particular distinctive feature, it is important to determine whether the child understands the words. If he or she does not, the feature properties may not be retained because the words will not be used in everyday speech. In other words, the child must possess a need to make a feature distinctive.

To check on the child's understanding, he or she is asked simple, either-or questions that can be responded to by pointing. If, for instance, a therapist is trying to teach a child the distinctive difference between the expressives *T* and *key* (front/back lingual contrast), the therapist must determine whether the pictures are relevant to the child (see Figure 14.3a). The child is asked:
"Which one opens the door?"
"Which one is a letter of the alphabet?"
"Which one goes into a lock?"
"Which one do you write?", etc.

MINIMAL WORD-PAIRS ORIENTATION

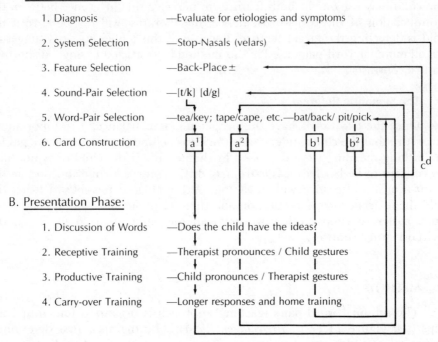

A. Preparation Phase:

  1. Diagnosis   —Evaluate for etiologies and symptoms

  2. System Selection   —Stop-Nasals (velars)

  3. Feature Selection   —Back-Place ±

  4. Sound-Pair Selection   —[t/k] [d/g]

  5. Word-Pair Selection   —tea/key; tape/cape, etc.—bat/back/ pit/pick

  6. Card Construction   a¹   a²   b¹   b²

B. Presentation Phase:

  1. Discussion of Words   —Does the child have the ideas?

  2. Receptive Training   —Therapist pronounces / Child gestures

  3. Productive Training   —Child pronounces / Therapist gestures

  4. Carry-over Training   —Longer responses and home training

FIGURE 14.2
Protocol procedure for organizing a minimal word-pairs therapy program. (a = change in word-pairs; b = change in position of contrast and/or sound-pair context; c = change in distinctive feature; d = change in sound system.) (*Source:* "Minimal Word-Pairs and Distinctive Feature Training" by S. E. Blache, in *Phonological Intervention: Concepts and Procedures* (p. 72), M. Crary (Ed.). 1982, San Diego: College-Hill Press, Inc. Copyright 1982 by College-Hill Press. Reprinted by permission.)

If it is known that the child can understand the questions and he or she points to the wrong picture, the child simply may not know the word ideas, or the pictures may be inappropriately drawn.

  If a child does not know the letters of the alphabet, *T* may be a poor choice. By using a cup and saucer with a tea bag, the therapist can use the same phonetic contrast with a different semantic referent, or [t] and [k] can be put into other pairs to serve the same function, i.e., to elicit the front/back lingual contrast. Word contrasts such as *tape/cape, ten/Ken,* and *told/cold* will serve just as well because the ultimate training goal is the distinctive feature.

Step 2: Discrimination Testing and Training

  Once the therapist is sure the child knows the ideas to be labeled phonetically, the child is examined for perceptual awareness of the distinctive

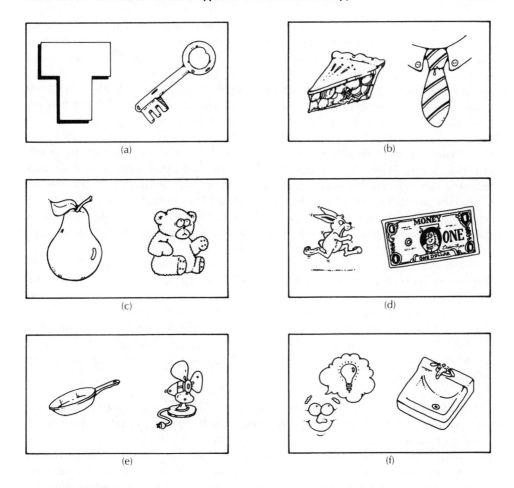

FIGURE 14.3
Exemplars illustrating six different distinctive feature contrasts. (a = front/back lingual; b = labial/lingual; c = voiced/voiceless; d = nasal/nonnasal; e = continued/interrupted; f = strident/mellow.) (*Source:* "Minimal Word-Pairs and Distinctive Feature Training" by S. E. Blache, in *Phonological Intervention: Concepts and Procedures* (p. 65), M. Crary (Ed.), 1982, San Diego: College-Hill Press, Inc. Copyright 1982 by College-Hill Press. Reprinted by permission.)

feature. The therapist speaks the two words, repeating them in random order. Each time the word is spoken, the child is asked to point to the word that has been said. If the child points correctly *seven consecutive times*, the therapist can be fairly sure that the child hears the distinctive feature difference. The probability of a child simply guessing the correct words is so low that this possibility can be discounted. However, it should be remembered there may be more than one perceptual cue for some phonemic distinctions, such as voiced–voiceless. For final consonants, vowel duration will be different in the voiced and voiceless context, so that cues may be provided even in the absence of the final phoneme. For example, the words *bat* and *bad* are produced as /bæt/ and /bæːd/ and may remain /bæ/ and /bæː/ when /t/ or /d/ is omitted.

Caution.   Children seem to have an almost standard reaction to this test. If the therapist uses a criterion much beyond seven consecutive correct responses, they tend to become bored with the task and may not attend. As attention wanders, discrimination errors will appear to occur. However, these errors are due to attention span and not discrimination ability. Once children demonstrate that they can perform correctly, seven times in a row, they have proved their skill. They are ready to move ahead to a more challenging task.

Program Modifications.   Sometimes a child will not be able to reach criterion levels. When this occurs, the therapist uses other word-pair contrasts with the same distinctive feature. If this happens repeatedly, poor discrimination skills are being revealed. The child should be encouraged to become a better listener through use of the minimal word-pairs as training items in a discrimination program. In this case, correct discrimination responses are reinforced, as with other auditory discrimination programs.

On occasion, a child will exhibit poor auditory memory span. The child does not remember significant linguistic information. In cases like this, the therapist pronounces one of the two words, but delays the visual presentation of the pictures. In the interim period, the child must remember the target word, and then demonstrate this retention when the two pictures are displayed. The delay times may be set to fit the needs of the individual child. Correct auditory memory responses are reinforced, as with other auditory memory programs.

Summary.   In the second step of the technique, the child is channeled into feature production training after demonstrating perceptual awareness, or the program is modified to strengthen auditory discrimination and/or auditory memory skills. The minimal word-pair that isolates the distinctive feature can be used in three ways: (a) discrimination testing, (b) discrimination training, and/or (c) auditory memory training. The important thing is to isolate the goal behavior, i.e., the feature to be perceived, discriminated, and/or retained.

Step 3: Production Training

There is a fourth use for the minimal word-pair: the elicitation of creative articulatory behavior—new sound gestures. Once the child demonstrates that he or she perceives the distinctive feature, the child is expected to demonstrate the use and control of the feature.

In this step, the child is told that he or she is to "be the teacher." The child is instructed to say the words, and the therapist is to point to the word that has been said. Due to the feature selection process, the child always can pronounce one of the words, but is unable to pronounce the alternate word. The child can be expected to exhibit the following standard pattern.

Demonstrating Deficit.   The child begins by pronouncing the word he or she can say. The therapist points to the word. Then the child attempts to say the word he or she is unable to produce correctly. The child expects the therapist's finger to move to the other picture. However, the second utterance sounds like the first. The therapist indicates this fact by touching the first picture again. The child, in most cases, will immediately point to the other picture, and tell the therapist he or she is wrong. The therapist then indicates that he/she heard the first word. The therapist then offers to help the child say the other word so that the finger will move. The therapist is helping the child "play the phonemic game."

Working at the Word Level.   Most children are motivated to get the finger to move to the other picture. The therapist then uses traditional cues to elicit the distinctive feature property. However, it is important to elicit a word response because a sound spoken in isolation is unnatural and too abstract. Furthermore, connected speech is extremely rapid. The sentence *Joe took father's shoe bench out*, a 17-segment expression, is generally said in less than 2 seconds. A sound spoken in isolation produces gestures of abnormal length. In the distinctive-feature approach, the child is being taught to say words that communicate meaning. When the therapist has cued the child properly, and the word is spoken correctly, the child often exhibits satisfaction in the accomplishment with a broad smile.

Immediate Reinforcement.   Immediately upon hearing the correct pronunciation of the feature, the therapist reinforces the child. This is done by a smile, praise, and the movement of the finger to the picture the child intended. The child is encouraged to practice the utterance while it is fresh in mind. The child then alternates the pronunciation of the two words. When the therapist is certain the child has the proper articulatory control, the program is expanded to ensure transfer into syntactical and social stiuations.

Isolating the Articulatory Goal.   It should be noted that the therapist must develop a sensitivity for the object of reinforcement, i.e., the distinctive feature. In this approach, a decision based on correct versus incorrect sound approximations is not accurate enough. The therapist must isolate the goal behavior with great precision. The child's creative attempts must be analyzed for their implications. If the utterance contains the desired property, it is reinforced. The therapist must think in terms of the features instead of the target sound.

Step 4: Carry-Over Training

Once the child demonstrates the ability to control the articulatory system and pronounce the desired word, the target word is put at the end of longer and longer expressions. Beginning with two-word expressions, the child is encouraged to say the target word in conjunction with the indefinite article *a*, and then the definite article *the*. This can be done by using an orthographic representation of the words *a* or *the* and placing them next to the minimal word-pair pictures. Both the target word and the distinctive-feature "lure" word are elicited in the practice session. The child practices saying "*a T*" and "*a key*." Using both minimal pair-words keeps the negative practice component in the task.

The indefinite article *a* is generally introduced before the definite article *the* because the former is less complex segmentally than the latter, i.e., V versus CV. If a child has difficulty at this stage, consideration should be given to modifying the program to include standard coarticulatory sequencing in the position of the definite and indefinite articles (McDonald, 1964). Words that end with all the basic sounds of American English are introduced in place of *a* or *the* preceding the target word and the lure. Therapists should concentrate on two considerations: (a) making the two-word expressions as natural as possible, and (b) reinforcing only the feature in the target word.

After the child pronounces two-word expressions, longer and longer utterances are tried. The three-word carrier *Touch the . . .* and the four-word carrier *Point to the . . .* permit the child to speak in a meaningful way and still practice the production of the feature. As the expressions become longer and longer, the child must remember to use the appropriate feature in an automatic way. This device has also been used in traditional therapy.

The Social Situation.   While the children are learning to talk in a meaningful way in the clinic, it is expected that they also practice at home. Each child has a word book containing all the target words that the child has learned. The parents are encouraged to set aside family time for the recitation of the words—generally at the end of the evening meal. The parents serve as motivators and monitors of the child's speech. At no time are the parents encouraged to correct the child's speech. Rather, the parents are instructed to praise the child for good word pronunciation. If the words are said incorrectly, the parents are asked to say nothing to the child, but are requested to report the situation to the clinician at the next therapy session.

Modifying Home Programs.   In general, parents are not equipped to perform a phonetic analysis on a particular utterance. They do not know when a creative utterance represents phonemic progress. After the parents report unusual articulations, the therapist analyzes the utterance(s) and informs the parents whether to reinforce or not. At the same time, parents are encouraged to provide positive reinforcement whenever possible. At the beginning of each therapy session, the clinician asks the parents about the child's progress. If parents lack the motivation or concern to help the child, an educational counseling program is instituted to develop better motivational reinforcement for the child and improve monitoring behavior on the part of the parent. Sometimes children learn skills in the clinic and do not use them at home. The involvement of parents is seen as crucial to avoid this type of carry-over problem.

Relationship to Current Approaches

The minimal word-pairs technique isn't really an alternative to current practice. Rather, it is an integration and streamlining of traditional techniques. The procedure highlights the importance of using a holistic approach to therapy. It stresses the psycholinguistic function of the feature, but also emphasizes the development of proper placement and auditory discrimination skills. The therapist serves as a representative of the linguistic culture and provides feedback as to the adequacy of phonetic skills—in a phonemic context.

Stimulation Versus Training.   The distinctive-feature approach is a stimulation program rather than a complete training program in that it provides a context in which learning can occur, but does not teach the child how to produce the sound. It is assumed that given the proper circumstances, children will seek to discover articulatory skills. This concept has its roots in Montessorian education. When the underlying problem is due to inadequate learning, the minimal word-pairs discovery process tends to be reinforcing in and of itself because the child can immediately use what he has learned for communication.

However, some children are prevented from developing natural articulatory skills by organic or structural problems. In such cases, the minimal word-pairs technique tends to be converted to a training program. The therapist implements management procedures to correct structural/organic defects. The basic program is modified to strengthen general motoric skills, improve auditory retention skills, and develop better listening habits, and when the child lacks the capacity to learn simply through discovery, reinforcement paradigms are introduced and/or augmented.

The distinctive feature encapsulated in the minimal word-pairs contrast is the cornerstone of the system. A distinctive-feature orientation forces the therapist to select one articulatory behavior at a time (feature) and teach the distinctive function of that feature.

Organizing the Distinctive-Feature Program

Before a distinctive-feature program is instituted, the therapist should check for a variety of factors that may necessitate modifications in the program. As a minimum, the therapist should check for a second language in the home, a regional dialect, a poor speech model, and the possibility that a child is using an idioglossia. In addition to this, each child should be evaluated for inadequate hearing and functionally inadequate articulatory structures. The therapist should have some indication of the child's intellectual capacity and the motivation to develop communication skills. Finally, it is often helpful to test the child's discrimination skills and auditory memory span. Deficits in any of these areas call for program modifications. Experience has shown that approximately two of every five children seen will require special programming.

Getting Started.   In the past, it has been popular to select a single distinctive feature for training and attempt to teach this feature in many different sound-pair contexts. The current approach restricts the feature selection process to specific sound classes. Developmental studies have shown that certain sound classes stabilize before others. Stops and nasals, for instance, stabilize in the child's repertoire before sibilants. The features are grouped by sound-pair contrast into six major sound classes: primitive, vocalic, stop/nasal, semivowel, continuant, sibilant. However, problems with only four of these classes tend to be seen in the age range between 4 years 9 months and 8 years. The earlier two classes represent children who have not begun to develop speech, or those that have significant problems with vowels. Both of these levels of development are expected to be completed by the third year. This discussion will concentrate on the four later-developing stages.

To develop a distinctive-feature program, the therapist must determine the level of development of the phonemic system. Once this is accomplished, sound-pairs and features are selected to rebuild or extend the existing phonemic system. Minimal word-pairs are selected and picture cards are drawn to elicit the desired distinctive features.

The Quick Test.   Level of development may be determined through the Quick Test (see Table 14.1). In this test, the child is asked to pronounce 67 words elicited through picture stimuli. The words represent the vocabulary items most commonly used in articulation testing. These 67 words represent a prevocalic, intervocalic, and postvocalic sampling of 25 consonantal and semivowel sounds (cf. Blache, 1978, Appendix J.) By design, each of the 25 sounds is tested one to three times. The child is graded on the number of times a sound is misarticulated, and the number is compared to the performance of other children of the same age. If the child misarticulates a sound more often than other children of the same age, the sound is considered defective—until evidence is exhibited to the contrary. This operation is repeated for each of the 25 sounds. This permits the formulation of some idea about the adequacy of the entire phonemic system.

Determining the Level of Development.   It is this overall pattern that is of greatest importance in the establishment of a level of phonemic development. The 25 sounds and the 67 words used to test those sounds are shown in Table 14.1. The sounds have been categorized and arranged in developmental order, i.e., stop/nasals then semivowels, continuants then sibilants. The therapist will determine what is the earliest sound system that needs stimulation.

Scoring Sounds.   To make this decision, the child is asked to pronounce the test words. Only one sound in each word is scored. The therapist notes the number of times the child misarticulates the sound. Referring to the appropriate age group, the therapist circles the symbol beneath the number of times the sound is in error. This is done for each of the 25 speech sounds. If a (*) is circled, it indicates a performance equivalent to that of the lower 5% of the age group. If a (?) is circled, it indicates a performance equivalent to that of the lower 6 to 10% of the age group. The (P) symbol indicates a performance that is appropriate for the child's age.

Estimating Phonemic Level.   After the performance on each of the 25 sounds has been evaluated, the therapist looks for two or more significant errors in the earliest sound class, the stop/nasals. If two or more significant errors are present, this is where therapy is begun. If no significant defect is found with the stop/nasal system, the therapist proceeds to the next developing sound system, i.e., the semivowel system. This operation is repeated until a level of development has been selected.

Mild Phonemic Problems.   In those cases where only one defective sound is found in a system, or there is a limited number of defective sounds, the therapeutic goal becomes one of sound stabilization rather than system reconstruction. In cases such as these, it is often helpful to deep-test the

TABLE 14.1
The Quick Test

				Age Groups				
Class	Symbol	Spelling	Test Words	4:9–4:11 Errors 0 1 2 3	5:0–5:11 0 1 2 3	6:0–6:11 0 1 2 3	7:0–7:11 0 1 2 3	8:0–8:11 0 1 2 3
	[m]	m	monkey, hammer, broom	p * * *	p * * *	p * * *	p * * *	p * * *
	[n]	n	knife, penny/money, moon	p * * *	p * * *	p * * *	p * * *	p * * *
	[ŋ]	ng	finger, ring	P P P	P P ?	P ? *	P ? *	P ? *
Stops and Nasals	[p]	p	pig, paper, cup	p * * *	p * * *	p * * *	p * * *	p * * *
	[t]	t	table, potato, boat	P P * *	P ? * *	P ? * *	P ? * *	P ? * *
	[k]	c,k	cat, cookie, duck	p * * *	p * * *	p * * *	p * * *	p * * *
	[b]	b	bicycle/bike, baby, bathtub	P ? * *	P ? * *	P ? * *	P ? * *	P ? * *
	[d]	d	dog, ladder, bed	P P * *	P P * *	P ? * *	P ? * *	P ? * *
	[g]	g	gun, wagon, egg	P ? * *	P ? * *	P * * *	P * * *	P * * *
	[hw]	wh	whistle	P P	P P	P P	P P	P ?
	[w]	w	window, flowers	P P *	P P *	P * *	P * *	P * *
Semivowels	[l]	l	lamp, balloon, ball	P P P ?	P P ? *	P * * *	P * * *	P * * *
	[r]	r	rabbit, carrot, car	P P P P	P P P ?	P P ? ?	P ? ? *	P * * *
	[j]	y	yellow, yoyo	P ? *	P * *	P * *	P * *	P *
	[h]	h	horse	P *	P *	P *	P *	P *
	[f]	f,ph	fan, telephone, leaf	P * * *	P * * *	P * * *	P * * *	P * * *
	[v]	v	vacuum, television/TV, stove	P P P ?	P P P *	P P P *	P P * *	P * * *
Continuants	[θ]	th	thumb, toothbrush, mouth	P P P P	P P P P	P P P P	P P P ?	P P P *
	[ð]	th	this/that, feathers, smooth	P P P ?	P P P ?	P P * *	P P * *	P * * *
	[tʃ]	ch	chair, matches, watch	P P P ?	P P ? ?	P ? * *	P ? * *	P * * *
	[dʒ]	j,g	jumping, pajamas/PJs, orange	P P P ?	P P ? *	P ? * *	P * * *	P * * *
	[s]	s,c	sun, glasses, house	P P P P	P P P P	P P P P	P P P ?	P P ? ?
Sibilants	[z]	z	zebra, scissors, eyes	P P P P	P P P P	P P P P	P P P ?	P P ? ?
	[ʃ]	sh	shoe, dishes, fish	P P P ?	P P ? *	P ? * *	P ? * *	P * * *
	[ʒ]	g	measure, beige	P P P	P P P	P P ?	P P *	P P *

Note: Speech sounds are tested only in the contexts given. (P = appropriate for age, i.e., *pass;* * = performance equal to the lower 5% of population, i.e., *failure;* ? = performance equal to lower 6 to 10% of population, i.e., *questionable.*).

defective sound in many different coarticulatory contexts. The therapist can then determine which features in the defective sound are most often in error and rank them. If there are several defective sounds, the earliest developing sound is evaluated first. A therapy program is designed for the particular sound. At the completion of the first speech sound program, the child's phonemic system is reevaluated and the former evaluation process repeated.

The Sound Systems.   After the completion of the Quick Test, the therapist has a good idea of where the child stands developmentally. Those children who have difficulty with two or more sounds in the stop/nasal system, [m n ŋ b d g p t k], are treated according to Therapeutic Model 1 (see Figure 14.4). Children with two or more errors in the semivowel system, [hw w l r j h], are taught with reference to Therapeutic Model 2 (see Figure 14.5). Children with difficulties with the continuant system, [f v θ ð tʃ dʒ], or the sibilant system, [s z ʃ ʒ], are treated in accordance with Models 3 and 4, respectively (see Figures 14.6 and 14.7). Before each of these models is discussed in detail, some general comments about the nature of the models are in order.

The Developmental Models.   Each model represents a progessive step in distinctive feature organization. Models 1, 3, and 4 represent an expansion of the consonantal system. Model 2 represents the stabilization of the semivowel system. It is envisioned that the consonantal structure and the semivowel structure are similar in character, but the sound systems are used sequentially in speech, and tend to be somewhat independent of one another.

Infantemes.   On each model, the distinctive-feature development has been illustrated by means of lines that separate the circles. The circles represent vague phonemic classes called *infantemes* (Albright & Albright, 1958). The *infanteme* is a set of motor-acoustic properties that are used to make words different *in the language of the child.* In other words, infantemes are childlike phonemes. When a child has incomplete mastery over the distinctive-feature system of the adult, the child appears to substitute one sound for another. Actually, when a child does not understand a distinctive feature, two or more sounds tend to be interchangeable. One of the sound elements is more probable than another, i.e., is more natural. This gives the appearance of a purposeful action of replacing one sound with another. However, careful examination of such behavior in repeated samples reveals confusion, rather than replacement. The two or more sounds tend to be in what linguists call *free variation.* Those sounds that are likely to be in free variation are grouped within the circle.

As will be noted in Model 1 (Figure 14.4), the voiceless, front-lingual infanteme has three free-varying elements, [t θ s]. Before the child understands the importance of continued production and dental airflow, these three sounds tend to be interchangeable. The sound element that is underlined is the most probable gesture to be stabilized, for it represents the most pertinent or natural utterance for the class. It can be seen that phonemes become progressively separated as we move through the models.

Acceptable Free Variation.   It can also be noted that the free-varying elements represent acceptable creative gestures for a given level of development.

For instance, if the child is learning the importance of the use of the lips versus the use of the tongue in a voiceless context, [p] may be contrasted with any of the three sounds in the front-lingual class. The child is more likely to use [t], but [θ] and [s] are also lingual utterances. As each system becomes better developed, greater rigor is applied when accepting variants. When the system is fully developed, as in the completion of Model 4, no free variation is expected; all the distinctive features have been learned. At this point the child's infantemes have become phonemes.

Order of Reconstruction.   Small arabic numerals may be noted next to the specific feature lines. These represent an optimal order for distinctive-feature selection. However, it is not necessary to teach each feature. The therapist begins by selecting the appropriate model for the child's level of development. The defective sounds in the center of the circles, as noted on the Quick Test, are circled in contrasting color. Each line that connects a defective infanteme to another infanteme is marked. After all the appropriate lines have been noted, the arabic numerals are recorded, from smallest to largest. This is the order of the first, provisional distinctive-feature program.

Maximal Contrast.   In general, the features are taught on a continuum beginning with the greatest physiological and acoustical contrast and moving to finer distinctions. This technique is called *maximal contrast*. The features and feature combinations have an inherent or natural hierarchy (Jakobson, 1941/1968) in which the pairs are ordered in such a way as to minimize changing the distinctive features. This is done by using similar sound-pair contrasts that are based on the same differential property. When therapy programs have been revised due to a lack of progress, carrier words are changed before sound-pairs, sound-pairs before features, and features before sound systems.

Interactive Therapy.   In interactive therapy the child is expected to develop initial command over a word utterance within a maximum period of 5 minutes. If progress has not been demonstrated by this point, another word-pair should be chosen and trained. Stimulation of the feature in a particular sound-pair contrast should continue in enough word-pair contexts until the therapist is confident the speech sounds are consistently differentiated.

Modifying a program within the confines of the models is strongly encouraged. If the therapist has a phonetic rationale for changing the prescribed order, he or she is generally thinking in distinctive-feature terms and considering the needs of a particular child. Therapeutic progress, of course, is the bench mark at all times. In this approach, top priority is given to rational rather than rote behavior for both the clinician and the child.

Synopsis.   Each line that has been noted represents a distinctive-feature contrast to be learned in a specific sound-pair context. The entire procedure is quite simple. It can be outlined as follows:

1.   Administer the Quick Test.
2.   Note the earliest sound system that has two or more errors.

3. Refer to the appropriate model and circle the defective sounds.
4. Note all the distinctive feature lines that join and connect to the defective sounds.
5. Note the arabic numerals on those lines to develop an order for training.
6. Apply the basic minimal word-pairs technique and monitor progress by means of the model.

These models are designed to help the therapist think in distinctive-feature terms. They yield a complex perspective for the individual speech sounds, provide a developmental sequencing for feature selection, and give a natural training order.

Model 1: The Stop/Nasal System. This system has nine infantemes developed through the comprehension and control of four distinctive features (see Figure 14.4). The nasal/nonnasal contrast and the voiced/voiceless contrast establish a three-point manner-of-articulation dimension, i.e., nasal, voice, voiceless.

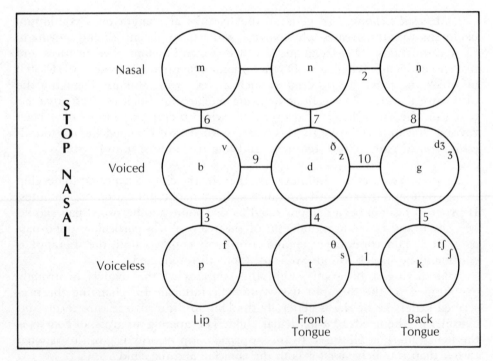

FIGURE 14.4

Model 1: The stop nasal system. The nine different infantemes of this system are organized by means of four different distinctive features; labial/lingual, front/back lingual, voiced/voiceless, and nasal/non-nasal. The arabic numerals represent the most typical training order. (*Source:* "Minimal Word-Pairs and Distinctive Feature Training" by S. E. Blache, in *Phonological Intervention: Concepts and Procedures* (p. 85), M. Crary (Ed.), 1982, San Diego: College-Hill Press, Inc. Copyright 1982 by College-Hill Press. Reprinted by permission.)

The labial/lingual contrast and the front/back lingual contrast establish a three-point place of articulation dimension, i.e., labial, front-lingual, back-lingual.

   Acoustic Standards.   In this level of development, the child is expected to be aware of the acoustic properties that represent the positioning of the velopharyngeal port mechanism and the vibratory state of the larynx. In addition to this, the child must be sensitive to those acoustic properties that signal place-of-articulation characteristics, i.e., formant transitions.

   Physiological Standards.   Physiologically, the child must develop control of sound gestures that could be characterized as labial, apico-lingual, and dorso-lingual in character. In other words, the child must use three distinctive positions to signal place characteristics. In addition to that, the child must be able to control voice onset time (VOT) with enough skill to make the presence or absence of voicing readily identifiable. Finally, the child must be able to open and close the velopharyngeal port with purposeful regularity.

Stop/Nasal Sound-Pair Order

No.	Pair	Feature	Sample Words
1.	[t – k]	front/back lingual	tea/key, tape/cape, ten/Ken
2.	[n – ŋ]	front/back lingual	win/wing, fan/fang, ton/tongue
3.	[p – b]	voiced/voiceless	pea/bee, pig/big, pat/bat
4.	[t – d]	voiced/voiceless	toe/doe, time/dime, tot/dot
5.	[k – g]	voiced/voiceless	curl/girl, coat/goat, cap/gap
6.	[b – m]	nasal/non-nasal	beet/meat, bat/mat, bike/Mike
7.	[d – n]	nasal/non-nasal	D/knee, deck/neck, dot/knot
8.	[g – ŋ]	nasal/non-nasal	wig/wing, bag/bang, log/long
9.	[b – d]	labial/lingual	big/dig, bark/dark, bow/dough
10.	[d – g]	front/back lingual	deer/gear, date/gate, doe/go

If significant deviations are found with [p t m n], the child's vowel system should be examined. Any vowel error is considered significant past 3 years of age. If significant vowel errors are apparent and/or the child does not distinguish between the lips and the tongue, refer to the early developmental programming described in *The Acquisition of Distinctive Features* (Blache, 1978, pp. 327–331).

   Model 2: The Semivowel System.   This system has six infantemes developed through the comprehension and control of four distinctive features (see Figure 14.5). The labial/lingual contrast and the front/back lingual contrast establish a three-point place-of-articulation dimension, i.e., labial, front-lingual and back-lingual. The voiced/voiceless contrast and the retroflex/nonretroflex contrast serve as the manner-of-articulation dimension.

   Acoustic Standards.   Acoustically, the semivowels have much in common with the diphthongs and continuants. At this stage the child is expected to be able to perceive formant changes that signal extreme vocal-tract closure in a front-mid-back position of the oral cavity (see Figure 14.5). In addition to that,

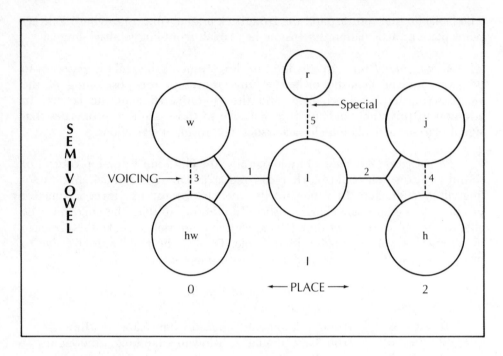

FIGURE 14.5

Model 2: The semivowel system. The six different infantemes of this system are organized by means of four different distinctive features; labial/lingual, front/back lingual, voiced/voiceless, and retroflex/nonretroflex. The arabic numerals represent the most typical training order. (*Source:* "Minimal Word-Pairs and Distinctive Feature Training" by S. E. Blache, in *Phonological Intervention: Concepts and Procedures* (p. 87), M. Crary (Ed.), 1982, San Diego: College-Hill Press, Inc. Copyright 1982 by College-Hill Press. Reprinted by permission.)

the child must be aware of the acoustic properties associated with the special tongue motions for the [r] sound and the vibratory state of the larynx.

Physiological Standards.   The child is expected to partially close, then open the vocal tract with enough regularity to signal labial closure, front-lingual closure and back-lingual closure. At the same time, the child is expected to be able to control laryngeal tone in conjunction with these movements. This must be done with enough regularity to signal a voiced/voiceless distinction. This latter component, however, is of limited importance to the language and seldom produces significant difficulties for this sound class. Finally, the child has to be able to curl the tongue in a rapid fashion with no lingual-alveolar contact.

Clinical Correlates.   The features are taught in a front-to-back direction, already observed with the stop/nasal class. Some 85% of the problems with this class tend to be internal in nature; i.e., sounds within the class tend to be confused with each other, rather than with sounds outside of the class. At times, some children will leave this system in an incomplete state of development and then develop the consonantal system in full. These children are sometimes referred to by the clinical label "lallers." This label is unfortunate because it does not specify the nature of the phonetic deviation. The often-heard statement "All I see are /l/, /r/, and /s/ problems" indicates that all /l/ or /s/ problems are alike. This may betray a lack of in-depth differential testing for causal agents and a sketchy understanding of phonetics—especially in the area of close transcription.

Semivowel Sound-Pair Order

No. Pair	Feature	Sample Words
1. [w/hw – l]	labial/lingual	wet/let, weed/lead, win/Lynn
2. [l – j/h]	front/back lingual	Lou/you, less/yes, limb/him
3. [w – hw]	voiced/voiceless	we/Whee!, nonsense words (optional)
4. [j – h]	voiced/voiceless	you/who, Yah!/hay, yellow/hello
5. [l – r]	retroflex/nonretroflex	led/red, low/row, list/wrist

Kantner and West (1969) indicate that there are nine different types of "r" sounds in American English. If one wishes to take such a microscopic view of this sound, the therapist has only to define the exact nature of the difference between the variants, and integrate these differences into the semivowel system. As will be noted, the models are very broad in nature. They are designed to illustrate the most prominent phonetic properties used in everyday communication. This should not prevent the therapist from developing finer models to eradicate unpleasant distortions. It should be noted that, at this microscopic level of training, the child is being trained to be more than a linguistic communicator. He or she is being trained to be a phonetician in the most subtle sense. Modifying pictures of speech sound targets to indicate correct versus incorrect approximations of the same word has been a traditional technique in the field and will not be expanded on here.

Model 3: The Continuant System.   This system has six infantemes appended to the previous nine infantemes of the stop/nasal system. These six new utterances are developed through the introduction of a new distinctive feature, continued/interrupted, and the generalization of place and manner features already observed in the stop/nasal system (see Figure 14.6; Figure 14.4).

Acoustic Standards.   The continuant system is acoustically similar to the stop/nasal class in that it makes use of voicing and place-of-articulation properties. This entire class has a prolonged voicing marker through a sustained noise signal. Acoustically, the child is expected to detect place-of-articulation characteristics on the basis of the dominant spectral features in conjunction with the presence or absence of a periodic tone.

Physiological Standards.   The child must learn to sustain a physical posture and force air through a particular vocal-tract constriction. Unlike the stop/nasals,

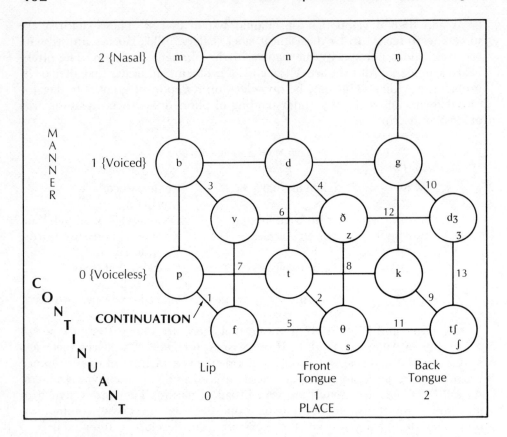

FIGURE 14.6
Model 3: The continuant system. The six new infantemes of the consonantal system are organized by means of four different distinctive features; continued/interrupted, labial/lingual, front/back lingual, and voiced/voiceless. The arabic numerals represent the most typical training order. (*Source:* "Minimal Word-Pairs and Distinctive Feature Training" by S. E. Blache, in *Phonological Intervention: Concepts and Procedures* (p. 88), M. Crary (Ed.), 1982, San Diego: College-Hill Press, Inc. Copyright 1982 by College-Hill Press. Reprinted by permission.)

the continuants require a dominant secondary vibrator (noise source) that results in sustained aspiration. At the same time, this effect must be maintained in the presence or absence of voicing. While the distinctive-feature properties common to the stop/nasal and continuant/noncontinuant system are very similar, it would be incorrect to consider them identical. The physiological and acoustical manifestations of voicing and place of articulation have more in common with each other within the respective systems than they do across the systems. This is one major reason why the distinctive features are taught within sound classes, rather than throughout the system, one feature at a time.

Clinical Correlates. Children who have not mastered the continuation feature (and the concomitant need to reevaluate voicing and place properties) tend to replace the continuants with the stop/nasal sounds. In process terminology, this is referred to as *stopping*. Children who exhibit this form of replacement have been called "baby talkers." While the speech is recognizable it retains many infantile characteristics. By the time this system has been fully stabilized, only the sibilants tend to be replaced or confused.

Unlike the stop/nasal development that required the learning of four distinctive features, the continuant system requires the acquisition of one new feature and the generalization of phonemic concepts that have been previously acquired. In essence, the development of the stop/nasals is seen primarily as feature acquisition; the development of continuants, primarily as feature generalization.

Continuant Sound-Pair Order

No. Pair	Feature	Sample Words
1. [p–f]	continuant/interrupted	pin/fin, pan/fan, pour/four
2. [t–θ]	continuant/interrupted	tree/three, tie/thigh, torn/thorn
3. [b–v]	continuant/interrupted	bee/*V*, base/vase, bat/vat
4. [d–ð]	continuant/interrupted	doze/those, ladder/lather, *D*/thee
5. [f–θ]	labial/lingual	free/three, fin/thin, fought/thought
6. [v–ð]	labial/lingual	*V*s/these, van/than, nonsense words
7. [f–v]	voiced/voiceless	fat/vat, fan/van, face/vase
8. [θ–ð]	voiced/voiceless	teeth/teethe, nonsense words
9. [k–tʃ]	continuant/interrupted	keys/cheese, kick/chick, cane/chain
10. [g–dʒ]	continuant/interrupted	Gail/jail, goose/juice, ghoul/jewel
11. [θ–tʃ]	front/back lingual	thief/chief, thick/chick, thin/chin
12. [ð–dʒ]	front/back lingual	nonsense words
13. [tʃ–dʒ]	voiced/voiceless	cello/jello, cherry/Jerry, chunk/junk

A careful examination of the training order of the distinctive features and sound-pairs will reveal two internal stages of stabilization. This training order presumes that children will introduce the continuation feature in the anterior place position. The anterior [f], [v], [θ] and [ð] sounds are integrated before the posterior affricates, [tʃ] and [dʒ]. Some children, however, will stabilize the latter sounds before the former.

Model 4: The Sibilant System.   The sibilant system has four infantemes appended to the previous stop/nasal/continuant system. These four new utterances are developed through the introduction of a new distinctive feature, strident/mellow, and the generalization of place and manner features already observed in the continuant system (see Figure 14.7; cf. Figure 14.6).

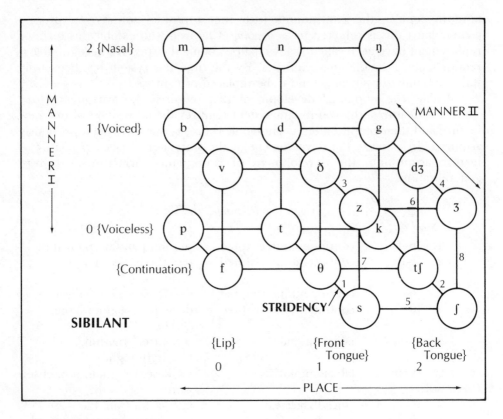

FIGURE 14.7
Model 4: The sibilant system. The four new infantemes of the consonantal system are organized by means of three different distinctive features; strident/mellow, front/back lingual, and voiced/voiceless. The arabic numerals represent the most typical training order. (*Source:* "Minimal Word-Pairs and Distinctive Feature Training" by S. E. Blache, in *Phonological Intervention: Concepts and Procedures* (p. 89), M. Crary (Ed.), 1982, San Diego: College-Hill Press, Inc. Copyright 1982 by College-Hill Press. Reprinted by permission.)

Acoustic Standards. The final step in the organizational process is reflected in Model 4. Acoustically, the sibilants require highly variable noise to make them distinct from their counterparts in the continuant system. Sibilants must vary in terms of frequency and intensity. This variability is detected by the ear as noisy and unpleasant. It has been given the name *stridency*. To hear this difference, compare a prolonged utterance of [θ:] and [s:]. The former is mellow; the latter is strident.

Physiological Standards. Stridency is produced by air being forced through constricted dental gaps. As the air passes through these small openings at a high rate of speed, the air particles bounce against each other in random fashion, resulting in a great deal of acoustic irregularity. When the tongue initiates or obstructs this air flow, the acoustic signal produced is less variable, and the sound is perceived as mellow.

Clinical Correlates.   The inability to stabilize the sibilant system has a clinical counterpart, i.e., lisping behavior. In Figure 14.7, it can be seen that the interdental lisp [θ/s] and the lateral lisp [ļ/s] or [ʃ/s] have distinctive-feature definitions. The former type of lisp is based on a stridency error; the latter, on place of articulation. Again, as with the [r], it is possible to develop more microscopic models to attack the [s] at the fine-transcription level. However, consideration should be given to the ultimate goal of the clinical program, the production of sound properties of sufficient quality to carry differential information in an undistracting manner.

Sibilant Sound-Pair Order

No. Pair	Feature	Sample Words
1. [θ–s]	strident/mellow	think/sink, thick/sick, thumb/sum
2. [tʃ–ʃ]	strident/mellow	chip/ship, chop/shop, chew/shoe
3. [ð–z]	strident/mellow	teethe/tease, nonsense words
4. [dʒ–ʒ]	strident/mellow	legion/lesion, nonsense words
5. [s–ʃ]	front/back lingual	sip/ship, seat/sheet, sell/shell
6. [z–ʒ]	front/back lingual	Caesar/seizure, nonsense words
7. [s–z]	voiced/voiceless	sip/zip, Sue/zoo, see/Z
8. [ʃ–ʒ]	voiced/voiceless	nonsense words

The stabilization of the sibilant system represents the completion of the consonantal system. At this stage, all the distinctive features should be salient and under formal motoric control. Sound substitutions are no longer observed because the child's infantemes have the same phonetic definition as the adult phonemes.

Individual Differences.   As in everything else, individual differences do exist. The models are not considered canonical but tentative in nature. At present, there are no data to support the concept of one sequential order of sound acquisition. What is apparent is a general unfolding organizational process. This natural unfolding is reflected in the sequential sound system models.

Review of Clinical Procedure.   To summarize, before the models are used, the therapist administers the Quick Test. He or she develops a hypothesis as to which training model is most appropriate. Because of the differential testing that has gone on beforehand, the therapist is prepared to modify the program for the individual. Using one of the models, the clinician determines which areas need to be rebuilt. He or she decides which distinctive features are the most likely candidates for therapy by noting the lines on the model that stabilize the defective sounds. The lines represent the distinctive features and have been numbered for optimal remedial order. After features have been chosen, minimal word-pairs are constructed. The child is taught to perceive and produce the distinctive features, which are incorporated into longer and longer verbal expressions. The words are practiced in different social settings. Throughout this entire process, the child is being taught a linguistic task—to make words different.

STRENGTHS AND LIMITATIONS

As has been alluded to before, this approach is primarily directed toward the functional articulation problem, i.e., the slow phonemic learner. The approach, which is flexible, must be modified to meet the particular needs of the individual child. This is particularly true of structurally or organically based problems. The distinctive feature and the minimal word-pair are given central focus; they are considered the keys for transforming a sound into a functional linguistic tool.

Although the approach is flexible, it does have certain natural limitations. The ability to perceive and produce the phonemic system is only one aspect of word production. Children not only have to make sounds, they must learn to sequence them over time. The distinctive-feature approach is not designed to aid in this aspect of training. While distinctive features are taught in prevocalic, intervocalic, and postvocalic positions, there is not a strong data base available to dictate when or how this phonemic sequencing process should be taught. It is assumed that the capacity to produce different phonemic utterances has priority over the ability to sequence phonemic utterances.

However, this does not mean that the latter ability is trivial. The priority of the capacity to generate the features over the capacity to sequence the features is a slight one. Some sequencing problems can be accounted for by an inability to generate the features, and these problems are not sequential problems at all. This is why the current approach was developed first. A second type of program is envisioned for sequential feature development within the word. However, more time is needed to research and develop such a program.

SUMMARY

Distinctive-feature theory provides the foundation for this program. Distinctive features are those components of phonemes that discriminate meaning. A failure in acquisition of a specific distinctive feature results in a phonological disorder that affects an entire class of speech sounds—all sounds that contain that feature as one of their component parts. For example, if a child does not acquire the voiceless feature, then all phonemes that include voicelessness in their composition will not be used, producing a phonological disorder that is perceived as defective speech.

Distinctive features are abstract concepts, yet their acquisition and use are essential to normal speech production. Teaching a child an abstract feature that he or she may lack presents a major challenge to the professional who hopes to help the child develop normal speech. The system explained here provides a method to teach features that is easy for children to learn and effective in its results. Essentially, the program uses pairs of words that are alike in every way except for one feature. These pairs of words are called minimal word-pairs. Examples are *pea* and *bee* which, when spoken, differ only by the voice-voiceless contrast in the initial consonant. Minimal word pairs are used to teach any feature requiring training. Meanings inherent in the words used bring the abstract nature of features to a level of concreteness which a child can grasp. An obvious strength of this procedure is that multiple sound errors may be corrected by teaching the correct use of a single missing feature that is responsible for the several errors.

As mentioned, minimal word-pairs that illustrate single distinctive-feature contrasts are used to stimulate the use of the necessary feature. Therapy is organized in steps permitting successive approximations toward correct productions, including discussion of words, auditory discrimination of the distinctive feature in the word-pairs, production training and carry-over. The program represents a holistic approach to therapy that integrates and streamlines elements of traditional methods.

REFERENCES

Albright, R., & Albright, J. (1958). Application of descriptive linguistics to child language. *Journal of Speech and Hearing Research, 1*(3), 257–261.

Blache, S. (1978). *The acquisition of distinctive features*. Baltimore: University Park Press.

Jakobson, R. (1962). Phoneme and phonology. In R. Jakobson (Ed. and Trans.), *Selected Writings. Vol. I: Phonological Studies*. The Hague: Mouton. (Original work published 1932)

Jakobson, R. (1968). *Child language, aphasia and phonological universals* (A. Keiler, Trans.) The Hague: Mouton (Original work published 1941)

Jakobson, R., Fant, G., & Halle, M. (1952). *Preliminaries to speech analysis: The distinctive features and their correlates*. Cambridge,: MIT Press.

Kantner, C., & West, R. (1969). *Phonetics: An introduction to the principles of phonetic science from the point of view of English speech*. New York: Harper and Brothers.

McDonald, E. (1964). *Articulation testing and treatment: A sensory-motor approach*. Pittsburgh: Stanwix House.

Appendix A

OROFACIAL EXAMINATION CHECKLIST

Client name: _____ Age: _____ Date: _____
Examiner: _____

    I. Facial Characteristics
        A. General appearance: normal color ____; normal symmetry ____;
            adenoid facies ____; other _____
        B. Frontal view
            1. eye spacing: normal (one eye apart) ____; hypertelorism
                ____; other _____
            2. zygomatic bones: normal ____; hypoplasia ____; other ____
            3. nasal area: septum (straight) ____; or deviated ____; nares
                ____; columella ____; septum/turbinate relationship ____;
                turbinate color ____; other notations _____
            4. vertical facial dimensions:
                a. upper (40% of face) ____; other notations _____
                b. lower (60% of face) ____; other notations _____
            5. lips: cupid's bow present ____; muscular union ____;
                neuromotor functioning—/i/ ____; /u/ ____; /p-p-p/ ____;
                other notations _____
        C. Profile
            1. normal (straight or convex) linear relationship between bridge
                of nose, to base of nose, to chin ____;

                retrusion $\begin{cases} \text{maxilla ____;} \\ \text{mandible ____;} \end{cases}$ protrusion $\begin{cases} \text{maxilla ____;} \\ \text{mandible ____;} \end{cases}$

            2. mandibular plane: normal ____; steep ____; flat ____
        D. General notations:

   II. Intraoral Characteristics
        A. Dentition
            1. general hygiene: good ____; needs improvement ____; car-
                ies ____; gingival hyperplasia or recession ____
            2. occlusal relationships ("bite on your back teeth" and sepa-
                rate cheek from teeth with tongue depressor)
                a. first molar contacts;
                    Class I—normal molar occlusion (mandibular molar is

Source: "Orofacial Examination Checklist" by R. M. Mason and C. Simon, 1977, *Language Speech & Hearing Services in the Schools, 8,* pp. 161–163. Copyright 1977 by the American Speech-Language-Hearing Association, Rockville, Maryland. Reprinted by permission.

one-half tooth ahead of maxillary molar) _____

Class I malocclusion (normal molar relationship with variations in other areas of dentition) _____

Class II malocclusion (maxillary ahead of mandibular first molar) _____;

Class III malocclusion (mandibular molar more than one-half tooth ahead of maxillary molar) _____

b. biting surfaces: normal vertical overlap (overbite) ____; excessive vertical overlap A____/ P____; normal horizontal overlap (overjet) ____; excessive horizontal overlap A ____/ P____; crossbite (mandibular tooth or teeth outside or wider than maxillary counterpart, or maxillary tooth or teeth inside mandibular counterpart) ____; notation of teeth involved ____; open bite (gap between biting surfaces) A____/ P____

c. sibilant production with teeth in occlusion: normal /s/ ____; /z/ ____; /f/ ____; /v/ ____

B. Hard palate ("extend your head backward")
1. midline coloration: normal (pink and white) ____; abnormal (blue tint) ____
2. lateral coloration: normal ____; torus palatinus (blue tint surrounding a raised midline bony growth) ____
3. posterior border and nasal spine: normal ____; short ____
4. general bony framework: normal____; submucous cleft ____; cleft ____; repaired cleft ____; other_____
5. palatal vault: normal relationship between maxillary arch/vault ____; narrow maxillary arch/high vault ____; wide maxillary arch/flat vault ____; other ____
6. general notations _____

C. Soft palate or velum (Examiner's eye level should be client's mouth level. Client's head erect, mouth three-fourths open, and tongue not extended out of mouth.)
1. midline muscle union (say "ah"): normal (whitish-pink tissue line) ____; submucous cleft (blue tint with A-type configuration during phonation) ____; cleft ____; repaired cleft ____
2. length: effective (closure of nasopharyngeal port possible during phonation) ____; ineffective (hypernasality noted) ____
3. velar dimple (where elevated soft palate buckles during phonation): normal 80% of total velar length (or 3-5 mm above tip of uvula) ____; other notations _____
4. velar elevation: normal (up to plane of hard palate) ____; reduced____; other _____
5. range of velar excursion (up and back stretching during phonation); excellent ____; moderate ____; minimal ____
6. presence of hypernasality during counting:
    60s ____; 70s ____; 80s ____; 90s ____
7. general notations: regarding air loss of unphonated sounds (nasal emission) and nasal resonance on phonated sounds _

D. Uvula
    1. shape: normal ____; bifid ____; other _____
    2. position: midline ____; lateral____
E. Fauces
    1. open isthmus ____; tonsillar obstruction of isthmus ____
    2. tonsil coloration: normal (pinkish) ____; inflamed ____
F. Pharynx
    1. depth between velar dimple and pharyngeal wall on "ah":
        normal ____; deep ____; other ____
    2. Passavant's pad: present during physiologic activity? ____
    3. adenoidal surgery (ask client); intact ____; removed ____;
        date of tonsil/adenoid removal _____
    4. gag reponse: positive ____; negative ____; weak ____
    5. general notations: _____
        _____

G. Tongue
    1. size: normal ____; macroglossia (rare) ____; microglossia ____
    2. diadochokinetic rate—an estimate of neuromotor matura-
        tion for speech (observe consistency and pattern of rapid
        movements during the 15-repetition sequence)
        a. normal movement patterns: tuh ____; luh ____; kuh
            ____; puh-tuh-kuh ____; describe variations _____
            _____

        b. mandibular assist: normal (until age seven and one-
            half) ____; possible neuromotor delay for speech (after
            seven and one half) ____
    3. lingual frenum: normal (tongue tip to alveolar ridge when
        mouth is one-half open) ____; short ____
    4. general notations: _____

III. General Observations and Other Findings

Appendix B
ACTIVITIES TO USE WITH CHILDREN

SOUND DISCRIMINATION

Pick and Poke (individual)

Randomly glue pictures of objects whose names contain target cognate sounds on a piece of poster board. Under each picture, punch three holes to represent the initial, medial, and final positions. (You may wish to paste reinforcers around the holes.) Mark the target sounds on one side edge of the board. Next to one (e.g., /k/), place a long piece of red yarn; next to the other, (e.g., /g/), a piece of green yarn. The ends of the yarn should be wrapped with masking tape to make it easier to poke with them and to keep them from unraveling. Poke the pieces of yarn through the edge of the board and glue them to the back.

To play, name the pictures one at a time. The child decides which sound was heard and pokes the appropriate piece of yarn through a hole under the picture.

Variation. Require the child to indicate which position the sound was heard in by selecting the appropriate hole.

Polly's Apron Pocket (individual/group)

Make an apron from construction paper or cloth. It should have at least one pocket. Give the child a group of flashcards with objects or words on them. The child places those cards containing the target sound in the apron pocket.

Variation. The apron will need three pockets. Instruct the child to place the flashcards in the pockets according to whether the target sound appears in the initial, medial, or final position.

STABILIZATION

Coffee Can (individual)

Decorate a coffee can and its plastic lid with contact paper. Punch holes in the lid. Thread pieces of yarn of different colors and different lengths through the holes, tying a knot at each end of each string. As the child pulls each string, he or she must sustain the target sound until the string stops at the other end.

Variation.   Have the child repeat a syllable rather than prolong an isolated sound.

The Bubble Blower (individual)

Draw a chart with a little girl in the corner blowing bubbles of three different sizes. In each bubble write the target sound or syllable. Give the child an ice-cream-stick pointer. As the child points to each bubble, he or she says the sound, changing intensity with the size of each bubble.

Syllable Dice (individual)

Construct two large blank cardboard dice and laminate them. Mark the dice with syllables made up of the target sound combined with various vowels. Use two different consonants for the two dice. The child rolls the dice and reads off the two-syllable combination shown.

Syllable Cups (individual)

Decorate styrofoam cups and write a target sound on the bottom (used as the top) of each one. Write vowels on ice-cream sticks. Have the child tap each cup with a vowel, repeating the syllable five times.

Duration Lines (individual)

Make a deck of cards with lines of various lengths on them. The child picks a card and repeats the target syllable for the "length" of the line on the card. If the child can do it, he or she gets to keep the card; if not, it goes back on the pile.

Froggy Jump (individual)

Draw a bunch of lily pads on one piece of poster board and a frog on another. Cut the frog out. On each lily pad, write a syllable using the target sound and a vowel. The child moves the frog from lily pad to lily pad, saying the repeating or alternating syllables.

Syllable Spin (individual)

Make a cardboard spinner divided into sections. Label each section with a syllable using the target and a vowel. Have the child spin and quickly say the syllable the spinner lands on.

Duration Cards (individual)

Construct index cards with patterns of long and short lines. For instance, one row would have a line all the way across the card; the second would have a line half way across; the next would have two short lines and a long line; and so forth. The child repeats the sound in a pattern matching each line on the card. Begin with a simple one-pattern sequence, and build up to three- and four-pattern sequences.

Automobile Strips (individual)

Cut strips of construction paper into long and short strips to represent long and short variations. Give the child a small model car to "drive" along the strips, making the appropriate vocalizations. Strips can be rearranged to make different patterns.

Hotdog (individual)

Draw an exaggeratedly long dog. Give the child an ice-cream stick to represent a bone. The child moves the bone out of the "hotdog" and sustains the target sound as the bone is moved from the dog's tail to its mouth.

Snoopy (individual)

Draw a picture of Snoopy and a chart showing a series of dishes of dog food. Cut out Snoopy and attach him to an ice-cream stick. The child moves Snoopy to each dog dish full of food. Targets can be written on Snoopy and on the dishes.

Variations. Use a series of doghouses and a different dog. Have the child move the dog from house to house. Or use Woodstock and a series of trees or a fish and a series of bowls.

Wiggly Worm (individual)

Draw a chart with a worm that goes up and down. Divide the worm into sections. The child moves his finger up and down the worm. He increases the sound in loudness as he moves up and decreases it as he moves down.

Mountain Road (individual)

Draw a scene with a series of mountains on it. The child moves a model car along the top of the mountains, changing the intensity of his vocalizations as he goes.

Uncover the Picture (individual)

Put a picture of an object such as a drum, butterfly, or a pair of glasses on a piece of poster board covered with contact paper. Cut up pieces of construction paper and tape them over the picture to conceal it. Have the child say his or her sound or word a given number of times. If it is said correctly, the child can take a piece of construction paper off in order to reveal the picture.

Dominoes (individual)

Make a set of dominoes with the target sound rather than dots. Have the child make the sound the number of times that it appears on the domino.

Variation. Use two different sounds on the domino set. This activity can be used with words as well.

Sound Tic-Tac-Toe (2 children)

Create a tic-tac-toe board with each section marked with a vowel. Each child has a series of markers with his or her target sound. As the child places a marker, he must say the syllable it makes. When a child wins, he must repeat all the syllables in the winning row.

Fishing for Sounds (individual/group)

Cut fish out of poster board and attach a safety pin through each one. Write target syllables on each fish. Create a "pole" from a string and a magnet. Have the children go fishing and say the targets they catch.

S-M-I-L-E (individual/group)

On a ditto draw round faces with eyes and nose. Do not put on the mouth. Have the child say five (or any preferred number) good sounds. After saying five good sounds, he can draw a smile on the face.

Variation.   Follow each single sound with a smile for a correct sound or a frown for an error. These activities can also be used with words.

The Kitty Cat (individual/group)

Cut a cat out of construction paper and place it on a flannel board. As the child says his sound a required number of times, he can place a construction paper spot on the cat. The cat's name should include the target sound.

Egg Carton Toss (individual/group)

Number the spaces in an egg carton. Have the child toss a paper clip into the carton. He or she must say the sound, word, or sentence the number of times indicated. Picture cards can be used to show the target word or sentence.

Paste an Apple on the Tree (individual/group)

Draw a ditto of a tree. Every time the child says five correct syllables or words, he or she may paste an apple on the tree. (Apples can be made from punches out of red construction paper.)

Variations.   Paste spots on a cow, petals on a flower, and so forth.

Animal Homes (individual/group)

Create a chart with pictures of a tree, a zoo cage, a pond, and a barn. Cut out pictures of animals that would live in one of these four places. Have each child choose an animal and place it in its home, while saying the animal's name. (Note: Many animal names have /s/ and /r/ sounds.)

Find the Target (individual/group)

Create 12 flashcards or pictures of objects whose names contain the target sound. First, the child is asked to name the object shown. Then the clinician displays the cards. If the target were /s/, the clinician might say, "I'm going to pretend that this piece of paper [a blank card] is soap. You close your eyes. I'll hide the soap under one of the other cards. You must guess which card the soap is under. Say, I*s* the *s*oap under the pen*c*il?" The child must ask the carrier question until he finds the soap. He looks under the cards himself.

Variation.   With a group, have the children each take one turn looking for the target. The one who finds it gets to hide it next, though the clinician supplies the carrier phrase.

Animal Cards (group)

Create a deck of cards with pictures of animals on them. The deck should include four matching pictures of each animal. Place the pack face down and have each child pick a card in turn. The object of the game is to get as many matches as possible.

Variations.   The child must say a syllable or word a given number of times, or say it and use it in a sentence, before he is allowed to pick a card. Or the child can be required to describe the card drawn, using at least one word with his or her sound.

Ladderboard (group)

Draw a ladder with each rung numbered. The numbers indicate the number of times the player is required to say his or her target sound or word. If it is said correctly, the child can move to the next rung. The object is to get to the top rung of the ladder.

Racetrack (group)

Create a racetrack divided into spaces on a piece of poster board. Each child is given a colored marker that represents his or her horse. In addition, each child has a stack of cards with pictures of names of objects using that child's sound (or word). In turn, each one rolls a die, moves the number of spaces shown on the die, draws that same number of cards, and says the sounds on the cards. If all the sounds are said correctly, the child's marker stays where it is. For each sound said incorrectly, the marker is moved back two spaces. Either the clinician or the other children judge the productions.

Variation.   Children at the sentence level can be required to put the target words into a sentence.

Spin the Arrow (group)

Construct a cardboard spinner divided into wedges. Write words around the edge of the circle and give each word a number between 1 and 10. Each child spins and says the word on which the spinner stopped the number of times indicated. If the child says it correctly, he or she receives that many points. The first child to reach a designated number of points wins. (The point value of the words should be based on their difficulty.)

Word Bingo (group)

On a ditto, draw enough nine-section bingo boards with pictures of objects in the sections that each child can have a different board. Each object name should use the target sound. Cut the pictures out of one copy and place them face down in a box. The clinician draws a picture from the box and the children look to see if they have that picture on their cards. If a child finds the picture, he or she says the word a required number of times or uses it in a sentence, and can then place a chip on the picture. The first child to fill a row going across, down, or diagonally wins.

Variations.　The first child to cover all nine sections wins.

Good Speech Land (group of 3 to 5)

Create a ditto with 30 blanks and a color key showing the colors red, green, black, orange, blue, and yellow. Copies should be given to the children the day before the game is to be played. The children are to fill in the blanks with words using their target sounds. Cut out small squares, triangles, and diamonds of construction paper in the six game colors. These should be pasted on a piece of poster board in 5 rows of 12 shapes each, with colors and shapes arranged at random. Label the top of the chart "Good Speech Land."

To play the game, give each child a marker. Each child places his or her marker at the end of one of the rows. One child is the caller. The caller sits facing away from the group with his or her word list and color key. The caller reads three words from the word list and the players move their markers one space for each word called. The caller then says a color from the color key. Any player whose marker is on that color must move the marker back to the beginning to start again. The others can keep moving ahead. The game proceeds this way until one player wins by reaching the top of the row—"Good Speech Land." That player becomes the new caller.

The Shopping Game (group)

Use poster board to create a spinner and a game board depicting four colored groups (red, blue, yellow, and green) of six stores each (florist, groceries, gifts, cards, pets, and so forth). Draw houses at the corners of the board to be starting points. The spinner should have 24 sections, representing the numbers 1 through 6 combined with each color. The first player spins and moves to the block of stores with the color indicated. He or she chooses one store to enter, then names an item that could be bought at that store. The name of the item must contain that player's target sound. He or she must say the name the number of times indicated on the spinner. Poker chips can be used as a reward, with the child receiving one chip for each time the word is said correctly. The winner is the child with the most chips at the end of the session.

CARRY-OVER

Around the Town (individual/group)

Create a board showing streets of your community with familiar stores and other buildings labeled. The child must tell a story about a trip to the bank, to the zoo, and so forth—what he or she would do or buy at each place.

Road Map (group)

Draw a map with made-up street and place names using the target sound. Make pairs of cards with place names from the map. Each child draws a card and moves a token to that place on the map. While moving on the roads, the child must say each street name correctly. If not, he or she does not keep the card and does not move. At the end of the session, the child with the greatest number of cards wins.

Variations.   Require the children to describe their paths or to answer questions about the destinations.

Password (group)

Make a set of cards picturing objects whose names contain the target sound. Each player is given a few cards. The first player says a carrier phrase that is a clue to the "password"—"I'm thinking of something hot." Other players guess the password, using full sentences such as "Are you thinking of the sun?" If the guess is wrong, the first player gives another clue. The player who guesses correctly gets the card and says a sentence using the password. The second player then gives a clue to his password. At the end of the session, the player with the most new cards wins.

Appendix C

Norms for syllable production in seconds/criterion count taken from oscillographic analyses of responses of 384 children, 24 boys and 24 girls, at each age shown. Scores represent time, in seconds, required for 20 repetitions of single syllables (that is, pʌ), 15 repetitions of bisyllables (that is, pʌtə), and 10 repetitions of pʌtəkə.

Age	pʌ	tʌ	kʌ	fʌ	lʌ	pʌtə	pʌkə	tʌkə	pʌtəkə
6 Mean	4.8	4.9	5.5	5.5	5.2	7.3	7.9	7.8	10.3
SD	0.8	1.0	0.9	1.0	0.9	2.0	2.1	1.8	3.1
7 Mean	4.8	4.9	5.3	5.4	5.3	7.6	8.0	8.0	10.0
SD	1.0	0.9	1.0	1.0	0.8	2.6	1.9	1.8	2.6
8 Mean	4.2	4.4	4.8	4.9	4.6	6.2	7.1	7.2	8.3
SD	0.7	0.7	0.7	1.0	0.6	1.8	1.5	1.4	2.1
9 Mean	4.0	4.1	4.6	4.6	4.5	5.9	6.6	6.6	7.7
SD	0.6	0.6	0.7	0.7	0.5	1.6	1.5	1.7	1.9
10 Mean	3.7	3.8	4.3	4.2	4.2	5.5	6.4	6.4	7.1
SD	0.4	0.4	0.5	0.5	0.5	1.5	1.4	1.2	1.5
11 Mean	3.6	3.6	4.0	4.0	3.8	4.8	5.8	5.8	6.5
SD	0.6	0.7	0.6	0.6	0.6	1.1	1.2	1.3	1.4
12 Mean	3.4	3.5	3.9	3.7	3.7	4.7	5.7	5.5	6.4
SD	0.4	0.5	0.6	0.4	0.5	1.2	1.5	1.1	1.6
13 Mean	3.3	3.3	3.7	3.6	3.5	4.2	5.1	5.1	5.7
SD	0.6	0.5	0.6	0.5	0.5	0.8	1.5	1.3	1.4

Source: "Time-by-Count Measurement of Diadochokinetic Syllable Rate" by S. G. Fletcher, 1972, *Journal of Speech and Hearing Research, 15*, p. 765. Copyright 1972 by the American Speech-Language-Hearing Association, Rockville, Maryland. Reprinted by permission. (The Fletcher Time By Count Test of Diadochokinetic Syllable Rate is available from C. C. Publications, Inc., P.O. Box 23699, Tigard, Oregon 97223-0108.)

Name Index

Subject Index

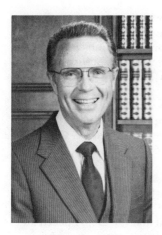

PARLEY W. NEWMAN is currently program chairman in the Area of Communicative Sciences and Disorders at Brigham Young University, where he has also served as coordinator of special education, chairman of the Department of Speech and Dramatic Arts, and professor of speech pathology. For 6 years he was associate secretary of the American Speech and Hearing Association, where he chaired ASHA's committees on ethical practice and organization structure. Dr. Newman received his Ph.D. from the State University of Iowa and his B.S. and M.S. from Utah State University. He is the author of numerous articles on speech pathology and professional affairs and has served as associate editor of *ASHA*, a journal of the American Speech and Hearing Association, and as an editorial consultant for the *Journal of Speech and Hearing Disorders.* He is a member and past president of the Utah Speech and Hearing Association and a fellow of the American Speech and Hearing Association. In 1971 Dr. Newman received the Master Teacher Award from Associated Students of Brigham Young University, and in 1965 the Presidental Citation to the Division of Handicapped Children and Youth of the U.S. Office of Education.

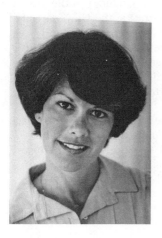

NANCY ACRA CREAGHEAD received her B.A. from Denison University, her M.S. from Purdue University, and her Ph.D. from the University of Cincinnati, where she is presently an associate professor of communication disorders. Dr. Creaghead has worked as a speech pathologist and as coordinator of speech services for the Cincinnati Speech and Hearing Center. She has been active in the American Speech-Language-Hearing Association and the Ohio Hearing Association, and is a past president and current chairman of the private practice committee of the Southwestern Ohio Speech-Language-Hearing Association. Dr. Creaghead has authored or co-authored numerous articles and gives frequent invited lectures on language disability, normal language development, and the development and assessment of pragmatic skills. She has received fellowships from the Vocational Rehabilitation Administration and Kappa Kappa Gamma, and was awarded the Southwestern Ohio Speech-Language-Hearing Association Honors of the Association in 1981.

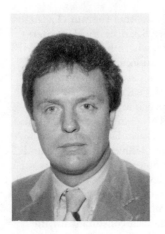

WAYNE A. SECORD, who worked for a number of years as a speech pathologist for the Ohio Public Schools, is currently an assistant professor of communication disorders at the University of Cincinnati. Dr. Secord received his B.S. and M.A. from The Ohio State University and his Ph.D. from the University of Cincinnati. He is the author of a book, *Eliciting Sounds: Techniques for Clinicians,* and of numerous language tests, including *T-MAC: Test of Minimal Articulation Competence, C-PAC: Clinical Probes of Articulation Consistency,* and *MILI: Multilevel Informal Language Inventory.* He serves as associate editor of *The Directive Teacher Magazine* and consulting test editor for the Charles E. Merrill Publishing Company, and is a member of the American Speech-Language-Hearing Association and the Ohio Speech and Hearing Association. Dr. Secord's current research interests include developing more efficient and effective diagnoistic and clinical procedures for individuals with severe speech-language disorders.

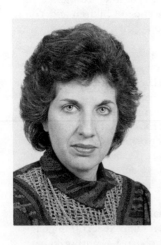

DOROTHY H. AIR received her B.S. and M.S. from Marquette University and her Ph.D. from the University of Cincinnati, where she is currently the associate director of audiology and speech pathology in the Medical Center. Before joining the staff at the University of Cincinnati, Dr. Air set up the speech pathology and audiology program at the Veterans Administration Hospital in Downey, Illinois, and served for several years as its director. Her professional memberships include the American Speech-Language-Hearing Association, the Ohio Speech and Hearing Association, and the Aphasiology Association of Ohio. She has served as chairman of the continuing education committees of both the Ohio Speech and Hearing Association and the Ohio Council of Speech and Hearing Executives. Dr. Air has given many presentations and workshops on auditory function, language disorders, and aphasia, and has been a lecturer for several Cincinnati hospitals.

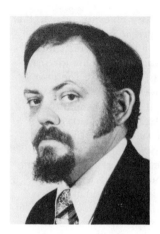

STEPHEN E. BLACHE received his B.A. and M.A. from the University of Massachusetts and his Ph.D. from Ohio University. He is currently an associate professor of communication disorders and sciences at Southern Illinois University at Carbondale, where he has also served as director of the Articulation Program. Dr. Blache is the author of a book, *The Acquisition of Distinctive Features*, and of a number of articles and book reviews. His memberships in professional associations include the American Speech-Language-Hearing Association and the Illinois Speech-Language-Hearing Association. He has served as associate editor of the *Journal of Speech and Hearing Research* and as an editorial consultant for the *Illinois Speech-Language-Hearing Journal*. Dr. Blache's current research projects include elaborations of the Blache Phonemic Inventory, which is a computerized system designed to simplify articulatory diagnosis, record keeping, and therapy planning. He has been identified by the American Council on Rural Special Education as one of the six national leaders in software design in speech/language pathology.

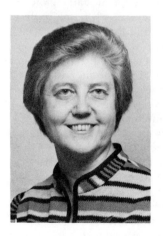

DORIS P. BRADLEY is currently a professor of speech and hearing sciences and chairperson of the Department of Speech and Hearing Sciences at the University of Southern Mississippi. She received her B.S. from the University of Southern Mississippi, her M.A. from the University of Florida, and her Ph.D. from the University of Pittsburgh. For 5 years, she was the head of clinical services at the Institute of Logopedics, Wichita State University. Dr. Bradley has authored or co-authored numerous articles on articulation disorders and therapy. She serves on the editorial board for communicative disorders of the *Journal of Continuing Education* and is a member of the professional advisory board and chairman of the publications committee of the National Society for Autistic Children. A member of numerous professional societies, Dr. Bradley has been especially active in the American Speech and Hearing Association and the American Cleft Palate Association.

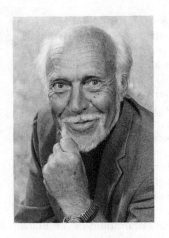

REUBEN COOPER is a professor emeritus of speech at Old Dominion University, where he founded the Department of Speech and served as its chairman for 14 years. He founded Old Dominion's Speech and Hearing Center in 1959 and was its director for the next 10 years. Professor Cooper received his B.S.S. and M.S. from the College of the City of New York and completed course work for the Ph.D. at Louisiana State University. He has published a number of articles in the field of articulation disorders, and is a member of the American Speech and Hearing Association and the American Cleft Palate Association and a fellow of the Speech and Hearing Association of Virginia. He has served as speech pathologist for the Eastern Virginia Cleft Palate and Oro-facial Clinic, as speech consultant to the Portsmouth Naval Hospital, and as a member of the Virginia Board of Examiners in Speech Pathology and Audiology. Professor Cooper has also taught English literature and composition and published several articles in that field.

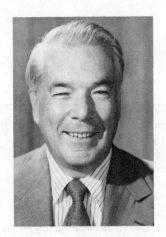

JOHN V. IRWIN, formerly the Pope M. Farrington Professor at Memphis State University, is now a professor emeritus a Memphis State and lives in Lexington, Kentucky. He received his B.A. from Ohio Wesleyan University, his M.A. from The Ohio State University, and his Ph.D. from the University of Wisconsin. For 16 years he was a professor of speech and director of the Speech and Hearing Clinics at the University of Wisconsin. He has contributed both to textbooks and to professional journals, and currently has a book, *Phonological Disorders: An Introduction*, in press. Dr. Irwin has served on many committees and site teams for both the U.S. Office of Education and the National Institutes of Health, and has been editor of *Acta Symbolica*. He is a fellow and former president of the American Speech-Language-Hearing Association and was awarded the Honors of the Association in 1970. He received the Honors of the Wisconsin Speech and Hearing Association in 1953 and the Citation for Distinguished Service of the Bureau for Education of the Handicapped in 1969.

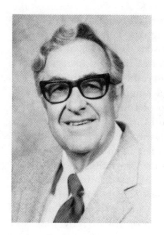

GORDON MORRIS LOW is a professor emeritus of communication disorders in the Department of Educational Psychology at Brigham Young University, where he served for a number of years as director of the Communication Disorders Center. He was formerly a professor of special education and codirector of the Communicative Disorders Clinic at San Francisco State College. Dr. Low received his B.S. and M.S. from the University of Utah and his Ph.D. from the University of Minnesota. He is a member of the American Speech and Hearing Association and a past president of the Utah Speech and Hearing Association and the Utah Federation of the Council for Exceptional Children. He has been active in public education, serving as president of the Provo City Board of Education and the Utah School Board Association. Dr. Low has co-authored a number of articles in the area of communication disorders, and with Mildred T. Ravsten has written the book *Resource Education for Children Having Communication-Learning Dysfunctions.*

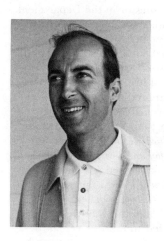

DONALD E. MOWRER received his B.A. and M.A. in speech pathology from the Florida State University and his doctorate from the College of Education at the Arizona State University, where he has been teaching in the Department of Speech since 1965. After receiving his master's degree, he was employed as an itinerant speech correctionist by four rural school districts in Ohio for 2 years, and later served as director of a Junior League speech clinic in Georgia. For 4 years, he worked in Arizona as a part-time public school correctionist and taught remedial reading at the high-school level. Dr. Mowrer's area of emphasis has been in the application of behavioral engineering strategies to the management of children's speech.

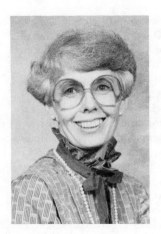

MILDRED T. RAVSTEN received her B.A. and M.C.H. in speech pathology from Brigham Young University, where she is currently an assistant professor of educational psychology and member of the core faculty of the Comprehensive Clinic. She served for a number of years as a consultant on speech and language development and disorders for the Bureau of Indian Affairs, the Ute Tribe Headstart Program, and the Uintah and Vernal school districts in Utah, and has worked as a speech therapist and teacher. Ms. Ravsten is a member of the American Speech-Language-Hearing Association and of the Utah Speech-Language-Hearing Association. She co-authored *Resource Education for Children Having Communicative-Learning Dysfunctions* with Gordon M. Low, and is currently engaged in research on the effectiveness of training procedures and skills assessment for clinicians and on the training of parents as facilitators of language development.

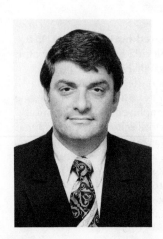

ALAN JAY WESTON is a professor in the Department of Speech Pathology and Audiology at the University of Wisconsin-Milwaukee, where he also served for a number of years as dean of the School of Allied Health Professions. Dr. Weston received his B.A. and M.A. from the University of Alabama and his Ph.D. from the University of Kansas. He has authored or co-authored numerous articles in the professional literature, as well as the *Paired Stimuli Kit* (with John V. Irwin) and several books, including *Survey of Allied Health Professions* and *Articulation Disorders: Evaluation and Therapy* (with Laurence Leonard). Dr. Weston has served as editor of *Allied Health and Behavioral Sciences* and as managing editor of *Acta Symbolica,* and has been a consultant to the National Institutes for Health and the U.S. Department of Education. He has received numerous research grants and was made a fellow of the American Speech-Language-Hearing Association in 1974.

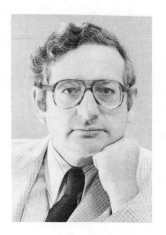

HARRIS WINITZ, who received his B.A. from the University of Vermont and his M.A. and Ph.D. from the University of Iowa, is currently a professor of speech science and psychology at the University of Missouri-Kansas City. Over a span of 25 years, Dr. Winitz has published numerous articles in the areas of phonetics, psycholinguistics, and articulation; his current research focuses on the relationship between auditory perception and articulation. He is also the author of several widely used textbooks, including *Articulatory Acquisition and Behavior* and *Phonetics: A Manual for Listening.* In 1981, he chaired, organized, and edited the proceedings of a major conference on native and second language acquisition sponsored by the New York Academy of Sciences. Dr. Winitz has served as editor of *Human Communication and Its Disorders: A Review* and as associate editor of the *Journal of Psycholinguistic Research* and the *Journal of Speech and Hearing Disorders.* He is a fellow of the American Speech and Hearing Association.

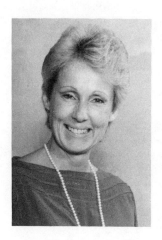

ANN STACE WOOD is a clinical speech and language pathologist in private practice in Cincinnati. She received her B.A. in English and speech from Miami University and her M.A. and Ph.D. in speech pathology from the University of Cincinnati. In addition to her private practice, Dr. Wood is a part-time instructor in aphasia at the University of Cincinnati and an adjunct affiliate staff member at the Jewish Hospital. She serves as a consultant for Doherty School, Clermont County Senior Services, and the Veterans Administration Hospital in Cincinnati. Her professional memberships include the American Speech and Hearing Association, the Ohio Speech and Hearing Association, the Aphasiology Association of Ohio, and the American Academy of Private Practice in Speech Pathology and Audiology.